The NEW

FROZEN SEAFOOD

HANDBOOK

A COMPLETE REFERENCE FOR THE SEAFOOD BUSINESS

The
NEW
FROZEN
SEAFOOD
HANDBOOK

A COMPLETE REFERENCE
FOR THE SEAFOOD BUSINESS

IAN
DORE

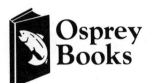

Osprey
Books

The New Frozen Seafood Handbook
A Complete Reference
for the Seafood Business

by Ian Dore

Published by
Osprey Books
6 West 18th Street
Huntington Station, NY 11746

Design by Lorraine Brod, Centerport, New York
Composition by New Age Typographers, Inc., Huntington, New York
Printed in the U.S.A.

Library of Congress Cataloging in Publication Data

Dore, Ian, 1941 –
        The new frozen seafood handbook : a complete reference for the
seafood business / Ian Dore
            p. cm. – (Osprey seafood handbooks)
        Rev. ed. of: Frozen seafood, the buyer's handbook. c1982.
        Bibliography: p.
        Includes index.
        ISBN 0-943738-26-1   : $69.00
        1. Frozen seafood – Purchasing.   I. Dore, Ian, 1941 –
        Frozen
seafood, the buyer's handbook.   II. Title.   III. Series.
    TX385.D67   1989
    641.3'92 – dc19   88-36828
                                                            CIP

Foreword

This book is based on *Frozen Seafood — the Buyer's Handbook* which was first published in 1982. It contains over twice as much information and has been completely revised and updated. The format, though, is the same: it is an encyclopedia of fish, shellfish and seafood products used in the U.S.A.

Because the entries are in alphabetical order, finding what you need is simple. However, some fish species have many names and it takes too much space to list each one separately. Therefore, if what you are looking for is not listed with its own entry, use the index to locate the word.

Commercially used names for fish and seafood are an important aspect of the industry and of this book. We have tried to find all names that are commonly used and to indicate which ones are likely to be legal and which ones are probably illegal. See the item Names for a full discussion. The U.S. Food and Drug Administration is the agency mainly responsible for determining how our foods should be labelled and named. However, the Customs service, the Department of Commerce and the Department of Agriculture all get involved from time to time. This book does not give you definitive answers; these can come only from the bureaucrats or, in the last resort, from the courts. Our intention is to provide as much information as possible on which you can base a judgement and, if necessary, a debate with the authorities.

Note on pack descriptions

Throughout this book the seafood industry's standard way of describing packs is used: the first figure represents the numbers of packages inside a master carton; the second figure gives the weight of each package.

For example, 10/5lb means there are ten packages of five pounds each, giving a master carton net weight of 50lbs; 12/3lbs shows there are twelve packages each of three pounds, for a master carton weight of 36lbs. 1/25lbs indicates a bulk pack (that is, one per master carton) of 25lbs.

This rule can be extended to define more complex packs also: for example, langostinos are frequently packed 4/12/12oz meaning that there are four inner packages each containing 12 pieces, each piece being 12oz in weight; so the total weight of the master carton is 48 units of 12oz each, which is 36lbs.

Fresh or Frozen Fish and Shellfish?

This book concentrates on frozen product, but also covers numerous items that are not usually available to the trade in frozen form. This helps to make it a one-volume reference and also provides information on many products which might, given market demand or changed harvesting methods, become available more widely. There is considerable prejudice in the U.S.A. in favor of "fresh" seafoods, fresh in this case meaning "not frozen." Like all prejudices, this one is based on ignorance. Distinguished food columnists and other formers of consumer opinion almost universally maintain the superiority of unfrozen fish over frozen. It is doubtful if many of them have ever given the alternatives a fair test.

Freshness is an aspect of quality not related to freezing. Unfrozen fish takes time, sometimes a lot of time, to reach the plate. Its quality, including its freshness, deteriorates rapidly over time. Even with the best handling – stable, cold temperatures, lots of ice which is removed and replenished every day or so – fish decomposes quite fast. Harold Wilson said a week is a long time in politics. It is also a long time in the storage life of a dead fish. Poor handling can reduce the shelf life to a matter of hours instead of days.

Nowadays, most frozen seafoods are processed soon after catching. Once frozen, the product maintains its quality, including its freshness, for a long time, making it possible to handle and distribute it to any place that has a freezer chest. Just as unfrozen fish must be handled properly, so must frozen product be handled and processed. Stale fish is not improved by freezing it. But good fish can be preserved as good fish by freezing.

The supermarket industry has in the last few years been particularly oriented to unfrozen product, often with poor bottom-line effects. There are clear signs that retailers now understand that good frozen fish is not only superior to stale, unfrozen product but also is much less wasteful, easier to inventory and more profitable to handle.

Raw fish in the form of sushi is an American craze which continues to grow. Sushi fans are horrified at the idea of eating frozen fish. Yet in Japan, where sushi originated, a great deal of the fish is frozen. This has two overwhelming advantages: it makes it possible to offer the essential wide variety of seafoods, all in top condition; and it removes the problem of parasites, which are destroyed after short periods in the freezer (see the items Parasites and Sushi). In fact, top hotel and restaurant groups in the U.S.A. specify only frozen fish if it is to be eaten raw. Anyone who cannot afford a lawsuit from a possibly parasitized customer should follow their example.

Successfully freezing fish for sushi is not easy. The fish must be fresh and be kept very cold and well iced before it is processed. It must be frozen immediately and held at low, stable temperatures. But such specifications are normal for any first-class freezing operation, of which there are many throughout the world. Fish frozen to the right specifications and properly handled after freezing will be almost as good as just-caught product – which is not available in the normal course of trade.

This is not to say that all frozen product is better. A few species do not freeze well. American lobster is one of them. Some frozen product is stale when it is processed. It is, of course, still stale when thawed and cooked. But a lot of "fresh" product is equally stale by the time it is eaten. One theme of this book is the importance of knowing your product and judging it for yourself. If you do that, the question of whether to use frozen or unfrozen product becomes moot: the important thing is to use good product, which your customers will want to keep buying.

ABALONE: *Haliotis rufescens,* red abalone, is the commonest California species. Also known as ormer. A large single shell mollusc that looks like a huge limpet. The meat is very expensive and highly regarded. Red abalone is the largest (it may reach 8lbs) and the most common, although no species is found in large quantities. Other Pacific coast abalone species include:

> *Haliotis corrugata* – pink abalone
> *Haliotis cracherodii* – black abalone
> *Haliotis fulgens* – green abalone
> *Haliotis kamtschatkana* – pinto abalone
> *Haliotis sorenseni* – white abalone.

The European abalone, *Haliotis tuberculata*, which is now found mainly in the Channel Islands and the Japanese abalone, *Haliotis discus*, are both similar to the California species. There are a number of abs in Australia, including greenlip, blacklip, brownlip and Roe's. New Zealand has *Haliotis iris*, known locally as paua which has a black covering on the flesh and is available mainly canned.

Pacific abalone eats kelp, so it is immune to the red tide which affects filter-feeding molluscs. It ranges from Baja California to Alaska, but stocks are small, partly because of over-fishing and partly because of the re-emergence of the sea otter as a significant predator. It is harvested by divers who pick them off the kelp one at a time.

California is the source of most U.S. abalone as well as being the major market area. Small quantities of abalone are landed in Alaska. Chile has also shipped abalone to the U.S.A., but this is a small, tough shellfish that bears little resemblance to the real thing. They are called "locos" in Chile. Usually canned, they are an inexpensive shellfish which is not an alternative to abalone.

Red abalone is now farmed quite successfully in California. Supplies may increase from other aquaculture work carried out in Europe, South America and Japan, although European and Japanese markets are at least as hungry for abalone as is California. Taiwan and China are cultivating local species of abalone and Australians are exploring prospects as well.

Frozen abalone meats are sold whole cleaned, or they may be beaten out and cut into steaks which are sometimes sold breaded, ready to cook. To prepare as steaks, the meaty foot is removed from the shell, cleaned of viscera and frill and sliced across the grain into round steaks, which are then pounded gently to soften the fibers. Abalone steaks must be cooked only very briefly, or the flesh toughens.

Because abalone steaks are one of the highest priced seafood products, there is considerable temptation to substitute other, cheaper products.

Cuttlefish is sometimes substituted for abalone steaks. The mantle (body flesh) of large cuttlefish may be cut into shapes resembling abalone. Cuttlefish is generally run through a meat tenderizer with needles. The needle pattern is quite distinctive. Another distinction between the two molluscs is that the cuttlefish has a membrane, small pieces of which may remain attached to the meat. Abalone steaks have no membrane. Giant squid is also used as a substitute for abalone. This similarly needs tenderizing so may have pin marks in the flesh.

ADDITIVES: Many substances are added to foods for flavor, for preservation or stabilization, for nutritional enhancement or for many other good reasons connected with enhancing, preserving and distributing the food supply. Additives have been tested possibly more than anything else we eat or drink. Without preservatives and anti-oxidants, much of our food would spoil too quickly. The amount and variety of our diet would worsen and many more people throughout the world would starve.

Even though freezing is a preservative process, some frozen foods require food additives. Generally, the more processed the food, the more likely it is to need and to contain some additives. Whole fish is gutted and frozen with no other process involved. Additives are seldom used. Fish fillets, however, are sometimes dipped in phosphate solutions to help them retain moisture when thawed and to improve their appearance by whitening them. Cooked product will almost certainly have some salt or spices added to give flavor. Highly processed products such as breaded portions will contain a number of additives including flavorings, preservatives, anti-caking agents and possibly nutritional enhancements in the breading, which is highly engineered to perform consistently in the varied environments of restaurant kitchens.

For more information on additives, see Dips and G.R.A.S. Various additives are mentioned individually.

ADEN TAILS: Also known as deep sea tails. Lobsterette may be the best term for this group of animals. See the description under Lobsterette.

Aden became the People's Democratic Republic of Yemen in 1967, but the small lobster tails exported from the region are still known as Aden tails or Aden dainties.

AHI: Hawaiian name for tuna, usually yellowfin.

A.K.C.: Short for Alaska king crab. See Crabs.

ALBACORE: See Tuna.

ALEWIFE *Scientific name: Alosa pseudoharengus:* Also called river herring; gaspareau is the French name often used in Canada and occasionally in the U.S.A. Gaspergoo is a corruption of the French word and is also heard occasionally.

Alewife is an anadromous North Atlantic herring, spawning in the rivers of New England and the Canadian Maritimes in April and May. Large numbers of the fish swim together into the streams of Rhode Island and Cape Cod where the fish is then caught easily with simple gear. Alewives are about ten inches long and are rather deeper in the body than regular herring. The flesh is dry and very bony, but fresh and salted alewives are eaten by a number of different ethnic groups.

The same fish lives in the Great Lakes, swimming up the tributary streams to spawn. The freshwater version of the species is small, usually around three inches long. Use is the same for the freshwater as for the anadromous alewife.

Alewife may be canned or pickled. Frozen product is generally whole (not gutted) and is used as raw material for further processing. Frozen alewife is often used for bait and for animal feed for zoos and aquaria.

ALLIGATOR: American alligators ceased to be on the "threatened" list in 1986. Since then, hunters and alligator farmers have provided an increasing supply of meat. Although most alligators are harvested for skins, the mild, boneless meat is also finding markets. Production is centered in Florida, with Louisiana and the other Gulf states also producing.

Tail meat is considered the best part. Other white meat comes from the jaws and loins. Leg and belly meat is darker and less favored.

AMBERJACK *Scientific name: Seriola dumerili:* Also called greater amberjack and Florida amberjack. A large member of the jack family, reaching as much as 100 pounds. Most fish handled commercially are between 10 and 40 pounds. The flesh is dark and oily and shelf life is short. Both appearance and freshness are improved if the fish is properly bled when it is first caught. This lightens the flesh color, reduces the off flavors caused by the oxidation of the blood and makes it possible to freeze the fillets, which are normally sold skin-on. In general, the fish is similar to mahi-mahi, although oilier and can be used in similar ways.

Amberjack is sometimes sold as a substitute for the similar but more expensive California yellowtail. Most fish are line-caught in the Gulf of Mexico. It ranges throughout the tropical and subtropical Atlantic from the Mediterranean to West Africa in the east and from Brazil to the Chesapeake in the west. In the summer, amberjack may be caught as far north as Cape Cod.

Although there are isolated reports of ciguatera in amberjack, this is not a problem outside the Caribbean islands. Parasitic worms are also quite common from time to time. Candling or simple inspection is usually sufficient to find them. They can then be removed easily with a knife.

ANADROMOUS FISH: Sea fish which migrate to freshwater rivers, streams and lakes to spawn. Salmon are the best known anadromous fish. Other examples are shad and alewife (river herring). Anadromous fish are vulnerable to pollution and to developments which may destroy the delicate and vital habitat in which these fish breed.

ANAEROBIC BACTERIA: Bacteria which multiply without oxygen. Canned and vacuum packed foods are vulnerable, since in both forms of packaging oxygen is excluded to deter spoilage of the product. Low-acid products in these forms of packaging are particularly at risk.

Botulinus is the best known anaerobic bacteria. The toxin that

15

this bug produces causes botulism, which is a very severe and sometimes fatal form of food poisoning. The risk of botulism is mainly in low-acid foods such as canned mushrooms, but it is an occasional hazard with vacuum packed and especially smoked items if they are improperly handled.

Correct processing and handling virtually guarantees that the product will be good; it is poor handling or production errors that lead to the spread of bacteria and consequent problems. Although there are fortunately very few instances of botulism, any occurrence gets widespread publicity.

ANCHOVY: A small sardine-like fish, mostly sold canned for human consumption.

There are numerous species of anchovy and anchoveta in both Atlantic and Pacific oceans. Main species are *Engraulis mordax* the northern anchovy from the Pacific and *Engraulis encrasicolus*, the European or Atlantic anchovy. For other species, see Names.

In California, anchovies used to be the basis of substantial fish-meal industry, but the decline of the fish stock put an end to that business and the small quantities now available are frozen whole for use as bait and for aquarium and zoo food. There are quantities available in both oceans for freezing. Sale as whitebait is possible. The fish is tasty, but needs to be handled with speed and care, since it will turn rancid very quickly.

ANGLERFISH: *Lophius americanus* and *Lophius piscatorius* are respectively goosefish and monkfish. Both are also known as anglerfish. For details, see Monkfish.

ANTARCTIC QUEEN: See Whiting.

ANTIBIOTICS: Some countries permit the use of antibiotics to preserve fish. This practice is not allowed in the U.S.A. Aureomycin, terramycin and tetracycline are among the antibiotics used in some countries. The purpose is to kill the bacteria which spoil the product. The reason for banning the use of antibiotics is simple: small quantities remaining on product will build resistance among people who eat the food, so making the drugs ineffective when they are needed to treat disease.

The absence of antibiotics is monitored by the regular F.D.A. inspection of imported foodstuffs.

A.O.A.C.: The Association of Official Analytical Chemists. Laboratory tests approved by A.O.A.C. are recognized by Federal and state courts as conclusive. Testing laboratories should always use A.O.A.C. methods when these are available.

AQUACULTURE: Fish farming is the fastest growing sector of the fishing industry and the great hope for the future of supplies of fish and shellfish.

Fish farming has been an important activity in parts of Asia for many centuries; carp, milkfish and shrimp are all grown as staple items. In the U.S., oysters have been farmed for many years following upon European tradition, which saw the start of oyster farming in Roman times. Trout is farmed on a large scale in the western mountain states and about 90 percent of production is now from Idaho. Nearly all the crawfish and domestic catfish used in the U.S.A. is farmed. The catfish industry particularly is an enormous success story with sales rising consistently and rapidly for a number of years. Catfish is a major cash crop in a number of southern states.

Aquaculture not only made headlines in the 1980s, it also produced a lot of fish and shellfish. Salmon has been the major breakthrough in fish farming. Norway led the way with cage-based techniques. A number of other countries, from Chile to northern Europe, have followed suit. Legal restrictions have been responsible for the late entrance of the U.S.A. into the business, though Canadian salmon farming on the Pacific coast has been a gold-rush type of activity.

Shrimp is the other aquaculture headliner. Asian countries, led by Taiwan and Thailand and now followed by China, are producing very large quantities of shrimp from ponds. In South America, Ecuador was the first, but is no longer the only country to market large tonnages of farmed shrimp. Shrimp markets have been transformed by the availability of farmed product.

Many other seafoods are now being farmed. Salmon technology is adapting to sea-going rainbow trout and even to cod. Turbot (the real one, not Greenland turbot) is also farmed now. Other flatfish will follow. Scallops and abalone have joined the traditional farmed shellfish – oysters, clams and mussels. Lobsters are not yet feasible, but the technical advances that the industry is making are such that almost any seafood might, in theory, be cultured one day.

The importance of fish farming to the seafood buyer lies in the potential for reliable and consistent supply that is offered by farming techniques and the associated marketing advantage that consistent product brings. But do not assume these advantages too readily. Farmed salmon is still harvested at certain seasons rather than year round. This is partly because of price fluctuations as wild fish are harvested; and partly because it is uneconomic to feed the fish during winter slow-growth periods. Shrimp ponds are harvested over very short periods and the harvest time can be forecast when the post-larvae shrimp are put in the ponds. A large proportion of the ponds in a region or country will be ready to harvest simultaneously. This problem will reduce as hatchery techniques improve and more shrimp are raised from hatchery eggs. Another problem that will probably not change is that of size. Most farmed shrimp are harvested at medium sizes. It is not worth keeping and feeding them to the very large counts that shrimp buyers used to prefer. Markets are adapting by using more, smaller shrimp.

Aquaculture is a fast changing business and an even faster changing technology. The reference section lists books and periodicals that help to keep you informed. See also Shrimp.

ARCTIC CHAR *Scientific name: Salvelinus alpinus:* A polar fish closely related to trout and salmon. It is found in the Arctic seas and in rivers and lakes where it breeds. The same fish comes from European and Siberian waters, as well as those of Canada and Alaska. There are some landlocked populations which spend their entire life cycles in fresh water, but the anadromous fish is generally preferred. It has red flesh and grows to as much as 30 pounds live weight.

The eating qualities of arctic char are excellent. Fish farmers are working hard on increasing the supply. Most fish available in the U.S. market is caught in late summer in northern Canada. It is generally available as dressed fish, frozen, graded 4/7lbs and 7/10lbs. A few larger fish will fetch premium prices, especially from smokers and if the flesh is deep red. (Flesh color varies with the fish's feed, but markets all prefer redder colors).

Char should be handled and treated like salmon. Many experts think it is superior. A. J. McClane in *Encyclopedia of Fish Cookery* writes "a fat fish with red flesh is in my opinion infinitely superior to salmon."

ARGENTINES: Another name for smelt, or smelt herring, or silverside. See Smelt.

ARROWTOOTH FLOUNDER, ARROWTOOTH SOLE: See Flatfish.

ATKA MACKEREL *Scientific name: Pleurogrammus monopterygius:* A greenling, not a mackerel. This is one of the four most abundant species of fish in the North Pacific. It is very common in Alaskan waters but hardly used at all in the U.S.A. A closely related species is extensively used in Japan. Exploitation of this resource is left to fishermen from Japan, Korea and the U.S.S.R.

Although Atka mackerel is occasionally sold salted in the U.S.A., it is generally regarded as a "trash fish." The flesh is fairly dark and oily and efforts to market it in the U.S. are unlikely in the immediate future. Meanwhile, the Japanese utilize a very similar Atka mackerel from their own waters in very large quantities in fresh, frozen and salted forms. This species is *Pleurogrammus azonus.*

Atka mackerel is a close relative of the lingcod, which is an important commercial species along the entire Pacific coast.

BACALAO: Dried salt cod. See Curing.

BACTERIA: Bacteria on foods cause spoilage and may cause illness. Viruses on foods may also cause illness. Fish and shellfish therefore must be clean. The Federal Food and Drug Administration (F.D.A.) is the agency responsible for monitoring and enforcing standards.

Much monitoring is still done by examining the product for *Escherichia coli* (*E. coli* for short) which is commonly found in the intestines of humans and other vertebrates. Its presence in salt or fresh water is an indication of fecal pollution which can cause diarrhea. Its presence is taken to indicate that other, more harmful organisms are also present. It is used as the benchmark because it is easy to identify.

No natural product is free of bacteria. The important point is that it should be free of the harmful ones. The F.D.A. does not allow shrimp to be sold if it contains any salmonella bacteria, *Vibrio cholera*, which causes cholera, or *Vibrio parahaemolyticus*. Staphylococcus, Shigella and other organisms are also monitored. There are few "standards" for these contaminants. The rule is that the product should be safe. The definition varies with the product.

This is not as strange as it sounds. Salmonella pathogens are easily destroyed by cooking. Therefore, their presence on a product which will be cooked is not as harmful as it is on cooked product. Similar considerations apply to other micro-organisms.

In general, a product will be rejected if it harbors 3.6 *E. coli* per gram of product, or a similar density of staph, or general coliforms exceeding 20 per gram or an aerobic plate count (that is all aerobic bacteria together) greater than 100,000 per gram. These standards are not universal and product could be rejected for carrying much lower levels of bacteria.

BAIRDII: Pronounced "bird-eye." The Latin name is *Chionoecetes bairdii* and the animal is the standard Alaskan snow crab. The name helps to distinguish it from the smaller snow crab of Alaska, *Chionoecetes opilio*. See Crabs for full information.

BARRACUDA *Scientific name: Sphyraena argentea:* An important game and food fish eaten fresh and dried on the west coast, in Mexico and in Central America. It ranges from northern California southwards. The fish grows to around 8 to 10 pounds. The flesh is firm and suitable for barbecuing and broiling. The fish tastes better if carefully bled when caught. Although most Pacific barracuda are sold fresh, frozen fillets are available. Again, bled fish makes a much better and longer lasting frozen product.
Sphyraena barracuda: The Atlantic barracuda is larger than the Pacific fish and is also highly prized for its sporting qualities. However, it is generally better not to eat it because it is one of the

species associated with ciguatera poisoning. See Seafood safety for further information on this subject. Although the incidence of ciguatera is low (as in any species), the chances of a major lawsuit arising from a single unfortunate incident are sufficient to deter commercial users from accepting the fish until a simple and reliable test for ciguatera is developed. Note that the Pacific barracuda has not been linked with ciguatera and is safe to eat.

Sphyraena sphyraena, the European barracuda, is a smaller species and is sometimes caught off the U.S. Atlantic coast. Barracuda is seldom traded in frozen form.

BARRAMUNDI *Scientific name: Lates calcarifer:* This is a very large catadromous fish from subtropical and tropical Australia and southeast Asia, prized by both sportsmen and commercial fishermen. Frozen fillets and steaks are occasionally imported into the U.S.A. Efforts to increase the resource through aquaculture and stocking are intensifying both in Australia and in Thailand, where barramundi grows very quickly and is known locally as seabass.

BASS: See also Striped bass and Sea trout. The name bass is applied to many quite different freshwater and marine fishes. Some of these are commercially valuable fresh, but are seldom traded in frozen form.

True bass (*Dicentrachus labrax*) is found in the eastern Atlantic and the Mediterranean and is an important game fish. It is not exploited commercially except for occasional local fresh sales. However, the sport fishery is economically important.

White seabass, *Cynoscion nobilis,* is a large Pacific game fish which is caught commercially in California and is not normally available frozen. It is called corvina in Mexico and is a drum, not a bass.

Smallmouth and largemouth bass are both important freshwater game fish.

Giant sea bass, *Stereolepsis gigas*, is a west coast species found mainly in California and Mexico where it grows slowly to as much as 500lbs. This species is also not exploited for commercial sale.

Black sea bass. *Centropristis striata* is a Florida reef fish, sometimes called blackfish or rock bass. It is sold fresh either whole or filleted.

Groupers are also called seabass. The F.D.A. seems to favor that name (see the Fishlist in Names). There are sea bass of different descriptions from all over the world. Striped bass, *Morone saxatilis*, which used to be an Atlantic species is now easier to find in the Pacific or from aquaculture. It is a protected species on the east coast, but a hybrid form, raised in ponds, is sometimes available. It looks and tastes very similar.

BATTERED: Product covered in batter. This is usually partly cooked ("pre-cooked") to set the batter before freezing. Batter serves the same purpose as breading. For a full discussion, see Portions.

BAY SCALLOPS: Generally, bay scallops are smaller than sea scallops. The market tends to describe any small scallop as bays. Calico scallops are also small, but much less expensive and tasty than genuine bay scallops. See Scallops.

BELLY BURN: A defect to look for on dressed and headless and dressed fish, especially salmon. If the entrails are left in the fish too long after the fish is caught ("too long" depends upon the fish, the water temperature, the air temperature and other factors) bacteria and enzymes in the gut create heat, which softens the bones and meat of the belly cavity wall. Belly burn is the condition where the rib bones protrude into the belly cavity. It usually indicates soft flesh and shows that the fish was not totally fresh when processed and frozen.

Belly burn is also caused by careless handling of the fish before freezing. For example, if fish is picked up by the belly wall flaps instead of by the tail, damage similar to typical belly burn may result.

Belly burn is a valid reason for rejecting fish for being less than top quality.

BELON: French word for European flat oyster *Ostrea edulis*.

BILLFISH: Sailfish, spearfish, marlin and swordfish.

BISQUE: A thick smooth soup usually based on lobster, shrimp or clam.

BISULFITES: See Sulfites.

BLACKCOD: See Sablefish.

BLACKFISH: See Tautog.

BLACKSPOT: See Melanosis.

BLANKS: Name given to cellos without labels inside the wraps. Normally packed 5/10, blanks have a bundle of labels placed separately in the outer carton. These labels are then placed with the cellos in a tray and overwrapped, weighed and priced by the retail store.

Pollock, hake or other inexpensive white fish is sometimes packed this way. The distributor may then sell the unlabelled cellos as cod, haddock or some other more desirable and expensive species or the retailer can similarly traypack and mislabel the wraps. This practice is most common in the mid-west, but occurs everywhere.

BLIND ROBINS: A smoked herring product.

BLOATERS: A Smoked herring product made from whole ungutted fish cold-smoked after dry salting. The bloater has little smoke flavor or color and a typical "gamey" taste. Bloaters used to be a popular item in Europe and the current interest in smoked products and exotic foods may lead to their appearance in specialty U.S. markets.

BLOCKLISTING: Automatic detention by the F.D.A. of certain products imported from specified origins or packers. In practice, this means that the importer has to prove that the product is acceptable before it can be admitted to the U.S.A. Blocklisting is applied to products, countries or regions with a particularly high record of rejection. See Rejection.

BLOWFISH: See Puffer.

BLUEBACK SALMON: Name given to both sockeye and coho salmon when canned. See Salmon.

BLUEFIN: See Tuna.

BLUEFISH *Scientific name: Pomatomus saltatrix:* An Atlantic relative of the mackerel that grows to as much as 25 pounds and three feet in length. Note that "Boston bluefish" is an illegal name used for Atlantic pollock, a very different fish. Bluefish is a voracious, fast moving fish prized by sport fishermen for its fighting qualities. Many sport fishermen do not care to eat the dark, oily flesh and either sell their catch to local dealers, or throw it back into the water.

Nevertheless, there is a good market for fresh dressed blues and also for fresh fillets. There is a growing business in smoked fillets which are excellent eating. The fish is difficult to store frozen because of the high oil content of the flesh, but frozen bluefish can be sold readily out of season if it has been properly handled and well wrapped to slow the onset of rancidity.

The fresh season, when bluefish is often available in large quantities, is winter time in Florida, spring along the southern part of the Atlantic coast and summer further north, where the fish reach southern Maine before heading back to warmer water.

Because bluefish spoils so rapidly, it must be gutted as soon as it is caught and handled quickly with plenty of ice, or frozen immediately after landing. Unfortunately, bluefish tends to be landed in erratic quantities mainly in small ports frequented by sport fishermen, with the result that quantities that are frozen tend to be the catch that the local dealer was unable to sell fresh. Consequently, frozen bluefish is more often than not an inferior product. If you have a year-round market and definitely can use frozen fillets, it is worth arranging to have fish processed and frozen for you according to specific standards, including storage temperatures of $-20°F$. or lower. Otherwise, handling this fish in frozen form is usually more trouble than it is worth.

The southern resource, especially in the Gulf of Mexico, is very large and not much fished. Prospects for increasing the supply of bluefish are good. It is an inexpensive and tasty fish which deserves to be more widely appreciated.

Small fish, known in the northeast as "snappers," are firmer fleshed and less oily than larger bluefish. These are preferred by many users.

Bluefish have had a lot of bad press in recent years, centering on PCB contamination in the mid-Atlantic region. State authorities advise against eating the fish too often. The warnings are grossly overstated. The original work indicating that the species might be contaminated was badly flawed. Although the mistake was realized soon afterwards, the original headlines left their mark. There have been no headlines setting the matter straight.

BLUE RUNNER: See Jacks.

BLUE WHITING *Scientific name: Micromesistius poutassou:* Also called Poutassou. A small deep-water member of the cod family found in the middle of the Atlantic. The fish is about ten inches long and the flesh is very soft. This abundant species is now fished by several European fleets. Despite the soft flesh the fish ultimately turn up in blocks and in other processed products. If taken advantage of, it could provide a large source of cheap protein. Blue whiting is difficult to catch and process, requiring sophisticated on-board equipment and knowledge.

The southern blue whiting, *Micromesistius australis*, is a similar but larger fish, found around the southern oceans from New Zealand to Chile. It has rather firmer flesh than the northern blue whiting and is available similarly in large quantities. There are large resources of this fish around the Falkland Islands. Some of this is used for fish blocks. Some marketers describe it as similar to hoki.

BONEFISH *Scientific name: Albula vulpes:* A prized sport fish, not traded commercially. It is found in warmer Atlantic and Pacific waters.

BONELESS FILLETS: Fillets from which the pinbones have been removed. Federal Grade Standards allow for the occasional small bone in Grade A fillets. (See Title 50, Chapter II, part 263.104 of the Code of Federal Regulations).

> Bone refers to a bone, or piece of bone, that exceeds either the dimension of 15mm in length or 0.355mm in diameter. Each area of one inch square (6.5cm) which contains a bone or a cluster of bones shall be regarded as one instance

of bones. The amount of bones is defined as follows:

Slight – 1 instance.
Moderate – 2 to 4 instances.
Excessive – over 4 instances

In other words, boneless fillets do not have to be completely boneless.

Normal cooking will soften most pinbones sufficiently to make them undetectable and some types of fish, particularly flatfish, are cut in such a way that there will not be any bones at all in the fillets. This may account for the popularity of sole and flounder with the consumer, who very definitely does not like bones in fish.

BONITO *Scientific name: Sarda sarda:* The virtually identical Pacific bonito is *Sarda chiliensis*. The striped bonito, *Sarda orientalis*, is found in both oceans. All three are very difficult to distinguish apart. Frigate mackerel, *Auxis thazard*, is biologically different, but for commercial purposes identical.

Bonito may be regarded either as a small tuna or as a large mackerel. It is found in all warmer waters of both coasts, growing to as much as three feet long and twelve pounds. The flesh is light gray-brown and oily. Bonito is often canned and mislabelled "light meat" tuna, a name not permitted under U.S. law for these species.

Frozen bonito is available headless and dressed, or occasionally steaked with skin on. It is a popular fish in southern U.S. coastal areas. It should be bled immediately after it is caught and then well-iced. The oily meat will spoil quickly if it is not handled with speed and care.

BORAX: A preservative used in some countries to improve the appearance of frozen product. Use of borax is illegal in the U.S.A.

BOSTON BLUEFISH: Also, Boston blue. These are illegal names frequently given to Atlantic pollock. It is a confusing practice since the fish is quite unlike bluefish.

BOSTON SCROD: Sometimes spelled schrod. This is not a fish, but a size designation. See Scrod.

BOTULISM: See Anaerobic bacteria.

BREADING: Flour-based covering used to coat fish, shrimp and other seafoods. The breading forms a jacket within which the product cooks gently. Breading helps to retain moisture in the product during cooking and also adds contrasting texture and flavor to the product. For a full discussion on breaded and similar items, see Portions.

BREAM: A name given to many different types of freshwater and marine fish. In commercial usage, sea bream is sometimes used as an alternative name for ocean perch (redfish). Scup (porgy) is sometimes incorrectly called bream. Otherwise, breams are not important in frozen trade. See also Bronze bream.

BRILL *Scientific name: Rhombus laevis:* A large European flatfish, very similar to genuine turbot. It grows to about 10lbs (turbot may reach 25 to 30) and is sold fresh, dressed. Similar to turbot in taste and usage, it is unlikely to be sold frozen. Most of the limited catch is readily absorbed fresh on local markets.

The name brill is occasionally applied to Pacific petrale sole, which is a totally different fish.

BROKERS: Sales agents representing suppliers who receive commissions on the sales made. Brokers do not take ownership of product, but introduce buyer to seller, leaving the seller to handle invoicing and shipping.

Brokers serve suppliers by providing sales, especially in areas remote from the supplier's own locality. Brokers serve their customers by offering a wide range of product from non-competing suppliers and by staying up to date on market conditions, making it easier for the customers to do their buying.

The U.S. seafood market is highly localized. The broker's knowledge of his own market area enables him to serve both buyer and seller.

Brokers also undertake retail merchandising work, which again is an important service to both the supplier and customer.

Suppliers of foodservice items such as breaded and battered portions, packers of many standard Alaskan and Canadian products and some domestic shrimp producers all regularly sell through regionally exclusive brokers. Most importers and other packers use brokers only intermittently and on non-exclusive terms, preferring to rely on their own telephone sales efforts.

Brokers can provide understanding of markets and trends over wide product areas and this expertise is valuable to suppliers as well as to users.

BRONZE BREAM: Freshwater bream reaching 15 to 20 pounds eaten widely in Europe. Small quantities are occasionally imported live into the U.S.A. It is unlikely to be traded as a frozen product.

BUCKLING: Hot-smoked herring. This is a popular item in Germany and other parts of Europe. Smoked gourmet products are becoming increasingly popular in the U.S.A. Buckling is a product which might be requested in the future.

BUFFALO: The name covers three species, all found abundantly in freshwater in the mid-west and South. *Ictiobus bubalus* is the smallmouth buffalo. *Ictiobus cyprinellus* is the bigmouth buffalo and *Ictiobus niger* is the black buffalo. Feeding habits and taste are similar to wild catfish, though the buffalo is generally much larger, reaching 30 to 50 pounds. Mostly, the fish is sold fresh. Frozen product is likely to be the residue of unsold product.

Properly handled, buffalo is an acceptable and inexpensive product, though the large number of bones will inevitably reduce its potential popularity. Proper freezing would make it more readily available.

BUTTERFISH *Scientific name: Peprilus triacanthus:* Also called harvestfish, dollar fish and silver dollar. A small, silver fish shaped like pompano or scup. It is caught inshore along the east coast between May and November. A very similar species, *Peprilus burti*, extends the range of the fish into the Gulf of Mexico. In

California another very similar species, *Peprilus simillimus*, is available virtually all year round. This fish is sometimes called Pacific pompano. European users of butterfish may sell them as pompano or the similar palometa.

Butterfish used to be regarded as "trash fish," fit only for pet food or bait, but it is now used as a table fish. The parasites that used to infest it seem to be less common, making the fish more palatable.

Japanese buyers take the major part of the frozen volume, packed whole (guts in), layered with polyethylene sheets between layers and carefully graded. For domestic consumption, headless dressed fish are used, especially by the retail trade, which tray-packs small butterfish. Smoked headless dressed butterfish is also becoming a significant item.

When you buy frozen butterfish, look for a 5kg or 10kg pack, whole fish, layered and graded. This is intended for the Japanese market, so is likely to be fish that was fresh when it was frozen. Butterfish has particularly poor keeping qualities, so avoid packs such as 25lb or 50lb blocks that may be product frozen as a last resort because the fish was not sold in fresh form.

Butterfish reach about 12 inches. Most are 6 to 9 inches. A six-inch fish is under 2 ounces. At 8 inches it will weigh a little over 4 ounces and will reach one pound at about 11 inches. Frozen, whole butterfish are graded in grams. Small is 80-105 grams (approximately 2.8 to 3.7 ounces). Medium fish go to 150 grams (5.28 ounces). Large are 150 to 200 grams (7 ounces) and extra large is anything bigger than 200 grams.

Butterfish are very good eating. The flesh is fat but white and delicate. The resource is also plentiful and supplies could be expanded.

In California, the name butterfish is sometimes applied to sablefish (black cod). This is particularly confusing since there is real butterfish available there. The two fishes are totally different in every way.

BUTTERFLY FILLETS: The two fillets from a single fish joined by the skin of the belly, making a double fillet with a shape a little like that of a butterfly.

BUTTERFLY SHRIMP: Also called fantail shrimp. Peeled and deveined shrimp with the shell left on the last (tail) segment. Shrimp in this form is used for breading. If the tail-fin segment with the shell remaining is not covered with the breading, the product is described as clean tail. Butterfly shrimp is necessarily deveined. Tail-on peeled undeveined shrimp is referred to as "tail-on round" shrimp. See Shrimp for more definitions of variations of these products.

CALAMARE, CALAMARI: Squid. These are the Italian words. "Calamari" is much easier to sell in the U.S.A. than "squid," which is a word that seems to frighten consumers. See Squid.

CALICO SCALLOP: A small scallop from Florida and the Carolinas, sometimes abundant in fall and winter when fresh scallops from other areas are scarce. See Scallops for full discussion.

C and F; C & F: See Delivery terms.

CAPELIN *Scientific name: Mallotus villosus:* A small, oily fish, very similar to a smelt, mainly from Arctic and sub-Arctic areas of the Atlantic and Pacific. Female capelin are prized in Japan for the roe. Canadian and Norwegian packers use machines for determining the sex of these small fish. The female capelin is frozen and exported for further processing, or the roe is removed and processed before shipment. Male capelin are fit chiefly for animal feed and are bought frozen whole in large blocks, mainly from Canada. Capelin are also used for the production of fishmeal. Capelin may be packed as smelts and are occasionally available smoked. However, the taste and texture are not particularly palatable.

CARP *Scientific name: Cyprinus carpio:* Carp is a freshwater fish that has been extensively farmed in Asia and Europe for many centuries and is a staple of both Chinese and Jewish cuisines. It was introduced into the United States in the 1870s and flourished, driving out more valuable species in some areas. Carp grow to large sizes but are usually harvested at 3 to 5 pounds. An increasing proportion of the supply is raised in ponds. The spring run of wild spawning fish is heavy, but fresh fish is available throughout the year.

The flesh is light tan (female fish) to reddish (male fish) and has a dark band of fat on each side which is generally removed.

Frozen fish is available whole, dressed or filleted. All forms are usually I.Q.F.

The grass carp, *Ctenopharyngodon idella*, sometimes called white amur, is becoming increasingly popular among fish farmers. These can be grown with catfish in catfish ponds, requiring no additional feed.

CATADROMOUS FISH: The name given to fish which live most of their lives in freshwater, but go to the sea to spawn. Eels are the best known example and some eels even have the ability to cross land to reach the sea. Barramundi are also catadromous. Catadromous is the converse of anadromous.

CATFISH: *Scientific names: Ictalurus punctatus* is the channel catfish, widely farmed in the U.S.A. *Ictalurus furcatus* is the blue catfish, which is larger and farmed to a lesser degree. The Brazilian catfish, caught in large quantities in the Amazon basin, is *Brachyplatysoma vaillanti*.

The two types of catfish widely available in the U.S.A. commercially are frozen Amazon catfish from Brazil, which is cheaper; and fresh or frozen farm-raised domestic catfish, which is premium product. Farmed product from other countries, such as Mexico, is not yet a market factor.

There are very many types of freshwater catfish, in the U.S.A. and around the world, ranging from the one-inch specimens used to clean the bottom of domestic fish-tanks, to the 300lb monsters of the Danube and the Mekong. There are numerous wild catfish species in the U.S.A., but in the commercial food business, freshwater catfish invariably means either the Brazil catfish or the very similar domestic farm-raised or channel catfish. Catfish farmers tend to distinguish their product by calling it channel catfish or farm-raised catfish. Both channel and Brazilian fish range up to about 1½lbs at harvest. The blue catfish is harvested at about 3lbs.

BRAZIL CATFISH: This is a high-volume low-price product which sells especially well through supermarkets. It is a standard item, almost a basic commodity. There are few problems with Brazil catfish, provided it is not allowed to get old in storage – catfish is fairly oily and turns rancid quickly. This business has matured into a quite stable, high-volume and year-round business.

When catfish is caught, it is headed, dressed, skinned and tail-trimmed. Catfish has a line of fat down the center of each side. This is usually removed when the fish is skinned and the fish is then described as "defatted." Almost all catfish is defatted. The fish processed to this stage is then frozen and made into products according to its size.

Most Brazil catfish is packed in 20/2½lb or 10/5lb printed polybags, most of which are printed with UPC codes to facilitate immediate retail sale.

Brazil catfish products include:

H&G: Headless dressed fish packed in the form in which it was frozen (see above). Grading is 6/8, 8/10, 10/12 and 12/14 ounces. Fish smaller than six ounces from Brazil are very unusual.

Steaks: Fish larger than about 14 ounces are sawn into steaks while frozen, at an even thickness of about three-eighths to one-half inch. Since the fish tapers towards the tail, this technique means that the weight of the individual steak gets less as the portions near the tail. The thinner tail section of each fish is not steaked but turned into tail fillets (see below). Steaks are not graded though they are usually described as 2/4 ounce, 2/5 ounce, or more properly and less frequently as "random." Steaks are packed into five pound boxes in layers, with poly film between the layers, or in 5lb polybags.

Tail fillets: When the steaks towards the tapered tail end of the fish become too small, the remaining piece is split into two halves vertically through the spine, making two "fillets" each containing part of the backbone. These are also packed 10/5lb boxes and are not graded, although like steaks a size range of 2/5 ounces is often quoted.

Side fillets: Sometimes the whole fish is split vertically through the backbone and then further divided into side fillets and tail fillets. Side fillets are graded in two ounce steps, 2/4, 4/6, 6/8, 8/10 and 10/12 ounces.

Catfish markets are volatile and because product type is determined by the size of the fish that is caught, the relationship between the prices for the different products may change. For example, one season the fish may all be small and packed as headless dressed. Consequently, steaks will be scarce and high priced. The following season the fish may be very large so headless dressed fish will not be packed and the price of this item will rise.

DOMESTIC FARM RAISED CATFISH: This is always priced substantially higher than Brazil catfish and achieves its higher value through consistency of supply and of quality – the wild product may vary considerably in taste depending upon what the fish is eating, but the farmed fish is artificially fed to produce, so far as possible, a standard flavor. Since there are occasional taste problems with the Brazilian product, many outlets prefer the guaranteed quality that the farming process gives them.

Note that one of the selling points for the farmed catfish is the absence of fishy flavor. There is no doubt that the American consumer prefers fish that do not taste fishy, so there is definite sense behind this claim.

Catfish farming is one of the major aquaculture success stories. Production, which is centered in Mississippi, Alabama and Arkansas, has been increasing rapidly for over a decade. The industry is well organized in its marketing, opening up new areas only when supplies are available. The U.S.A. is now covered. The industry's advantages over the wild Brazilian product include reliability and consistency of supply. This strategy is effective since it ensures product for menus on a year round basis.

Channel catfish is shipped either fresh or frozen. It is processed in automated plants where it is delivered live in tankers, then killed and processed in a very short time. Headless, dressed, skinless fish predominates. Frozen fish is I.Q.F., individually polywrapped, usually packed 1/15lbs and graded in ounces 2/5, 5/7, 7/9, 9/11, 11/13, 13/15 and 15/17. Note that farmed catfish is marketed in smaller sizes than can be shipped from Brazil.

Frozen I.Q.F. fillets, which should be cut without the nuggets, are usually packed in 10lb or 15lb boxes and graded in ounces 2/3, 3/5, 5/7, 7/9, 9/12 and 12 up. Boneless fillets are cut from the skinned, dressed fish. Fillets are sometimes further processed into strips, which are cross-cuts of the fillets and nuggets, which are the belly strips.

Nuggets range from ½oz to 3½ozs and are not graded. They are used for appetizers or kabobs.

Steaks are cut to customer specification from larger frozen carcasses.

The catfish industry offers a great deal of promotional assistance to users of their products and if you are one of these users, or are considering using catfish, you should take advantage of what is offered. Although catfish may not sound like an exciting topic, the unique growth of this aquaculture industry is a point of great pride for those involved and is a story that you can use most effectively as part of your marketing of the product.

Because catfish is grown in agricultural areas, government regards it as part of the farming industry, rather than the fishing industry. Consequently, if you need information on production, sales or regulations, the U.S. Department of Agriculture is the lead agency, not the National Marine Fisheries Service.

OCEAN CATFISH: *Scientific name: Anarhichas denticulatus:* Also called wolffish. A deepwater North Atlantic fish reaching 30lbs. The flesh is firm and sweet tasting and used in parts of Europe as a substitute for genuine Dover sole. A single fillet is cut from the lower side of the fish and is always boneless. Ocean cat is landed in the northeast and imported from Canada, Norway and the U.K.

Product forms are 10/5lb cello fillets, usually one per wrap; layer pack fillets, usually of large size; and fish blocks, most of which are thawed and used as fillets.

Many offers of cello cat are inferior fish, especially hake, which is far softer. Mention of pinbones, in or out, is an indication of substituted product, since properly prepared ocean cat has no pinbones anyway.

Norwegian product is almost certainly genuine; product from the U.K. very rarely so.

SEA CATFISH: *Scientific name: Arius felis:* Also called hardhead catfish. This is an abundant, small marine fish caught mainly in the Gulf of Mexico as an incidental catch with shrimp.

The meat is light colored and mild. The species ranges up the Atlantic coast as far as Cape Cod. The sea cat grows to about 1lb and has poisonous spines on the fins, which make it difficult to handle. It is generally too small for efficient machine processing. It is thought to be a large resource.

CAVALLA: See Kingfish.

CAVIAR: Sturgeon eggs preserved with salt. Caviar must be handled and transported fresh at refrigerated temperatures between 25°F. and 30°F. Freezing destroys the cell structure of the sturgeon eggs and turns this incredibly expensive product into mush. Lumpfish and whitefish eggs are often used to make a substitute product called black caviar, lumpfish caviar, or anything else that can mislead the purchaser into thinking he has bought real caviar at a cheap price. Be aware that legally, the word "caviar" may be used only in reference to sturgeon roe. The alternative products are like serving lightly fried pork fat instead of fillet mignon with the excuse that "it is all meat…"

Caviar comes in many grades and types. All of it is expensive. New technology for freezing caviar is not yet proved in the marketplace. For further details, see *Fresh Seafood – the Commercial Buyer's Guide* published by Osprey Books, 6 West 18th Street, Huntington Station, NY 11746.

CELLO WRAPS: See Packing styles.

CEPHALOPOD: Squid, octopus and cuttlefish are the commercially utilized cephalopods, which are molluscs with heads and arms.

CERO *Scientific name: Scomberomorus regalis:* Similar to king mackerel and Spanish mackerel. It is fairly common around Florida, the Caribbean and the northern coast of South America. See Spanish mackerel for usage.

CEVICHE: See Seviche.

CHAR: See Arctic char.

CHERRYSTONE: See Clams.

CHIKUWA: Broiled surimi product. See Surimi.

CHINOOK: See Salmon.

CHOWDERS: A thick stew-like soup usually based on clams. A number of processors sell frozen chowder concentrates, formulated so that the end user adds water, milk, cream or tomato juice according to preference.

Manhattan style chowders are made with tomato juice. New England style chowders are white chowders made with milk or cream.

Chowder concentrates are generally packed in half-pint, pint or quart containers for retail sale and in half-gallon or gallon containers for institutional use. Most packers use plastic tubs and case sizes vary widely.

Each processor has his own formulation for chowder base and recipes vary in type of clams used, in thickening material and in spices and flavorings. Since both retail and restaurant customers will become accustomed to a particular taste of the chowder served them, it is important to ensure consistency of supply so that customers receive familiar product each time they return.

The word is also used as a size designation for large quahogs (hard clam) suitable for using to make chowders. See Clams.

CHUB: *Scientific name: Coregonus spp:* Also called cisco and lake herring. A small freshwater fish from the Great Lakes region, this soft-fleshed and rather bony fish is usually sold smoked, either dressed or in chunks. It is seldom sold frozen.

CHUM: See Salmon.

C.I.F.: See Delivery terms.

C.I.F.R.: See Delivery terms.

CIGUATERA: A specific poisoning from certain tropical fish, ciguatera is caused by a toxin in the flesh of the fish and is totally unconnected with the freshness, staleness or handling of the fish.

Ciguatera is largely restricted to the West Indies and the South Pacific. Although it is rarely fatal, the effects are extremely unpleasant. There is no treatment or antidote.

The toxin is produced in vegetarian fish eating a particular plankton. These fish are eaten by other fish, which in turn may be eaten by humans. The incidence of the toxin is rare. It is concentrated in the viscera and fat of affected fish and it is found only occasionally. Nevertheless, it cannot be detected easily so the best course is not to eat species which might be affected. Because of this, certain fish are largely avoided: barracuda in the Caribbean, for example. The toxin has been found in over 400 species, many of which are not used for human food. Ciguatera occurs only in reef areas in the tropics. See also Seafood safety.

CISCO *Scientific name: Coregonus spp:* Also called lake herring and tullibee. A freshwater lake fish found in New England and Canada. Usual size is about 1½lbs and 15 inches in length, though the fish may grow to as much as seven pounds. There are a number of different species, all very similar and virtually indistinguishable to the user. Frozen dressed cisco is imported from Canada and minced blocks of the fish are also available.

CLAMS: A wide variety of bivalve molluscs (shellfish with two shells) ranging from the small softshell clam of the northeast to the huge geoduck (pronounced "gooey-duck") of the Pacific northwest. The frozen clam business is an adjunct of the much larger trade in fresh, live clams and the structure of the fresh business determines the operations of trade in frozen clams and clam products.

Under the Federal Shellfish Sanitation Program, all clams, mussels and oysters sold in the U.S.A. must originate from a licensed shipper. (See Shellfish Sanitation Program for details of how this works). Most clams are fished close to shore by individuals using primitive tools (not necessarily from choice but because conservation regulations use this technique to limit landings) so clams are landed in small quantities at many, many places around the coast. Grading, packing and nomenclature are highly localized.

Clams are fished along the northern parts of both the Pacific and Atlantic coasts, although most of the business is based upon

Atlantic clams, which are frequently shipped to the west coast fresh as well as frozen. Pollution severely limits harvests, especially in New England. While depuration could expand supplies, the technique is not universally accepted. Some experts believe that the best conservation techniques require the control and eventual ending of pollution rather than the use of palliative or avoidance measures.

There are substantial resources of clams that are not currently exploited for various reasons. Alaska in particular has large stocks which cannot be harvested because of the prevalence of red tide and the difficulty of monitoring the region.

SOFTSHELL CLAMS: *Scientific name: Mya arenaria:* Also called Ipswich clams, belly clams, fryers and steamers. The term "Ipswich" can apply to both live or breaded clams.

Softshell clams are the steamers and fryers of New England and Maryland. The clam is oval shaped and the siphon protrudes beyond the shell. Soft shell clams are found from Maryland all the way north into the Canadian Maritimes, where there are large unexploited reserves. Northern clams tend to be smaller than those from the south. Some consumers prefer large clams, some prefer small – there is no quality implication in the size. Softshell clams are found on the Pacific coast, mainly in Washington, but not in exploitable quantities.

Live softshell clams are sold by the bushel (8 gallons) and fresh shucked meats are sold in gallons (usually metal cans bearing the license number of the establishment where they were shucked). Clams in the shell are used for clambakes and for steamed clams; shucked meats are fried. They are generally too expensive to be used for chowders, clam cakes or similar recipes calling for minced clams.

Frozen softshell clam meats are usually breaded and I.Q.F., packed in four or six ounce portions ready for the fryer. 24/4oz and 18/6oz are usual packs. Prices may be quoted per case rather than per pound or portion. These clams are often called "whole fryers" or "Ipswich clams" to distinguish them from breaded clam strips (see below). Softshell clams are not frozen whole (with shell).

Razor clams are also shucked and fried, but as these are comparatively limited in quantity, they are not offered in frozen form.

QUAHOG: *Scientific name: Mercenaria mercenaria:* Also called hard shell clam and chowder hog. The American Fisheries Society prefers the name "northern quahog." There are other spellings used such as quauhog.

The quahog is the single species of hardshell clam that is sold fresh on the east coast. The shell of the quahog was the Indian raw material for wampum, used as money. The clam's size determines its usage – generally quahogs get tougher as they get bigger – and its price. The approximate size definitions and usages of quahogs are as follows:

Littlenecks count about 450 to 600 to a bushel which weighs about 60lbs. Littlenecks should be no more than two inches across. They are served mainly raw on the half shell, and sometimes steamed. Littlenecks are the most expensive grade of quahog.

Cherrystones count 300 to 400 to the 60lb bushel and are also eaten raw on the half shell in many areas, though considered rather large for this purpose in New England. They are about three inches across. Cherries are also used for clams casino and similar cooked dishes.

Topnecks count about 200 to the bushel. They are liked in some markets for clams casino and similar purposes and may be used for stuffed clams.

Quahogs or chowder clams are the largest, up to 125 per bushel. They are used for baked stuffed clams and are minced for chowders, clam cakes and other clam products.

Pumpkins are huge chowder clams. Some shippers will separate out the really big animals and sell them separately.

Note that there is no consistency to these grades or counts: the counts given here are an approximation from experience. Every region, and in some regions every shipper, has its own definition of each of these sizes, and purchasing live clams requires you to know your supplier. Local names vary as well as the counts: quahog is seldom used as a name in New Jersey. In parts of Connecticut the smallest size is termed a cherrystone and the next largest a littleneck, so reversing the usual names. Topnecks are used in New York and Philadelphia, but many other places have never heard the name used.

SURF CLAM: *Scientific name: Spisula solidissima:* The official name (from the American Fisheries Society) is Atlantic surf-clam. Other names sometimes used include hen clam, skimmer and bar clam. This is a large, deepwater clam, used for processed products such as stuffed clams, breaded strips and chowder. It is available year round and ranges along the whole Atlantic coast of the U.S.A. The meat is white but tougher and less tasty than the quahog.

OCEAN QUAHOG *Scientific name: Arctica islandica:* Also called mahogany clam and black quahog. The American Fisheries Society name is mahogany clam.

The mahogany is tough and the meat is much darker than quahog meat. If the bellies are discarded before the clam is chopped, the product is lighter and more acceptable. This may still be a little dark for chowders made with milk or cream, New England style, but is perfectly good for most other uses.

MANILA CLAM *Scientific name: Venerupis japonica:* This is an eastern Pacific clam accidentally introduced into the U.S.A. in the 1930s. It is similar to the Atlantic quahog, but darker and smaller. The meat is a little tough for use by the half-shell trade. Harvested in Washington and British Columbia, these clams are purged and frozen whole and packed in polybags. They are inexpensive and excellent for uses such as clam sauce for pasta or as steamed clams. Markets are increasing as buyers discover their convenience and low price.

Manila clams are farmed on a very large scale in Japan. Supplies could no doubt be increased substantially in the U.S.A.

PACIFIC LITTLENECK *Scientific name: Protothaca staminea:* Also called native littleneck. This is another northwest clam which resembles the Atlantic quahog. It is best used for steaming or in sauces and chowders, much like the manila clam. The resource is quite small and almost all the harvest is from the state of Washington.

Two other clams which are similar in appearance and range on the west coast are the pismo clam (*Tivela stultorum*) and the butter clam (*Saxidomus giganteus*). These are used much as the manila clam.

GEODUCK: *Scientific name: Panopea abrupta:* This is the largest clam. It looks rather like the Atlantic softshell clam, with its protruding siphon. Some specimens reach ten pounds and are nine inches long, with meats weighing up to five pounds. Japanese buyers generally take most of the harvest. Most of the harvest comes from Washington, but beds in British Columbia and Alaska are less exploited.

ARCTIC SURFCLAM: *Scientific name: Mactromeris polynyma:* This polar clam is highly regarded in Japan. Also known as Stimpson's surf clam, large stocks were located in northern Canada. The clam is small and the meat turns red when cooked, making it generally unacceptable for the U.S. market.

FROZEN HARDSHELL CLAM PRODUCTS: **Chopped or minced clams:**

This is a staple product used for chowders, clam cakes, stuffed clams and the like. There are two important aspects to the specification – how much meat and what type of clam is used. These two points are discussed in detail below.

Some packers distinguish between chopped and minced clams. The distinction is unclear. Most chopped or minced clams are put through a grinder with ⅜ inch diameter holes. Smaller holes make a rather mushy product; larger holes produce some bigger chunks that may not cook sufficiently.

The whole animal, except for the shell, is minced, unless the mantles are used separately for clam strips (see below). The stomachs are discarded if they are full of (algae) feed which makes the product dark colored and mushy. This is often the case with mahogany clams.

Chopped clams for institutional use are usually packed in half-gallon milk cartons which hold four pounds of product. Six, eight or twelve of these may make up an outer carton. One gallon (eight pound) milk cartons are less frequently used; plastic tubs holding four or five pounds are quite common. For processing use, such as for canned chowder production, larger containers like 15lb pillow packs are available. Retail packs are half-pint, one pint and one quart containers, mostly plastic tubs.

The percentage of clam meat in chopped clams is a vital component of the specification. When clams are shucked, they are drained and the clam juice collected. This juice may be frozen or bottled for sale as clam juice (see below) or it may be added back into the chopped clams.

Meat percentage in chopped clams varies from 50 per cent (that is half meat and half juice) described as 50/50, to 70 percent meat, described as 70/30, to dry pack which in theory contains no juice, but in practice will thaw out to about 90 to 92 percent meat (there is always some juice in the meat tissue and this will drain out on thawing. See Defrosting methods.

Obviously, the drier the pack the more it will cost, but this does not mean that a dry pack is automatically superior to a 50/50 pack. A user making clam chowder, for example, will probably add clam juice to the recipe, and may prefer to buy a "wet" pack rather than having to buy and store two separate ingredients. Stuffed clams also need juice to moisten and flavor the product, so in this case as well it may be more convenient to use a wetter combination pack.

The relative advantages of the different packs therefore depend on what the customer is going to do with the product and also on what he is used to handling. While a 75/25 pack will suit most people for most uses, no one pack is universally preferred.

Follow your customers' requirements and make sure that the pack is correctly labelled – that the contents meet the description. It is also a worthwhile precaution, when ordering, to specify the meat percentage. For example, order "70 percent meat" rather than "70/30", since the 70/30 description leaves an untrustworthy supplier the opportunity to maintain that his particular definition of 70/30 is 70 percent juice and 30 percent meat, the reverse of what you want.

The regular chowder quahog is too expensive and not plentiful enough to use for chopped clams and where it is used it is a premium product carrying a very high price. Most chopped clams are surf clams or mahogany clams.

Confusion arises when sellers describe their product as quahogs, when the mahogany or ocean clam, not the traditional quahog, is used. You should always press for full information on this point and it is useful to have the Latin names as a check. These are given above with the descriptions of each clam.

Clam juice:

This is usually sold pasteurized in bottles for retail use and unpasteurized frozen for institutional purposes, in half or one gallon containers, or 5lb plastic tubs – packed similarly to chopped clams. Clam juice is used to improve the flavor of chowders, clam cakes, stuffed clams and similar products. As mentioned in the section on chopped clams, it is often bought as a constituent of the chopped clam product and not kept and used separately.

Clam strips; stripped clams:

Outside New England and the middle Atlantic states, "fried clams" means breaded clam strips. This is an important frozen seafood item, either as raw unbreaded strips, or breaded strips, which may be either raw or precooked.

Inside the shell, the clam consists of a mantle (the fleshy part), muscles to operate the two shells, and soft parts (the stomach and other organs). Strips are made only from the mantle, which is spread out and cut into strips about ¼ to ⅜ inch wide and up to four inches long.

Unbreaded clam strips are packed the same way as chopped clams in 5lb, half-gallon and gallon containers. Strips should be dry pack – there is no obvious benefit in having juice. Breaded clams may be packed in 5lb or 6lb boxes, or 24/4 ounce or 18/6 ounce portions. Strips are made from surf clams and also from the mahogany clam.

It is possible to make acceptable clam strips from squid, although this is done less often than is rumored. Squid has a similar texture to a clam strip, but a clam flavor has to be added to the breading to make the dish acceptable.

Whole frozen clams:

West coast manila, butter and pismo clams are sometimes frozen whole and packed in polybags for retail sale. There is a potential risk with this product: if it is allowed to thaw and then to warm up, instead of being kept cold after thawing, the bacteria growth rate could be very high. However, if clams are frozen and handled properly, the texture remains practically unaltered and the frozen whole clam can be a very good product. It is ideal for steaming, for sauces and for adding to clambakes. Because of the risk of bacterial growth, frozen whole clams should be thoroughly cooked.

Stuffed clams:

Chopped clam meat mixed with a bread stuffing and cooked on the clam's half shell. This is a popular bar and snack item and is available from a number of packers in the north-east. Most "stuffies" are packed in trays or bags of one dozen, with the number of dozens per outer case varying from packer to packer. Retail packs containing two stuffies are also available. Some packers use artificial shells instead of real clam shells and others use scallop shells. You may wish to test local consumer acceptance for the different types of shell.

Stuffed clams are an easy item for a restaurant or bar to make, and carry a high profit margin when made on site. Chopped clams are the basic raw material. There are enough different recipes to allow any seller to offer an individualized product. It is of course essential to have a supply of clean and sterilized empty shells of consistent size. Artificial shells and scallop shells, which are easier to clean than clam shells, are often used although consumer preference seems to be for the genuine shell. Provided shells are available, it is easy to maintain the item at all times on menus.

The chopped clams used for stuffies need some juice to moisten the mixture. A 75/25 pack is generally considered the best for this purpose. Alternatively stuffies can be made using both dry-pack chopped clams and clam juice if the user wishes or has other need to stock both items.

Other clam products:

Chowder is listed as a separate item.

Clam cakes are not normally available frozen, although retail packs appear from time to time.

Clams casino and similar half-shell products are generally better made on site and frozen institutional products have not been successful.

For further information on clams, read the items on Depuration and the Shellfish Sanitation Program.

CLEAN TAIL: Breaded tail-on shrimp where the breading does not cover the shell-protected final tail segment. This design makes it cleaner when eating the shrimp with the fingers. See Shrimp.

CLUMPING: Individually quick frozen (I.Q.F.) product where some of the contents of a pack are stuck together. This is usually caused when the product warms slightly during distribution so that the glaze surrounding each piece sticks to glaze on other pieces as the temperature reduces to correct levels. Clumping is an indication that product was not handled properly. The texture may be inferior because of temperature changes in the product. If storage temperatures have fluctuated, shelf life is likely to be shorter and oily products will go rancid much faster.

CLUSTERS: See Crab. Clusters consist of the legs and claw from one side of the snow crab (or similar crab) frozen as one piece, without the top shell, cleaned of viscera.

COBIA *Scientific name: Rachycentron canadum:* Also called (incorrectly) ling and crabeater. Cobia is found off Florida and in the Gulf of Mexico. It is also fished in the Indian Ocean. Mainly caught by game fishermen (it may reach 100 pounds and is prized for its fighting qualities), the cobia is sometimes marketed as frozen fillets, usually skinless since the skin is tough. These fillets can be sliced and broiled or baked, much like mahi-mahi which it resembles in flavor and texture.

COCKLE: Small, clam-like molluscs. Not normally used in the U.S.A., but popular in Europe and Asia.

COD *Scientific names: Gadus morhua* is Atlantic cod. *Gadus macrocephalus* is Pacific cod.

The Fishlist (see Names) uses "cod" for both Atlantic and Pacific species. In addition, it allows Atlantic cod for *Gadus morhua* and Pacific cod and Alaska cod for *Gadus macrocephalus*. The term "true cod," which is frequently applied to the Pacific variety, is not approved and should not be used.

There are various other codfish, such as tom cod, morid cod and arctic cod. None of these other species is a significant fishery product. Sablefish is sometimes called "black cod." It is nothing like cod. Lingcod is not a cod and also not at all like one.

Cod is one of the most important commercial fishes and is a mainstay of the seafood industry. It is a large, deep water, round white fish, providing thick, meaty and well-flavored fillets. Cod is fished in the North Atlantic and in the North Pacific. The two cods are virtually identical, but the Pacific variety has flesh that is a little softer and has a slightly higher water content. Therefore, it is considered marginally inferior to the Atlantic product.

Despite the similarity of codfish from Atlantic and Pacific, each is put into a largely different range of products and this tends to highlight the differences between them.

ATLANTIC COD: The 100 to 200 pound codfish that were common a century ago and that played an important part in the attraction of early settlers to North America, have been fished out and the average size now is probably around 10lbs, although fish of 30lbs are not uncommon.

In the U.S.A., Atlantic cod is landed head-on, gutted and the Boston market grades them fresh as follows:

small	under 1½lbs
scrod	1½ to 2½lbs
market	2½ to 10lbs
large	10 to 25lbs
jumbo	25lbs and up

Size ranges in most other ports follow these steps.

A great deal of cod is frozen in the U.S.A. and even more frozen cod is imported from eastern Canada. Iceland, Norway, Denmark, the U.K., Germany and Poland are among other suppliers. There are market perceptions of the quality of frozen cod – and perhaps of frozen fish generally – from different origins. For Atlantic cod, domestic fish is at or close to the base. It is acceptable quality, but not the best or near the best. Canadian fish is thought to be a little better, often selling for several cents a pound more. Cod from Iceland, Norway and Denmark often sells at premiums of 20 percent and more over the domestic fish price, because the buyers believe the products to be superior in quality in all respects. These countries built up reputations both for particular brands and for their countries as origins for very fresh fish, top quality processing, good weights and general reliable excellence.

How far all this is true and how far it is produced by skillful propaganda, is a matter of opinion. Whether the differences are important to you and your customers depends on your own business and you must judge it on the basis of your own needs and experience.

In between the basic domestic U.S. product and the prized Nordic origins there are numerous other suppliers with less well defined images. You should examine brands and products offered and make your own judgements on each.

Products of Atlantic cod:

Fish blocks/Grade A blocks: Cod blocks were once the most widely used type of fish block. Although pollock now has that distinction, cod is still a vital part of the block industry and therefore of the entire portion and breaded fish markets.

For the U.S.A., blocks are mostly made from boneless and skinless fillets. (Blocks with pinbones are made and used in Europe). See Fish blocks for full details.

Cello wrap fillets are usually packed 10/5lb, six wraps per five pound inner box. The premium size is one to two (1/2) fillets per wrap; the second grade, usually selling for less, is two to three (2/3) fillets per wrap. Avoid higher counts as they probably consist largely of pieces instead of whole fillets.

Cello cod is the standard cod pack for both institutional and retail trades. If customers ask for pinbone cod they mean cello wrap fillets with pinbones, and if they ask for boneless cod they mean cello wrap fillets without pinbones. Note that boneless packs are usually stencilled "boneless" but that packs with pinbone ("pinbone-in" or "pbi") are generally marked "skinless," with no specific reference to the bones. You may find that a supplier offering boneless fish at an attractive price delivers cartons bearing no words on them about the presence or otherwise of bones. He is actually using pinbone-in fish and relying on the fact that pinbones nearly always soften in cooking and become undetectable. You will be better off if you know what you are using so look for this tactic and resist it.

Layer pack cod fillets may be skin-on or skinless, boneless or pinbone-in. 10lb, 14lb and 15lb packs are the most frequently offered; six, five, four or three to the master carton. Customary grading is 4/8 ounce, 8/12, 12/16, 16/24, 24/32 and 32-up ounces. Larger sizes particularly vary in specification according to the packer and the available fish. Nowadays, anything over 16 ounces may be called "jumbo" cod and terms like "small jumbos" are applied to 12/16 ounce fillets. As always, grades expressed in ounces are preferable to having debates about the definitions of descriptive terms like "jumbo".

Dressed cod: Scrod and market fish may be packed as landed, either dressed or headed and frozen.

Cod may be frozen in single layers, or be I.Q.F. The domestic market for dressed fish is limited except in Puerto Rico. If you buy this item, check carefully for deterioration since there are still packers who only freeze fish which did not sell while it was in fresh form.

Salt cod; bacalao: The U.S.A. produces small but increasing amounts of salt cod mainly for export. Canada is a very large producer. Salting is the traditional way of preserving fish and is an important component of Portuguese, Spanish and Italian cuisine. Cod is of course not the only fish salted: any large, round, white fish is usable and ling, pollock, haddock and cusk are all salted.

Modern salt cod needs freezing or refrigeration, as the cure is now for flavoring rather than for preserving the fish. Split fish in 1lb or 2lb retail polybags, and boneless fillets in 1lb bags or 1lb wooden boxes are the usual packs. Salt cod is an expensive product, the U.S. market is expanding.

Dried salt cod; stockfish: Hard dried fish. For full description see Curing.

Smoked cod: Cod may be brined then hot smoked in exactly the same way as haddock is processed to make finnans. A yellow dye is often used to meet market expectations of the color. Some of the smoked haddock or finnan haddock sold in the U.S.A. is smoked cod. The two are very hard to distinguish, except by examination of the skin – haddock has a "thumb-mark" near the nape on each side and a black lateral line. Cod and Atlantic pollock have white lateral lines.

Frozen smoked cod fillets are imported from Scotland in 15lb wooden boxes, graded by count of fillets per box, such as 5/7 count, 7/9 count. This item may be marked "smoked fillets" and is usually cod, but might also be pollock. "Smoked" fish can be prepared using a liquid smoke dip instead of a smoking kiln.

Cod steaks are rare in the U.S.A., but are sometimes available packed 6/5lb or 10/5lb boxes, or in a bulk pack. Cod steaks are seldom graded, but the thickness required should be specified. 1½ inches is normal. (See also U.S. Grade Standards).

PACIFIC COD: Also called true cod, the Pacific cod is caught from Oregon to Alaska. Japan and Korea supply large quantities. Russian vessels also catch a great deal of this fish. Pacific cod is smaller than Atlantic cod – most fish are around 7 to 8 pounds – but otherwise it is very similar indeed. U.S. vessels will catch increasing volumes of it in the future since regulations have changed to encourage greater use by American fishermen of the resources within the 200-mile limit.

Products of Pacific cod: Like Atlantic cod, Pacific cod is used to produce fish blocks, smoked cod and increasing amounts of salted cod. Unlike Atlantic cod, it is seldom made into cellos, though these are available from Asian suppliers from time to time. A large part of the catch of Pacific cod is processed into I.Q.F. fillets. These are almost always skinless and boneless.

The Japanese pack of this product is the standard and their normal grading is in ounces: 2/4, 4/8, 8/16 and 16/32. 25lb boxes, each fillet polywrapped, are also standard. Some packers use polylined cartons instead of individually wrapping the fillets.

Some domestic packers grade and pack in a similar manner to the Japanese. Many others use 10lb boxes instead of 25lbs and strap together four of these for a 4/10 pack. Others, unfortunately, are less concerned about the size grading and ship the fillets randomly packed or ungraded. This is customary with a number of west coast groundfish species. They do not vary much in size, but the range of possible cod fillet sizes makes ungraded product unacceptable for many market uses. Grading is required if product is to be sold at the market price.

Korean and other origin Pacific cod is generally packed in the same way as the Japanese product. Some Asian supplies are frozen at sea headless and dressed then thawed and filleted on land. Such product may be a little inferior to once frozen fillets.

COD CHEEKS: The face muscles of large codfish are considered a delicacy by fishermen, who may remove them for their own use if there is time on the trip back to port with their catch. There is a widespread belief that cod cheeks substituted for scallops. For the most part this is not economically feasible. The industry is used to substituting one product for another, but only if it makes a profit thereby.

CODEX ALIMENTARIUS: An international system of food industry rules and standards which are established by multinational committees working under the administration of two United Nations agencies. The agencies are the Food and Agriculture Organization (F.A.O.) and the World Health Organization (W.H.O.). The standards are advisory but may be adopted wholly or partially by governments. The U.S.A. is closely involved in the development of many of the Codex documents. Processors who follow Codex recommendations will produce wholesome, clean food which is likely to be acceptable in most countries.

COHO: Silver salmon. A Pacific salmon averaging eight to ten pounds when caught. See Salmon.

COLEY: Also coalfish and saithe. Names used in the U.K. for Atlantic pollock. Imported product may occasionally be labelled with one of these names.

COMMON NAMES: See Names.

CONCENTRATES: Chowder base or bisque base which requires the addition of water or other dilutants before serving. Most frozen chowders sold are concentrates, requiring approximately equal quantities of water, milk, cream or tomato juice to be added by the chef.

CONCH: Also called scungili, sea snail, whelk, dog-whelk. These are large sea-snails. There are two different types, one from the Caribbean area, especially the Bahamas and the other from the Northern part of the Atlantic coastline. The two types are different in appearance and in the way they are processed.
Bahama or Caribbean conch *Scientific name: Strombus gigas:* Called queen conch or pink conch. It is taken from the shell, eviscerated and washed, then frozen in 5lb boxes, 10 to a master carton. Product is sometimes offered uncleaned, similarly packed. Uncleaned and partially cleaned Caribbean conch can be a problem to handle and is best avoided unless you are sure that you have a use for it. It is cheaper than the fully cleaned pack, but normally only sells when there is no cleaned conch available. Car-

ibbean conch is whiter and larger than Rhode Island type conch and most users are not willing to substitute one for the other, either way, so the two conches are not particularly competitive with one another in the marketplace.

New England conch consists of two species: *Busycon carica* is the knobbed whelk and *Busycotypus canaliculatus* is the channeled whelk. Both range from Cape Cod to Florida with the majority of the catch taken in Rhode Island and southern Massachusetts where they are usually called snails or scungili. The species are also found in the Pacific. Channeled snails may bring a better price than knobbed whelks as the meat is lighter in color. The animal is normally cooked before being shelled and cleaned. The meats are often packed in bags and frozen and a few packers vacuum pack the bags. There is no standard size bag or outer carton for this product. Conch is perhaps the only shellfish which becomes more tender with extended cooking. It needs several hours boiling, or alternatively plenty of beating with a mallet, to make it soft enough to eat. The cooked conch originating in Rhode Island and other parts of the north-east invariably requires further cooking before use. The processor in this case cooks the conch to facilitate its removal from the shell, not to prepare the meat for the user. Full cooking also reduces the yield substantially, so the saleable weight for the processor is less if the conch is fully cooked. Be aware that every supplier will swear to you that his conch is not only fully cooked, but it is the only such genuinely described product on the market. Before you repeat such descriptions to your own customers, make sure you try to eat the conch yourself. The chances of the shellfish actually being fully cooked are remote. It may, however, be sufficiently cooked for certain uses, such as scungili salad where the marinade softens the flesh or for pasta sauce which will involve it being cooked further anyway. Some Rhode Island conch is now packed raw, which at least avoids the problem of misrepresentation of the amount of cooking. Raw conch goes sour if it is not absolutely fresh when frozen. Cooked conch dehydrates rapidly, which is the reason for vacuum packing. Both Caribbean and Rhode Island conches are packed by large numbers of small producers and there is little consistency with many of the labels. Check your shipments to ensure that the quality is acceptable. Look for signs of sourness, dehydration and for remnants of viscera. If you buy cooked product, check the tenderness or toughness, and be aware that if you have to cook conch the smell is awful and the shrinkage can be high.

CONGER EEL *Scientific name: Conger oceanicus:* There are similar species in most of the world's oceans. *Conger conger* is the European conger eel. *Conger verreauxi* is the Australia/New Zealand species. All are fairly large (the European fish reaches almost 100lbs). The meat is firm and white, but not much used. Conger steaks are sold in some parts of Europe. It is a cheap fish which could be marketed, although the "eel" in the name would not help.

CONSERVATION: See Fisheries management.

CONSIGNMENT: See Delivery terms.

COONSTRIPE: A northern shrimp caught from Oregon to Alaska. It is sometimes frozen raw, heads on, for export to Japan but is mostly sold cooked and peeled with other northern shrimp. See Shrimp.

CORVINA: Drums from the Pacific coast of South America. Skinless corvina fillets are available from Ecuador, Peru and Chile. The flesh is white and firm and well flavored, but supplies are erratic so it is difficult to build up trade.

CRABS: The following types of crabs, all commercially important in the U.S.A., are discussed individually below, in alphabetical order as follows:

Blue crab	Red crab
Blue softshell crab	Rock crab
Dungeness crab	Snow crab
King crab	Stone crab

Products made from each crab are mentioned under the name of the crab and are also cross-referenced throughout this book.

BLUE CRABS: *Scientific name: Callinectes sapidus:* An abundant small crab caught along the entire Atlantic coast from Massachusetts southward into the Gulf of Mexico. The newly moulted blue crab is the softshell crab widely used in restaurants (see below). Blue crabs, which are named for the bluish tint on the claws when the crab is alive (all crabs turn red when they are cooked), are sold alive in bushel baskets, or are cooked and sold fresh, or the meat is picked and sold fresh, pasteurized or frozen. In some areas blue crab meat is also canned. Picked meat is packed in 8, 12 or 16oz containers and is mostly now pasteurized and refrigerated, since this technique retains the flavor and texture much better than freezing does and still allows a shelf life of at least six weeks. There are a number of packs:

Jumbo lump is made up of the two large pieces of meat in the backfin.

Backfin or lump should be the same as jumbo but contains some smaller pieces.

Flake meat or body meat are the smaller pieces from the body. Also called special, regular or deluxe.

Claw meat is the meat from the claws, which is browner and a little more fibrous than the body meat.

Minced meat is removed from the shell by a mechanical process which minces the meat.

Cocktail claws are the table-ready claws with the tip of the claw shell left on. Note that there are no standard definitions for blue crab products. The expensive jumbo lump meat is particularly likely to be mixed with other body meat to reduce the cost. The backfin lumps should ideally be the size of a quarter. It is essential to know your supplier and to monitor the product carefully if you need this pack.

SOFT SHELL CRABS : are the just-moulted stage of the blue crab, when the crab has shed its old shell and is beginning to grow a new one. Harvesting should take place within an hour or two of moulting since the process only lasts a few hours. Clean the crabs by removing the apron, which is the triangular or T-shaped flap folded under the bottom shell. Remove the gills, stomach and intestine from behind the head inside the top shell and cut the "face" off behind the eyes. The rest of the crab is edible. They are sometimes breaded before being frozen. Fresh soft shell crabs

53

are shipped all over the country, but the major part of the catch is frozen, since the shelf life of the live crab is very short. The trade in softshell crabs is substantial. The industry expanded geographically in recent years. Blue crabs are now fished all around the Atlantic and Gulf coasts from Maryland southwards. At one time the crab was largely produced from the Chesapeake and adjacent areas. Also, processors can now hold hard-shell crabs until they moult, harvesting them as the much more valuable softshells. This new technique has added greatly to the supply. Softshell crabs are graded by width of the shell from side to side. The names are universally used; however, the sizes may differ markedly from shipper to shipper. The following is offered as a reasonable standard:

Mediums	3½ to 4 inches
Hotels	4 to 4½ inches
Primes	4½ to 5 inches
Jumbos	5 to 5½ inches
Whales or slabs	over 5½ inches

Different parts of the market require different sizes of crab. There is no quality distinction between the different sizes. The most important feature is that the shell is truly soft. Crabs that are beginning to harden are called buckrams.

DUNGENESS CRAB: *Scientific name: Cancer magister:* Dungeness crabs come from the north west and are one of the best crabs to eat. They are found from Baja California to the Aleutians. Northern California, Oregon and Washington generally produce most of the catch, which fluctuates widely from year to year. They reach up to 4lbs, with most of the inshore ("bay") crabs between one and two pounds. Whole cooked, brine frozen crabs wrapped in parchment or in printed polybags sell well along the west coast, particularly before September and after February when the fresh crab is out of season. Fresh crab is clearly superior to a frozen one, so it always finds the market preference. Dungeness crabs from Alaska and British Columbia extend the season so that it is virtually year-round for restaurants and markets willing to pay high prices. Dungeness crabs are hardly used at all east of the Mississippi and supplies are rarely sufficient for any packer to become interested in developing further market areas. Whole cooked crabs are usually packed in dozens, or sometimes 24, per carton. Some shippers pack them in 50lb boxes. Grading is either 1½/2½ and 2½/3½lbs per crab, or in half-pound steps. Cooked sections (half the crab without the top shell and viscera) are sometimes available in bulk packs of 100lbs. These are intended for meat extraction by canners and are generally cooked in unsalted water. Dungeness crab meat is packed in 5lb cold-pack cans and frozen. Cases are 6/5lbs. The standard pack has 50 percent body meat and 50 percent leg meat. Other packs have 60 percent body meat. Meat from the top joint of the legs, called the merus, is packed separately in 5lb cans and called fryer legs.

KING CRAB: Large spider crabs found in the northernmost waters of the Pacific, from Alaska to northern Japan. There are three species:

Paralithodes camtschatica	Red king crab
Paralithodes platypus	Blue king crab
Paralithodes brevipes	Deepwater or brown king crab

King crabs average 6 to 8 pounds each, but in Alaska, where the crabs are bigger than in Japan, they sometimes grow as large as 20 pounds. The U.S. market is supplied largely by domestic product, all of it from Alaska. The U.S.S.R. has become a significant supplier since the introduction of conservation rules in the 200-mile zone and the negotiation of a bilateral agreement between the two countries. Small quantities of a closely related species, *Lithodes antarctica*, are imported from Chile and Argentina. This is sometimes repacked as Alaskan king crab. The crab is smaller than the Alaskan species and the processing and packing are generally inferior. The inclusion of "Alaska" in the name commonly used in the market helped to establish the domestic product as the exclusive "genuine" king crab. No doubt, as demand increases beyond the already limited supply and as processing techniques in South America improve, the alternative products will begin to gain market acceptance. The present position is that only the Alaskan product is fully accepted and appreciated by the buyers. King crab is landed whole, immediately cooked, then split and cleaned by removing the gills and viscera and discarding the top shell. The tail shell is also separated at this stage. The remaining two pieces, which are made up of the legs and claw on one side connected by the shoulders, are called sections. These sections are the basic raw material from which all other king crab products are made. All products, therefore, are cooked before processing and freezing. Brine freezing and blast freezing are the two methods used for freezing king crab, and each method has its supporters. Brine freezing produces a moister product, but one that may taste too salty, while blast freezing may accelerate dehydration and give a less moist product. In practice, both methods give excellent results if done properly. As consumers get more health-conscious, the strongly salted flavor of brine-frozen product may become a disadvantage. King crab meat is normally plate frozen in cartons.

Products of king crab: The following section describes a wide range of products that are made from king crab. At this time, few of them are readily available. The market now uses legs and claws almost exclusively. The very high cost of meat products deters all but a few users and the low-end competition from surimi-based imitations has also hurt sales. King crab meat is a low-volume product and merus meat is hardly seen. Even such once-standard items as split legs are now mostly made only to special order. These descriptions and outline specifications are printed in case the price of king crab falls and again permits manufacturing on a larger scale.

Fancy legs and claws: Each crab has six walking legs, one large ("killer") claw and one small ("feeder") claw. Packs of legs and claws should be in these same proportions as the whole crab. Legs should be complete with both shoulder and walking tip. The exposed meat at the shoulder should be well glazed and each leg and claw should be lightly glazed overall.

Meat content of legs and claws should be at least 50 percent of the weight.

The usual pack of legs and claws is 1/20lb polylined cartons, with the packer's plant number stencilled or printed on them. The glazed products should weigh 23lbs to allow for the weight of the glaze and give 20lbs net weight of product. You may find boxes containing 20lbs of glazed product: these are underweight and usually the "overweight" is removed by someone in the distribution chain.

Grading may be "ocean run", that is, ungraded, or expressed in counts of legs per 10lbs. The largest legs, sometimes called jumbos, are 8/12 count. Regular product is in the region of 14/16 count. Different packers have various count standards, depending partly on where their plants are situated, since in some areas the crab size is more consistent than in others. To check the grading, set aside the claws, count the legs, allowing for broken legs, then divide the number by two to give the count per 10lbs. Generally, the larger the legs, the higher the price.

Legs and claws are a very substantial volume item in food service markets and are now a staple of the food business in the U.S.A. There are a number of things you should check when receiving shipment of legs and claws, to ensure that the product is good quality. Shell color should be fairly uniform and shells should be clean, without barnacles or black spots. (Barnacles should be cleaned off by the processor, not included with the weight of the crab; black spots are melanosis and are a likely cause for complaint from your customers). The shell should be lightly glazed all over to protect the product and the walking tips of the legs should be intact.

The shoulder end, where the meat is exposed, should be heavily glazed, since dehydration is rapid on exposed meat. Signs of dehydration (freezer burn) are yellowing and then honeycombing of the meat, which takes on a spongy appearance. If dehydration advances, the meat becomes spongy even while frozen and the legs will feel light for their size. A yellowish membrane encloses the shoulder of a live crab so it is important to distinguish between naturally yellow parts of the crab and the discoloration due to dehydration and the onset of rancidity.

Fancy legs: These are exactly as legs and claws, but without the claws. The same comments apply throughout.

Large claws with arm: Killer claws. These are packed with the arm attached and should contain about 40 percent meat. The same boxes are used as for legs and claws, but sometimes 25lbs instead of 20lbs will be packed into one carton. Quality considerations apply as for legs and claws.

Small claws with arm: Feeder claws. Like the previous item, these are cooked claws with the arm attached, but the feeder claw is the smaller of the two. These will contain only about 30 percent meat and so are cheaper than large claws, or legs and claws. Small claws are generally packed in 25lb boxes. Quality considerations apply as for legs and claws.

Split legs, or split legs and claws: Legs, or legs and claws, cut in half lengthwise, through the diameter of the leg section, so that the meat is exposed. Split legs are an expensive product, since the legs are ready for use, and also require careful handling and glazing by the processor so that the meat stays in place in the shells. Split legs alone are a more desirable and attractive pack than split legs and claws, but most of the product available includes the split claws. This product is not generally available except by special order.

In the past, it was possible to buy split legs graded according to length, so that all the pieces were approximately the same size. The cost of producing this reduced its appeal.

Quality considerations are similar to those for legs and claws, and, in addition, it is very important that the cutting is accurate, so that the two split legs halves are equal in thickness. Packs are usually 1/25lb polylined cartons. Twelve ounce retail packs were once available.

Other king crab products: There are numerous less than perfect king crab products offered and some of these are worth attention. For example, broken legs and claws vary from product lacking only the walking tip, to product consisting only of shoulders and tips (the merus sections sold to Japan at a substantial price). A good broken leg is cheaper than a fancy grade, but is just as good in use. As with all such product, it is essential to examine each shipment in detail – you can be sure that consistency will not be a feature.

Whole tails are sometimes available, but these are of little value to most users. It is necessary to have labor to remove the meat from the shells.

If you take reasonable care in checking what you buy, there are definite bargains found in number two (second quality) king crab product. Take care not to encourage customers to plan on the intermittent bargains as a constant factor.

Whole merus meat or all-leg meat: The merus is the largest segment of each of the crab's six walking legs and is the segment closest to the shoulder. Whole pieces of meat from merus sections are roughly cylindrical in shape, red colored and between four and eight inches long. 5lb blocks of merus meat are packed six per master carton. Often, the 5lb block is split into two pieces each of 2½lbs. Merus meat is the most expensive of the king crab products and indeed is one of the most expensive seafood products of any type.

Fancy meat; 60/40 meat; regular meat: The most widely used king crab meat pack is also packed 6/5lbs, or 6/2/2½lbs, in the same way as the merus meat. Fancy meat should consist of three layers within each block. The bottom layer is 25 percent of the weight and consists of merus meat. Up to 70 percent of this layer may be broken merus meat. The top layer is 20 percent by weight and is red meat. The remaining 55 percent is the center layer and consists of large pieces of white meat and should not include tail meat or meat from the walking tips of the legs.

The 60/40 designation, which is universally used as shorthand to specify king crab meat, means that there should be 40 percent leg meat (the top and bottom layers) and 60 percent body meat (the center layer) as target proportions. It is desirable to have more leg meat and less body meat, so nobody will complain if the percentage of leg meat in practice is higher than the 40 percent requested and specified. It is for this reason that packers aim at a 45/55 split, to ensure that there is a minimum of 40 percent leg meat in the product.

Salad meat: This is a cheaper pack and consists of smaller chunks of white and red meat mixed together. Salad meat chunks should be greater than ⅜th inch square, though this is a very difficult specification to check exactly.

Shred meat: This consists of the smallest pieces of meat from the body of the crab, together with any small fragments broken from the leg pieces. It is not offered very often.

Minced meat; rice meat: Mixed meat put through a ricer to give it a uniform texture, for use in stuffings and similar applications. This is the cheapest king crab meat product. It is important that the mincing is not too fine, otherwise the meat loses all texture and thaws to a mushy consistency which is not acceptable.

Tail meat: The king crab has a triangular "purse" on the underside of the shell and the meat in this tail is extracted and sold separately, as tail meat. Whole tail meat is extremely tough, but has good flavor and when chopped is an excellent inexpensive product for sandwiches or salad mixtures. Some packers mince the tail meat before freezing it, but this tends to be too finely chopped for most uses and becomes an alternative to rice meat.

Tail meat is cheap, but it is genuine king crab meat, which makes it worth the effort of using for appropriate applications.

Note on packs of king crab meat products: Alaskan king crab products, shell items as well as meat, should have the packer's plant number clearly printed on the outer carton. Alaskan king crab meat products are always packed in 30lb master cartons, usually 6/5 but sometimes 6/2/2½. Retail packs of four and six ounces in printed boxes are offered, but at current prices for crab meat, the retail market is very slender.

All king crab meat products should be polywrapped and placed in an inner carton, to give the best possible protection for these expensive items. You should insist on this packaging and refuse meat that is polywrapped only, without an inner carton. The price of the product can stand the small additional cost of an inner carton and you cannot afford to risk dehydration of expensive inventory.

Crab meat may be picked from fresh sections or shaken from frozen sections, then refrozen into blocks. The quality differences between the two techniques are not normally distinguishable. Both packs are frozen into "long johns" of 15lbs, then sawn into 2½ or 5lb blocks for final packing. The uneven ends of the long johns are packed separately and offered as sliced meat, or are made into a retail pack with random weights.

RED CRAB: A deepwater crab resembling a small snow crab, found off New England. The resource is a large one, but the crab lives in very deep water and is difficult to catch and handle. It is also quite difficult to process satisfactorily because of its small size. Red crab is made into meat, and into cocktail claws. The taste and texture are very good and the color is also attractive, being a deeper red than snow crab. The small scale of operations does not permit much market exposure or development.

ROCK CRAB AND JONAH CRAB: Jonah crab (*Cancer borealis*) and rock crab (*Cancer irroratus*) are similar, small crabs found along much of the east coast. The Jonah crab is larger and has thicker legs, but the easiest way to distinguish them is that the Jonah has black tips on its claws. Neither species is very popular with fishermen or with consumers. They are small, so eating their meat requires considerable work. Their claws are usually large enough to provide reasonable eating, but the crabs are not caught in large enough numbers to justify producing a claw pack.

However, the meat is good and some New England packers are prepared to pick the crabs and sell fresh or pasteurized meat. The resources are thought to be large. It is now possible to sell softshell rock crabs. There is some potential to develop a market for this product, which is vacuum packed and frozen. Softshell rock crabs could substitute for softshell blue crabs during the winter when the blues are scarce.

SNOW CRAB: *Scientific names:*

Chionecetes bairdii is the larger Pacific species, commonly called bairdii;

Chionecetes opilio is the smaller Pacific species, commonly called opilio;

Chionecetes tanneri is the Canadian Atlantic species, commonly called tanner or queen crab.

Snow or tanner crabs come from the North Pacific and from Canadian waters in the North Atlantic. The name queen crab is mainly used in Canada. The largest snow crab is the Alaskan bairdii crab (pronounced "bird-eye"). The Canadian snow crab is similar in size to opilio and some new smaller resources are now fished. Bairdii produces clusters (see below) of about 10 to 16 ounces; opilio clusters are generally around eight ounces. Canadian snow crab produces clusters of 6 to 8 ounces from the larger crab and as little as 3 to 5 ounces from the smaller one.

Alaskan snow crab is the most expensive. It is also superior in taste to the Canadian crab; in fact, many users prefer the taste and texture of Alaskan snow crab meat to that of king crab meat. However, king crab has the reputation with the consumer, and snow crab, whatever its intrinsic quality, sells for much less money than king crab.

Clusters: Snow crab clusters are the equivalent of king crab sections, that is the three legs and one claw from one side of the crab joined at the shoulder; gills, viscera and top shell removed. Alaskan clusters are usually packed with the claw, but may be sold without. Canadian snow crab is invariably claw on. Clusters are packed in 25lb boxes, polylined. Size grading is in ounces, commonly 5/8 ounces and 8 ounces up.

Snow crab cocktail claws: Cooked claws are scored around the top so that the shell cap may be removed easily. These sell as "snap-and-eat" claws. They are packed in 2lb or 3lb bags or boxes, usually six per master carton. Sometimes the cap is removed and the exposed tip of meat is heavily glazed for protection. Gradings are 8/12 count per pound, 12/16, 16/24 and 24/32. Alaskan and Canadian product is similarly prepared and packed, but the Alaskan product is more expensive.

Single legs: The clusters may be cut at the shoulder and the legs sold as separate pieces. This is never a particularly popular pack, probably because the small size of the snow crab makes a cluster a suitable portion.

Snow crab meat: Alaskan snow crab meat is packed in similar manner to king crab meat (see above). Merus (all leg meat) packs are also produced. Specification and packing are much the same as for Alaskan king crab and the snow meat is similarly offered in 60/40 form. Like king crab meat, Alaskan snow crab meat is no longer a significant product.

Canadian and Japanese snow crab meat is still available. It is usually packed in 70/30 percentage and the merus pieces are much smaller than those of the Alaskan crab. These snow crab origins invariably sell for substantially less than Alaskan products with similar names.

Salad meat and rice meat are produced. The Canadians sell a minced crabmeat which is finely ground so that it defrosts almost to a paste. It is a good, cheap product for adding flavor without texture to numerous applications, especially for further processing. Minced product is particularly useful for stuffings and soups or bisques. For purposes requiring some texture to the crab, it can be used if a suitable filler such as a firm white fish is added to it.

STONE CRABS: These are found almost exclusively along the Gulf Coast of Florida and only the claws are used. The claws are removed and the crab is thrown back into the water in the belief or hope that it will regenerate the lost limbs. The claws are cooked and packed in 3lb or 5lb bags, 8 or 12 per master carton. Gradings vary, but the largest claws may be 2/4 per lb and the smallest about 16/20.

A small quantity of product from Chile and other parts of South America is imported. The stone crab there is very similar in taste and texture, but has a less shiny shell than the Florida crab.

Stone crabs from all sources have very hard shells, from which feature they derive their name.

OTHER CRABS: Worldwide, there are an enormous number of crab species, some of which are harvested for local sale. Others are frozen or canned and may appear on the U.S. market. There are also several potential crab resources which may be exploited in the future. Among these is the Korean hair crab of the North Pacific (*Erimacrus eisenbecki*). This species sells for high prices when shipped live to Japan. F.D.A. requires it to be labelled as "Korean variety crabmeat" or "Kegani crabmeat." There are also reports of substantial crab stocks around the Falkland Islands.

CRAYFISH AND CRAWFISH: Crayfish is another name for spiny lobster. See Lobster. It is also the name for species of freshwater crustaceans, very similar to clawed lobsters in appearance, but mostly growing to only a few ounces. The crayfish is also called crawfish, which is its official name in Louisiana, the source of most U.S. production. It has a wide variety of other names such as crawdad and mud bug. The major species in the U.S.A. are:

Procambarus clarkii	Red swamp crawfish
Procambarus blandingii	White swamp crawfish
Pacifastacus leniusculus	Pacific crawfish

There are many other species which are not exploited commercially. European species (*Astacus astacus* is the major one) are also very similar and there are many species from Australia. One of these reaches 8 pounds.

The market for these small animals is increasing rapidly. Increasing quantities are farmed in Louisiana, Texas and other southern states. Developers are looking to Mexico, Central America, Europe and Australia for further farming opportunities.

An increasing part of the catch is sold frozen. As supplies increase, it is probable that there will be more frozen crawfish available. Even farmed, the harvest is seasonal, mainly between December and June, with peak supplies in April and May. The animals burrow into the mud under the ponds in the summer, so even farmed fish are not available. Year round supplies are dependent on freezing, or on aquaculture developing in other parts of the world with different seasons.

A wide range of products is available. Whole uncooked fish may be frozen, purged or unpurged. Purging empties the digestive vein and makes the animal much more attractive when served. However, the process is expensive and is not done by many packers. Uncooked crawfish must be frozen to very low temperatures and carefully glazed. Cooked whole crawfish are also frozen.

Many users prefer peeled meats. The crawfish are cooked and then peeled. The product is sold either with or without the yellow digestive gland, known as fat, which contains most of the flavor. Those familiar with Cajun cuisine like the fat. Others prefer the cleaner appearance of the tailmeat without it. The fat turns rancid quickly so careful handling is essential. Sometimes the meats and fat are sold separately.

Melanosis is a potential problem if crawfish are not handled properly. The darkening of the shell spreads quickly to the meat, making it unattractive.

Frozen prepared dishes are increasingly available, but the most spectacular new product is softshell crawfish, invented in the mid 1980s. The yield on this product for the producer is much higher than the 14 percent meat from processed tails. Only the digestive organs and the two small "stones" which store calcium are removed. The rest of the softshell animal is edible and saleable. Japan is an important market, but the U.S. market is growing very fast. Most softshell crawfish are frozen, packed in dozens. Counts are 21, 31 and 41 to the pound.

Producers are expecting substantial profits from softshell crawfish. It appears that crawfish moult mainly between 10 a.m. and 3 p.m. These "bankers hours" are thought to be a good omen.

CREDIT AND CREDIT CONTROL: Normal credit terms for frozen seafood are thirty days from invoice date. Invoices are usually issued on the day of shipment. Few suppliers offer discounts for prompt or early payment. If you are able to pay faster than other people, you should negotiate a discount case by case or supplier by supplier.

Fresh seafood is customarily sold on seven-day terms, or on the basis of settlement at the end of week, which effectively is three to four day terms.

As a buyer you want all the credit you can get so that the suppliers help to finance your inventory. As a seller you have to take very considerable care to extend credit only to customers you are certain will pay their bills when due.

Credit is not handled very professionally in the seafood business, probably because the small size of many suppliers allows the proprietor to know his customers personally and to develop a personal relationship with them. The high cost of money in the 1980s has severely affected seafood users and a more conventional approach is needed. Lack of attention to giving credit can mean losses from bad debts and margins are not great enough to absorb many such losses.

Your credit profile on each customer should include how long he has been in business; his corporate structure (are you billing a corporation or an individual?); his net worth and how it is structured; his credit lines; his bank reference and if his banking relationship is less than two years old; a reference from his previous bankers; and at least three trade references.

If the customer is small or new, check on his previous history. You may find this new business was opened by someone with a record of failures. Net worth is important as an indicator of whether you will get paid – it shows if there are assets that in the event of bankruptcy might be sold to pay the creditors. A wise rule is not to extend credit of more than ten percent of net worth. If the figures available to you are old when you check, ask for a statement. Remember, it is your money that is at risk, not the customer's.

Trade references help you decide whether the customer pays promptly, whether he has a habit of taking deductions, and what sort of volume he buys. Try to find out who else the customer uses as a supplier, in addition to the names he gives you. Often, the names you research for yourself will have more revealing information than those you are given by the customer, since he is of course concerned to show you his best aspects.

Above all, use independent reports from Dun and Bradstreet, the New York Board of Trade of the Wholesale Seafood Merchants, Seafood Credit Corporation, and anyone else, especially local groups, who may have information. If there are local groups covering the food business, join them and participate as fully as you can. Timely information is worth a great deal and advance word of failing customers can save you much.

Since you may buy from and sell to the same business at different times and because the whole seafood business is permeated with gossip, your credit package should include "street knowledge" of the other business. Be sure to check. It is easy to find gossip repeated, but that is not confirmation, that is repeated gossip. Facts can be checked and it is facts that determine your business decisions.

CREVALLE JACK *Scientific name: Caranx hippos:* Also called jack crevalle, toro, cavalla and horse crevally. A species shaped like a pompano and reaching 40lbs. Most are fished at between two and six pounds and are found throughout the warmer waters of the world. In the U.S.A. it is only exploited to a limited extent in Florida, but the available resource is very large in Florida and Gulf waters. The flesh is solid and rather dark, with reddish fat. Cutting off the tail to bleed the fish immediately after it is caught improves the meat, making it lighter and moister. Frozen fish are sold whole in 25lb and 50lb boxes. Larger fish are sometimes smoked. Markets could be developed for this fish, which is readily and inexpensively available.

CROAKER *Scientific name: Micropogonias undulatus:* This is the Atlantic croaker, known also as hardhead, which is a name the Fishlist (see Names) does not encourage. It is a small fish between eight and 25 ounces landed in large quantities on the Gulf coast and historically on the Mid-Atlantic coast. It is frozen whole in blocks for bait and zoo food and is sold headless dressed, or filleted and I.Q.F. for traypacking for retail sale in the south. The species extends down most of the South American coast. Imported croaker is sometimes available to supplement domestic supplies. Brazil, Uruguay and Argentina catch the major quantities.

Availability varies greatly. There are cycles of abundance followed by years without a great deal of fish. Overall, it is a common and cheap fish with an excellent flavor and texture. The market is mainly along the east and Gulf coast from New York southwards. The flesh is oily but succulent.

Atlantic croaker is also a possible raw material for surimi.

Croakers are found throughout the world (they are so-called because they have a bladder in the throat with which they make a frog-like noise). Large quantities of several species are landed in the western Pacific and Indian oceans. F.A.O records catches exceeding half a million tons a year.

CRUSTACEA: Shellfish with external skeletons and jointed legs. There are 25,000 different species (some of them are land-based). The commercially important ones are lobsters, crayfish, shrimp and crabs.

CURING: Salting and smoking. Before refrigeration, curing was the most practical way to preserve foods. Modern curing techniques aim to give a pleasing flavor to food rather than to preserve it. Smoked and salted fish are often frozen for longer shelf-life.

Some of the cures are briefly defined as follows:

Amarelo: Portuguese cure. Salt content about 18%. Yellow color.

Branco: Portuguese cure. Salt content about 20%. White color.

Dry salting: See Kench, below.

Fall: Light salt, pickle cure, 45% to 48% moisture.

Gaspe: Light salt, pickle cure, 34% to 36% moisture.

Hard: Dry-salted; dried to moisture content 40% or less.

Heavy salted fish: Has about 40% salt (dry weight basis) and moisture content with a range of definitions, in Canada, as follows:

> Extra hard dried – less than 35% moisture
> Hard dried – up to 40%
> Dry – 40% to 42%
> Semi-dry – 42% to 50%
> Ordinary cure – 44% to 50%
> Soft dried – 50% to 54%

Heavy salted soft cure fish have about 17% salt (dry weight basis) and about 47% moisture.

Kench: Dry salting: Split fish and salt in alternate layers, allowing the moisture to drain. This is a basic curing method.

Labrador: Heavy salt (about 18%); 42% to 50% moisture.

Pickle cure: Wet salting: the fish are salted in a container so that they are cured or pickled in the liquid that forms.

Shore: Light salt, kench cure. About 12% salt and 32% to 36% moisture.

Soft: Dry salted, dried to over 40% moisture.

The following are some examples of dried fish:

Stockfish: Unsalted fish dried in cold air. Fish is headed, gutted and hung to dry in the sun.

Dried salted codfish (also called bacalao and klipfish): Salted fish is washed, salted again and dried (see Saltfish below). Keeps well in cool, dry areas. See Cod.

Saltfish: Headed, gutted with the larger part of the backbone removed. The fish is cleaned and washed then preserved with dry salt for three weeks. Sold whole or in fillets, it keeps well in cool temperatures.

See also Smoking.

CUSK *Scientific name: Brosme brosme:* A cod-like fish which reaches a size of 2 to 3 feet and 20 to 30 pounds. Small quantities are caught in the colder parts of the North Atlantic. The flesh is white and firm and the cusk is often salted. It is also packed in cellos and sold as ocean catfish.

Cusk is the American and Canadian name. In Europe it is usually called tusk.

CUSK EEL: See Kingklip.

CUTTLEFISH: Also called inkfish and sepia, which is the German name (and similar to the Italian name, which is spelled seppia). A close relative of squid, sepia is shorter, wider and far less common. It is mainly used in Portuguese and Mediterranean style cuisines and sells to a limited market in the U.S.A. Sales tend to concentrate around Christmas.

Large sepia of two to three pounds from France or Portugal supply the premium end of the market. Smaller sizes are less desirable. Cheaper and much smaller sepia (as small as two ounces) are imported from Korea, Thailand and other Asian countries.

Sepia is washed to remove the slime, then packed and frozen whole. Size grading varies from packer to packer. The ink is used in cooking so evisceration, which destroys the ink sac, is a negative feature – users prefer to buy their cuttlefish whole. Like squid, cuttlefish are voracious feeders and it is not unusual to find whole fish undigested in the stomachs of larger cuttlefish.

Cuttlefish is sometimes used as a substitute for abalone. See Abalone.

DAINTY TAILS: See Lobsterette.

DARK CHUM: The poorest description of chum salmon, so called because of its dark grey to black skin and greyish flesh. See Salmon.

DECOMPOSITION: See Inspection and Defect action level.

DEEP SEA TAILS: See Lobsterette.

DEFATTED: The term mainly applies to blocks and fillets of South American whiting, which has a layer of fat under the skin. This fat remains on skinless fillets unless the skinning knives are set to cut deeply enough to remove it. If the fat is removed, the yield is lower and so the cost is higher.

The fat on the whiting is an unappealing brown and causes the fillets to look less attractive. Because whiting fat turns rancid quickly, the life of defatted product is longer. Note that in New England, the subcutaneous fat and connective tissue of flounder and cod is deliberately left on, but this is a shiny silver layer which actually improves the appearance of the fillet.

Use of defatted fillets for block manufacture results in an obviously preferable block of solid white fish flesh, without streaks of brown fat.

DEFECT ACTION LEVEL: The F.D.A. has set standards of defects for a number of seafood products. If these levels are found, the food is automatically rejected. However, lower levels do not mean automatic acceptance.

The following gives current levels for natural or unavoidable defects in seafood for human use that present no health hazard.

Defect action level for fresh or frozen fish or fillets weighing 3 pounds or less: Decomposition in 5 percent or more of the fish or fillets in the sample (but not less than 5 fish) show Class III decomposition over at least 25 percent of their areas; or

20 percent or more of the fish or fillets in the sample, (but not less than 5 fish) show Class II decomposition over at least 25 percent of their areas;

The percentage of fish or fillets showing Class II decomposition as above, plus 4 times the percentage of those showing Class III decomposition as above equals at least 20 percent and there are at least 5 decomposed fish or fillets in the sample.

Classes of decomposition:
- No odor of decomposition
- Slight odor of decomposition
- Definite odor of decomposition

Defect action levels for tullibees, ciscoes, inconnus, chubs and freshwater whitefish: 50 parasitic cysts per 100 pounds (whole or fillets) provided that the 20 percent of the fish examined are infested.

Defect action levels for blue fin and other fresh water herring: 60 cysts per 100 fish (fish 1 pound or less) or 100 pounds of fish (fish over 1 pound) provided that 20 percent of the fish examined are infested.

Defect action levels for red fish and ocean perch: 3 percent of the fillets examined contain 1 or more copepods accompanied by pus pockets.

Defect action levels for shrimp, fresh or frozen, raw, headless, peeled or breaded: Decomposed as determined by organoleptic examination: 5 percent Class III or 20 percent Class II (See above or if percentage of Class II shrimp plus 4 times percent of Class III, equals 20 percent).

Defect action levels for salmon, canned: Decomposition: A defective can is defined as one that contains Class II or Class III decomposition (for definitions see above). Two Class III defective cans, regardless of lot and container size; or

2 to 30 Class II and/or Class III defective cans as required by sampling plan based on lot size and container size.

Defect action level for calico scallops: If 20 percent or more of calico scallops are contaminated with nematodes, the scallops should be recommended for seizure. All samples should consist of 10-one pound sub-sample. Samples should not be frozen because the scallop meat will become opaque. (Source: F.D.A.)

DEFROSTING METHODS: The following is taken from Title 50 of the Code of Federal Regulations. It gives thawing procedures for frozen foods and for shrimp. Correct thawing is essential for an accurate determination of drained weights.

Regulatory tolerances for net weight are established under the provisions of the Federal Food, Drug and Cosmetic Act, as amended.

The following procedures are based on the Thirteenth Edition of the Official Methods of Analysis of the Association of Official Analytical Chemists.

Net Weight of Frozen Seafoods – Procedure: Set scale on firm support and level. Adjust zero load indicator or rest point and check sensitivity.

Glazed seafoods: Remove package from low temperature storage, open immediately, and place contents under gentle spray of cold water. Agitate carefully so product is not broken. Spray until all ice glaze that can be seen or felt is removed. Transfer product to circular no. 8 sieve, 20cm (8 inches) diameter for product less than or equal to 0.9kg (2lb) and 20cm (12 inches) for a product greater than 0.9kg (2lb). Without shifting product, incline sieve at angle of 17-20° to facilitate drainage and drain exactly 2 minutes (stop watch). Immediately transfer product to tared pan (B) and weigh (A). Weight of product = A - B.

Modified AOAC methods for determining the net weight of frozen peeled shrimp blocks and package: Equipment needed:
- Container of sufficient size and capacity so as to completely submerge the product. Wire mesh basket large enough to contain contents of package and with opening small enough to retain all pieces. Expanded metal test-tube basket or equivalent, fully lined with standard 16 mesh per linear inch insect screen, mesh bags or other suitable containers are also satisfactory.
- Balance. Sensitive to 0.011 ounce or 0.25 grams.
- Sieve. U.S. standard #8 wire sieve 12 inches diameter (30 centimeters).
- Thermometer.
- Stop watch.

Procedures: Place contents of individual package in wire mesh basket and immerse in container of fresh water so that top of basket extends above water level. Introduce water at 80°F. ± 5°F. (26°C. ± 3°C.) at bottom of container at flow rate of 1 to 3 quarts or liters per minute. As soon as the product thaws so that the glaze can be removed and the shrimp separated easily, transfer all material to a 12 inch (30 centimeters) No. 8 sieve, distributing evenly. Tilt the sieve to above 20 degrees and drain for exactly two minutes. Immediately transfer shrimp to a tared container and weigh.

"Drained weight" of cooked shrimp is determined by the following AOAC 18.018 method modified: Weigh product free of all wrapping and record weight. Place product in a container containing an amount of fresh potable water 80°F. ± 5°F. (26°C. ± 3°C.) equal to 8 times the declared weight of the product. If product is block frozen, turn block over several times during thawing. If frozen shrimp are caked together they may be parted manually provided they are not injured in the process. When all the ice has melted, empty the shrimp into a 12 inch (30 centimeters) No. 8 sieve, distributing evenly. Tilt the sieve to about 20° and drain for exactly two minutes. Immediately transfer shrimp to a tared container and weigh.

Source: Federal Register, May 20, 1982, amended Oct. 1, 1986.

For more information on net weights and thawing, see Economic fraud in the seafood business.

DEHYDRATION: See Freezer burn.

DELANEY CLAUSE: A Federal provision stating that no substance which might cause cancer may be added to food. The additive does not have to be a proven carcinogen, just a suspected one.

DELIVERY TERMS: In domestic trade, goods are usually sold either "f.o.b." or "delivered." In this context, f.o.b. means that the sale is made at the current location of the goods. This is a bad term, because in international trade f.o.b. has a specific and quite different meaning (see below). Generally, it is better to specify "ex-warehouse" or "in-warehouse" depending upon whether a release or a transfer is required.

Product is transferred when the warehouse changes title of the goods from the seller to the buyer who pays storage charges from the date they are next due. A product is released when the warehouse gives the goods to a specific carrier on behalf of the buyer (the carrier is often the buyer's own truck).

Product transferred is billed immediately, as the transfer gives the buyer immediate control over the goods. Releases are usually billed when the goods are physically picked up. If further storage charges are due between the time of the transaction and the actual removal of the goods, the seller will continue to be responsible for the cost, since the goods are still his property.

As far as possible, buy on delivered terms, making the seller responsible for freight charges to your destination. If the product is poor and has to be returned, you will not be liable to pay a freight bill for product you could not use.

In international trade a number of delivery terms are used. These are all specifically defined by the International Chamber of Commerce. The following brief definitions may assist you to understand your importer.

F.A.S.: Free alongside ship. Seller delivers goods to the dock beside the vessel. Buyer pays the costs of loading the vessel, and all charges from that point.

F.O.B.: Free on board. Seller delivers goods on to the vessel for the buyer.

C & F: Cost and freight. The seller delivers the goods on to the vessel and prepays the freight to the stated destination point. The buyer pays subsequent charges, including the cost of insuring the goods.

C.I.F.: Cost, insurance and freight. C & F plus the insurance is paid by the seller.

C.I.F.R.: C.I.F. and insurance against rejection is paid by the seller (see Rejection).

Note that in all cases, the freight covers the cost of getting the goods to the destination. The cost of removing them from the vessel and responsibility for Customs clearance, duties, taxes etc., rests with the buyer.

CONSIGNMENT is not exactly a delivery term, but has similar implications. A packer may ship his product to a destination for an importer or agent to sell on his behalf. Typically, the importer pays the shipper up to 80 percent of the expected selling price of the goods; then, when the goods are sold, the excess over that amount is split between importer and shipper to an agreed formula.

Consignment deals are good for an importer because his risk of actually losing money is slight. They are also good for the exporter who feels he is participating in the market and sharing in any speculative profits that the importer would otherwise earn entirely. In practice, some consignment deals encourage the importation of product that the market does not need, which distorts prices. With such transactions, both parties probably suffer.

It is useful for buyers to know when importers have consignment product to sell, since importers may be less interested in selling at the highest possible price than in fast turnover at a reasonable level of profit. This helps the buyer negotiate keener prices.

DEPURATION: The practice of cleansing bacteria from live shellfish to make them safe to eat.

Clams and oysters are often eaten raw and whole. Clams, oysters and mussels are often eaten whole with very little cooking.

Because many more bacteria are present in the digestive tract than in the flesh, there is a considerable risk of infection if shellfish containing harmful bacteria are eaten whole and with little or no cooking.

In order to protect both consumers and the shellfish industry, the F.D.A. operates the Shellfish Sanitation Program with the active participation of all states where shellfish are produced. Part of this program regulates the use of depuration facilities.

Clams, oysters and mussels are all filter feeders (so are scallops, but we do not eat the digestive tract of scallops, only the muscle). Filter feeders live on algae which they trap by pumping water through their bodies and filtering out the nutrients they require. Along with the algae, the shellfish also absorb bacteria. The amount varies according to what is in the water. Water contaminated with sewage, for example, gives the shellfish a great deal of food, but because of the number and the nature of the bacteria ingested from such water by the molluscs it is harmful to humans who feed on the shellfish. It is therefore important that all the shellfish eaten are either taken from waters which contain little or no pollutants or they are cleaned in such a way that they lose the bacteria which might harm the consumer.

Shellfish either digest bacteria or excrete them in a period of 24 to 48 hours. If they are placed in clean water which is kept sterile for that length of time, they will lose the bacteria they absorbed and be clean and safe to eat. This is the simple basis of depuration.

Depuration is allowed to be used on shellfish taken from waters that exceed the permitted bacteria level for direct consumption. Depuration therefore makes it possible for shellfish in contaminated areas to be fished and sold and so increases the supply for the consumer. For a variety of reasons, the process is little used in the U.S.A., although sanctioned by the F.D.A. and subject to its supervision and regulation.

In the north-western part of Spain, there are a number of huge depuration plants processing annually hundreds of thousands of tons of mussels and oysters for sale throughout Europe. All shellfish are processed through these plants, not just those from contaminated areas, so consumer confidence in Spanish shellfish is firm. Spain's success as Europe's major supplier of live shellfish attests to the effectiveness of their system.

In Spain, most plants use large-scale chlorination of the water to ensure cleanliness. Much smaller systems, using ultra-violet light, ozone or biological filters, are available and the depuration process can work economically on a very small scale, as well as with very large volumes.

The major advantage of depuration is that it makes available large resources of shellfish that at present cannot be used. A secondary advantage is that if all shellfish were to be cleaned, the monitoring of the industry would simplify because it would be concentrated into fewer locations for testing.

Fishermen tend to be suspicious of depuration, which would certainly change the business dramatically if depuration were done on a large scale. Some shellfish shippers are also opposed on the grounds that depuration would reduce the need to clean up coastal waters and cleanup is more important. Some health officials state that depuration will remove bacteria but not viruses, so giving a false sense of security. Overall, the political will to establish depuration plants is largely lacking. However, plants in a number of states have been operating for some years with success. Interest is increasing as clams, mussels and oysters become more expensive and as traditional fishing areas become more polluted.

Depuration has to be done properly. This means that ultra-violet sanitizing lights must be changed at regular intervals, other bactericides must be used correctly and monitored carefully and that the water temperature and salinity must be adjusted so that the animals actively pump the clean water through their systems. The process is quite expensive, requiring capital expenditure on plant and laboratory facilities as well as time (it takes at least two days to purify oysters, for example). The final problem is marketing: convincing customers that the product is worth the additional cost and being able to label the product as purified.

Despite the problems and the traditional lethargy about depuration, it seems that the trend is towards increasing use of the developing technology. In the longer term, this should increase supplies, add to consumer confidence and help the industry all around.

DEVEIN: To remove the sand vein (intestine) from the tail section of a shrimp, lobster or other crustacean.

DILL SALMON: See Gravlax.

DIPS: A number of similar chemicals used in processing seafoods to help retain moisture and sometimes to improve the appearance by whitening. Sodium tripolyphosphate, sodium or potassium pyrophosphate and other phosphate compounds are among the chemicals used. The use of these or any other additives should be listed on the label of each inner pack.

Fillets dipped in polyphosphates drip less than undipped fillets, both as fresh product and on thawing after freezing. Dips also reduce the gaping of fillets when thawed. Scallops are frequently dipped, since they both drip and darken if left alone.

The use of dips is long established and is harmless so far as is known. It is, or course, common in other parts of the food industry also. There are two problems to keep in mind. The first is that dips may be used without mention on the label and this is illegal. The second is that, very occasionally, a packer will use an excessive concentration of dip. Imported peeled shrimp and imported scallops are the most likely items to suffer in this way. Excessive use of phosphates makes the product tough, sometimes to a point where it will seem not to cook. Phosphates are easy to use and this processing error is fortunately rare. Excessive phosphates can also mask off-odors. A piece of fish which smells acceptable before cooking, but smells badly during and after cooking, was probably over-treated. This is one reason why you should cook a small sample of fish when inspecting it.

Other chemicals are also used. Sulfites prevent blackening (melanosis) of shrimp. The residual levels of sulfites are strictly controlled and monitored by the F.D.A., particularly because there is a small segment of the population (suffering from asthma) who are strongly allergic to sulfites. For this reason, the chemical is already banned from use on salads in salad bars. Its use is likely to be more restricted in the future. For other chemicals, see the appropriate entries.

DOGFISH: Also called dog shark, huss and flake. None of these other names are approved in the Fishlist. (See Names.)

Dogfish are small members of the shark family with white, sweet flesh. The difficulties of handling account for the general lack of interest among American producers for this product, even though the fish is popular and well used in many European countries.

There are two main species. *Squalus acanthias* is the spiny dogfish, found on both coasts. *Mustelus canis* is the smooth dogfish of the Atlantic. Both species are abundant and increasing quantities are caught and processed for export to Europe. Much more is available if domestic markets develop. Skinless, boneless dogfish backs are cheap to produce and the flesh is firm, sweet and well flavored. The difficulty with dogfish is selling the name. In the 1940s, dogfish was canned and sold as "gray fish," a name that is also unattractive.

Smooth dogfish reach about 12lbs and the spiny dogfish about 7lbs. Back fillets are generally between 1lb and 5lbs. Like all sharks dogfish lack urinary tracts and excrete body wastes through the skin. The fish therefore must be handled with great care and speed to prevent spoilage of the flesh through the development of uric acid, which has a strong ammonia smell. Few U.S. processors handle dogfish correctly, which is why their product sells in Europe only when alternative supplies are exhausted.

Dogfish under the name of "rock salmon" used to be a staple of the fish and chip trade in Britain, until well-intentioned bureaucrats decided that the name was misleading and had it banned. Consumers did not recognize the new names of "flake" and "huss" and so were protected from a cheap source of nutritious protein. The point of this is not to debate naming conventions but to make it clear that dogfish was a well regarded seafood when marketed in a way acceptable to the consumer.

You can find skinned backs intended for export graded in 200gm and 500gm steps, packed in 10kg, 20kg or 28lb boxes, either I.Q.F or layer packed. Dogfish is cheap and good, is always boneless and is worth trying.

In Germany, the bellyflaps are smoked as "schillerlocken." There is a world market also for the dried or frozen tails, which can be made into shark fin soup.

DOG SALMON: Chum salmon. See Salmon.

DOLLY VARDEN *Scientific name: Salvelinus malma:* See Arctic char. This is not the same fish as Arctic char, but is very similar. Marketing of the two fish is the same.

DOLPHIN: Porpoise. This is a mammal, not a fish. It is protected by law and is not used for food in the U.S.A.

DOLPHIN FISH: It avoids any confusion with the animal dolphin if this fish is called by its Hawaiian name, mahi-mahi. This name is approved by the F.D.A. Selling the fish as dolphin is asking to get your business picketed. It is, after all, totally different. See Mahi-mahi.

DORIES: There are three distinct types of dories you might find traded:
John Dory: *Zeus faber,* the European John Dory and *Zenopsis ocellata*, the very similar American John Dory are probably the best. When available, these fish are generally sold fresh. The meat is white, firm and fine tasting. The French call it St. Pierre, which is St. Peter.
Smooth oreo dory, *Pseudocyttus maculatus*, is a deepwater species from the southern oceans. New Zealand first marketed the fish in the northern hemisphere, but it is also available from Australian, South African and South American waters. Some of this supply is via Korean, Russian and other factory ships which fish throughout the open oceans.

Smooth oreo dory has firm, white fillets suitable for cooking by most methods. It is available in 22lbs (10kg) shatterpacks. New Zealand processing quality is invariably good. Other origins, however, may pack it as a substitute for (and labelled as) orange roughy.
Black oreo dory, *Allocyttus spp.* is a smaller fish producing thinner fillets with a greater tendency to dry out. They are less white when cooked than the smooth oreo fillets. 2/4 ounce fillets are about standard, usually produced from fish that was frozen at sea in headless and gutted form.

DOVER SOLE, GENUINE *Scientific name: Solea vulgaris:* European Dover sole is probably the most expensive of all flatfish and is the original true sole. As such, it is the foundation of French fish cookery. The flesh is very firm and white and often cooked on the bone for the best yield and flavor. It is vastly superior to the Pacific fish with the same name.

Imports come from Holland, Belgium, Denmark, the U.K. and France and are normally individually polybagged, I.Q.F. and packed in 25lb or 50lb boxes. The fish is invariably dressed and scaled. Grading is in ounces:

Small	10/12. 12/14. 14/16 and 12/16
Selects	16/20, 20/24 and 24/28
Large	28/32, 32/36 and 36/40

The select sizes are preferred.

DOVER SOLE, PACIFIC *Scientific name: Microstomus pacificus:* A flatfish caught from southern California to Alaska. It averages 2 to 2½lbs and is legally marketed as sole or Dover sole, in skinless and boneless fillet form. See Flatfish.

DRAWN: Eviscerated; gutted.

DRESSED: Same as Drawn.

DRUM: There are many quite different varieties of drum. For information on some of them see Sea trout, Corvina and Croaker.
Freshwater drum, *Alpodinotus grunniens,* is sometimes available frozen whole or dressed. It is a small fish from the Great Lakes and Mississippi regions, harvested mostly at about 1lb.
Black drum *Scientific name: Pogonias cromis:* A Gulf and Atlantic species with rather coarse flesh. The species often contains parasites so should be cooked thoroughly. It is also better if it is bled. Black drum is popular in Chinese cuisine and may be offered as an inferior substitute for red drum (red fish).

DUBLIN BAY PRAWN: See Lobsterette.

DUNGENESS CRAB: See Crabs.

ECONOMIC FRAUD IN THE SEAFOOD BUSINESS:

There are three types of economic fraud in seafood:

Substituting an inferior product for one that sells at a higher price: Actions like selling swordfish but supplying shark or invoicing for crabmeat but shipping a surimi imitation constitute deliberate substitution and conscious fraud.

There are many products which may be targeted for substitution. Almost any fish or shellfish which is in short supply or fetches a high price is vulnerable. Throughout this book, possible substitutions for items covered are mentioned in the appropriate section.

Substitutions may occur in whole fish. These are the easiest to spot because all of its identification features are intact. Pomfret, though, can sometimes be passed off as pompano. There are a number of good snappers that are sold as "red snapper" although that designation is reserved for *Lutjanus campechanus*. Headless, dressed fish is harder to identify, because fins and heads are important identifying features. Outside the northwest, comparatively few people can identify the different species of Pacific salmon.

Fillets, even with the skin on, become harder still to identify. Haddock has a characteristic black lateral line and "thumb print" mark, while cod, pollock and related fish have a white line and no thumb print. Skinned cod and haddock fillets are indistinguishable without the aid of scientific tests such as iso-electric focussing.

If you have used the help available in this book and in the many others suggested in the Reference section at the end but are still in dispute over how to identify seafoods, scientifically valid analysis is the answer. In the unlikely event that you have a whole fish, there are many good scientists at museums, research institutions and universities who can identify it. Thanks to the work of the Smithsonian's Austin Williams, lobsters can be identified accurately from the tail alone. But if you have to go further, there are now two analytical techniques which can provide accurate identification of samples.

The first is iso-electric focussing, which is described fully in a separate heading later in this book. The second is the use of monoclonal antibodies. These are prepared from samples of positively identified species and give totally accurate results on cooked as well as raw product.

Laboratory tests such as these can provide conclusive identification if needed.

Packaging can also increase the confusion. Many cartons are printed with a list of possible products. When the carton is packed, the actual contents are checked off. Check marks can be changed. (They might also innocently be wrong). Some cello packs are unlabelled (called blank cellos). The labels are loose in the carton for the retailer to enclose under the tray wrap. Such labels can be changed by unscrupulous dealers anywhere along the distribution chain.

Chinese white shrimp and domestic white shrimp are virtually indistinguishable, but the market prefers the domestic product by as much as $1 per pound on medium to large sizes. It is quite easy and very profitable to convert Chinese shrimp into U.S. product, but definitely illegal.

Be aware that as markets and supplies change, so does the substitution business. The only protection is to know your product thoroughly, check it carefully and use known, reliable suppliers.

See also Names.

Deliberate short weight or short shipment: There are two aspects to this type of economic fraud. The simpler one, and the easier one to combat, is the short weight shipment. There are various techniques. A full pallet of cartons may be delivered strapped or even wrapped. But it is possible for an entire carton to be missing from the center of a pallet, without it being apparent from the external appearance and layout of the cartons. The protection is simple (although time-consuming). Unload the pallets and count the cartons.

On a smaller scale, the same approach applies to individual cartons. It is possible to remove an inner 5lb box from a carton containing ten 5lb boxes (leaving nine boxes in the carton). If the top layer of boxes appears complete, the carton appears to be full. But it feels lighter than the other cartons which contain the correct 50lbs. Again, the solution is to handle every box. Any warehouseman should be able to tell whether cartons weigh less than others in the same shipment.

It is easy to remove one or two lobster tails from a 10lb box, leaving the box looking as though it is full. The same applies to crab clusters and similarly bulk-packed product. This sort of stealing is really quite difficult to detect, unless buyers make a habit of checking everything that comes in.

Always check cartons without straps, or which have been retaped. These deficiencies may be symptoms of pilferage or even substitution during distribution.

The worldwide use of the metric system has created another opportunity for shortweighting. 2-kilo boxes may look the same as 5lb boxes, but contain 12 percent less product. Even if a box is labelled 2 kilos, which is 4.4 pounds, unscrupulous dealers may change the marks on the box, or even maintain that 2 kilos equals 5 pounds.

Short weight is easier with fresh fish, of course, since the boxes include ice which has to be rinsed off before the product can be weighed. This book focuses on frozen product, but watch for this problem with fresh fish and shellfish.

The more complex part of the short weight scam is the excessive use of glaze – ice protection which is necessary to maintain the quality of frozen product. Glaze is a protective coating of ice which prevents dehydration. The weight of the glaze should not be included in the net weight of the product.

Excessive ice is not restricted to the outside of a product. For example, lobster tails may have water injected under the shell – between the shell and the meat – to make the tails appear to be heavier than they really are. This not only adds weight, which is billed as expensive lobster tail rather than as inexpensive ice, it may also be sufficient to increase the apparent weight of a tail enough so that it fits into the next larger size classification, worth more per pound.

Lobster tails, and other product sold in the shell, are a special case. Adding water to a product by dipping it into a chemical solution is much more common. Phosphate-based chemicals are widely used in food processing. They have a slightly preservative effect. On fish fillets they whiten the meat. Phosphates also improve the retention of natural moisture, preventing some drip loss after thawing. (See Dips for further information). Unfortunately, phosphate dips can be abused to make the product absorb additional water. This works for a wide range of products. Scallops are the most easily affected. Other products that may be dipped include fish fillets and shrimp.

The F.D.A. defines the additional water absorbed by dipped product as an adulterant. If you buy fish, you do not want to pay for water; the definition seems entirely reasonable.

The problem is to determine the net weight without glaze, since most seafoods will drip their own moisture for days. Definitions of net weight and drained weight, and disputes about them, are a continual problem throughout the industry.

Properly refrigerated fresh products may lose as much as 10 percent of their weight in three days through natural drip loss. It is possible to take a 5lb block of scallops and let it thaw overnight at room temperature, and find in the morning that there is only 4lb of product left. If the same scallops are left for another day, there may only be 3lb of product. There are users who will then complain that their scallops were short weight by an enormous amount and refuse to pay for them as billed. Scallops are an extreme example, because they lose natural moisture by dripping continuously until almost the whole scallop has disappeared. This will happen with fresh as well as frozen product, though the damage done to cell walls by freezing makes the situation worse for frozen product.

Thawing methods: It is very clear that the way an item is defrosted greatly affects the apparent net weight, so there needs to be a recognized and generally accepted way of thawing and checking the weights of products.

Firstly, it should generally be accepted by reasonable people that the product when frozen should contain no less than the labelled net weight of product. It is then necessary to determine at a later date whether this amount was in fact packed.

Much work has been done by the American Shrimp Canners Association, which have established quite complex guidelines for checking the weights of blocks of frozen peeled shrimp. The techniques were worked out by first freezing a known amount of product and then comparing the net weights given by different thawing methods with the actual weight of the product when-frozen so that the most accurate thawing method could be defined. The method is complex because the temperature of thawing water used and many other factors have to be carefully controlled if the answer is to be right. But it is possible to freeze a known weight of peeled shrimp, store it for a time, then defrost and check the weight and determine the original weight frozen. Unfortunately, this work applies only to peeled shrimp and while it probably is applicable to other products, the necessary experimental work has not been done.

The Association of Official Analytical Chemists also have guidelines for determining weights and these are reasonable for most product.

The Code of Federal Regulations, Title 50, lays down defrost methods for a number of common products and provides the standards used by most of the seafood industry. The standards are not perfect, but they have the advantage that the National Marine Fisheries Service will perform tests as specified, for a fee, and any parties in dispute will accept that the tests are objective, and performed by an independent third party. For full specifications of these tests, see Defrosting methods.

Whatever the tests used, it is always worth telling suppliers, and if necessary also customers, which tests will be accepted as proof of net weights. There are plenty of traders who will do scientifically invalid tests for weight and make claims on suppliers, either to void deals or to make themselves extra margins. If the rules are specified and agreed before business is completed, many problems can be avoided and disputes can be settled amicably and fairly.

If the effect of incorrect thawing is fully understood – the effect being that you can defrost product down to very little, whatever its original weight – and the proper tests and methods are understood and utilized, a great many problems can be avoided.

Inferior quality or size: 21/25 shrimp costs more per pound than 26/30 shrimp. But how many people bother to check that a box of 21/25s has between 105 and 125 whole tails? It is quite easy for the next smaller size to be substituted. Even easier is offering 31/40 count as 31/35s. Wherever precise size grading is critical to price and value, there is the possibility of fraud. Lobster tails, mentioned above in the context of under-shell glaze, are similarly "up-sized" for additional profit for the seller.

As with any economic fraud, it is only going to happen when there is an economic reason for doing it. The relationship between prices for different sizes of shrimp varies a great deal. But whenever there is a major differential between adjacent sizes (and such differentials can sometimes exceed $1 per lb) there is an opportunity for someone to remark a box as the next larger size in order to make the extra, substantial profit.

Check sizes of product. Count randomly selected boxes of shrimp and lobster tails. Weigh individual fillets as well as counting the number in a container. Vigilance is the best defense.

Inferior quality is harder to pin down because it covers a huge range of possibilities. Again, though, the best defense is to examine product, check it out very carefully and apply as much experience as possible to judging its quality and value.

Workmanship affects quality, appearance and, therefore, value and price. Fillets with ragged edges, pieces of skin, blood clots, parasites, belly membranes or extraneous material are less appealing to customers, and, because they have to be trimmed and cleaned up, less economical to use. You have to be aware of the quality of workmanship that you expect and pay for.

Watch out for rat-packing – the practice of putting good quality, nice looking product at the top of the container, while hiding inferior product underneath. Always look through the whole container, not just at the top.

Freshness is as vital for frozen fish as it is for unfrozen product. Smell is the best tool to use to determine whether the product was fresh before it was processed (and whether, for that matter, it still is). If thawed fish or shellfish smells stale, it certainly is. Fatty frozen fish is particularly likely to turn rancid in storage (see Rancidity) and this condition is easy to detect by smell. Freezer burn (see separate entry) is dehydration of the product, recognizable from the yellowish, cottony appearance of the "burned" sections. Belly burn, bruising, gaping, net marks, poor filleting and all the various ways quality can be affected for the worse must be checked. See the section on quality and the associated entries on the various conditions and terms.

The deliberate supply of poor quality fish at the price of good quality fish is as much a fraud as the deliberate supply of a cheaper species.

The only way to guard against these problems is to know the product and inspect it carefully. Write down specifications and adhere to them. Examine product before you accept it. Follow markets and prices: a deal that is too good to be true probably is.

EEL *Scientific name: Anguilla rostrata:* Also called American eel and freshwater eel. The juveniles are called glass eels and elvers. The American eel, which is very similar to the European eel *Anguilla anguilla* and the Japanese or Asian eel *Anguilla japonicus*, is mainly exploited for export trade, although there are domestic sales around Christmas. Virginia and the Chesapeake are the main catching areas, although eels can be caught along the whole of the Atlantic and Gulf coasts as well as in freshwater areas which have outlets to the ocean. Most of the catch is shipped alive to both domestic and overseas markets.

Eels may grow as large as 20lbs, but most of the harvest is brown (or yellow) eels, which are small because that is the stage when the mature fish are returning to freshwater to grow. Brown eels are generally 1 to 3lbs, which is a popular size for European markets. Silver eels, which are eels heading for the spawning grounds, tend to be much larger. Glass eels, the transparent immature eels and elvers, which are pigmented immature eels, are caught in estuaries as they return to the rivers to grow. Most of these are shipped alive to overseas markets.

Frozen eels are available either whole, or headless and dressed. Eels that are frozen whole must be kept alive for long enough to allow them to purge themselves of food before being killed and frozen. Whole eels are sometimes frozen alive in bags. The animals intertwine, which makes them difficult to thaw and handle. A better alternative processing method involves stunning them and freezing them individually. This process makes them a better buy for smokers, who are major buyers of eels.

Eels are catadromous. American and European eels both breed and spawn in the Sargasso Sea area of the middle Atlantic.

Frozen eels are also available from New Zealand. The longfinned eel, *Anguilla dieffenbachii*, can grow as long as five feet. The shortfin eel, *Anguilla australis*, reaches over three feet. This species is also found in Australia. Eel resources are generally greater than the demand. Consumer prejudice against these snake-shaped fish is unlikely to permit any major market to develop in the U.S.A., despite the excellence of smoked eel.

There are several eel-like fish sometimes called eels, including conger eel, which may grow to 85lbs and is sometimes eaten in Europe. See Conger Eel.

EELPOUT: See Ocean pout.

ELVERS: Baby eels, up to about three inches in length. Elvers are a delicacy in some Asian countries and are also exported live to be grown in aquaculture operations. See Eel.

ENGLISH SOLE *Scientific name: Parophrys vetulus:* A west coast flatfish marketed as fillets along with other soles and flounders. It has rather soft flesh without much flavor. See Flatfish.

FALLS: Fall chum. A poor grade of chum salmon. See Salmon.

F.A.S.: See Delivery terms.

FAT FISH: Oily fish. Fish which contain fat throughout the body tissue. Examples of fat fish are herring, mackerel, tuna, butterfish, trout and salmon. These fish differ from lean or white fish which have the fat mainly in the liver. Fat fish are generally, but not always, darker. Fat fish are better for broiling and other intense-heat cooking methods.

The fattest parts of most fish include the belly walls and the darker meat along the lateral line. Oily fish often have a layer of fat just under the skin. All fish store fat in the liver.

Fish oils and fats are good for you: they contain the omega-3 fatty acids which are widely believed to help prevent heart attacks and other diseases. However, contaminants such as PCBs are concentrated in the fat and the liver although their presence is, thankfully, rare. See Seafood safety for more details.

FEDERAL INSPECTION: Meat and poultry are inspected by the Federal government. Seafood is not. Mandatory inspection of seafood products has been a political issue for many years. Proponents claim it would increase consumer confidence. Opponents insist that seafood has a very safe and clean record and that inspection would cost too much. The issue is complex, but political pressures seem likely to achieve mandatory inspection of seafood.

The U.S. Department of Commerce through the National Marine Fisheries Service (N.M.F.S.) operates a voluntary inspection service which is paid for by companies who participate. This program offers product and plant inspection to U.S. Grade standards. For more details, see the entry U.S. Grade Standards.

Mandatory inspection, if and when it happens, will probably be based on a technique known as Hazard Analysis of Critical Control Points, or HACCP. Meat and poultry inspection examines the product to determine if it is contaminated in any way. HACCP determines the areas where contaminants might originate and controls and monitors those to reduce the hazards. It is a much more modern and reliable system. For details, see Inspection.

FILLETS: U.S. Grade Standards (Title 50, U.S. Code) define fillets as "slices of practically boneless fish flesh of irregular size and shape, which are removed from the carcass by cuts made parallel to the backbone and sections of such fillets cut so as to facilitate packing."

A fillet is the side muscle of a fish, with or without the skin. Most fish yield about 30 to 40 percent of the total live weight in the form of fillets. Most fish fillets contain pinbones or other small bones. For a definition of "boneless fillets" see the entry Boneless fillets.

There are a number of ways to cut fillets, partly depending on the fish itself and partly depending on the intended use of the fillet. From a cod-like fish, a full fillet should be trimmed of nape, belly bones and any membranes, especially around the belly area. To make the same fillet boneless, the pinbones must be removed. J-cut and V-cut are the alternatives. V-cut takes longer but gives a better yield.

Fish like red snapper give a different shape fillet, usually without pinbones. If these fish are large, the fillet is very thick. Snapper fillets are often cut into different shapes – the whole fillet is then described as a "natural" fillet while the pieces are called "cuts."

Smaller flatfish like flounder and sole should be trimmed of the frill round the outside edge. These fish do not have pinbones, so there is no risk of bones if the frill is properly removed. Larger fillets may be divided down the lateral line, so that the fish yields two pieces from each side instead of just one.

Large flatfish like halibut are more often steaked than filleted. If a fillet is made it is called a fletch. The fletch then is further divided into boneless portions or boneless steaks.

Butterfly fillets are made from smaller fish like herring and mackerel. The two fillets are kept joined by the skin of the belly.

FILTER FEEDERS: Molluscs such as clams, mussels, scallops and oysters. These shellfish pump water through their digestive systems and absorb the nutrients they need from the water. See also Depuration.

FINGER PACKS: Shrimp or other small items laid in rows in a block and frozen. This looks attractive and sometimes sells for a small premium.

FINISHED COUNT: This term applies to peeled shrimp. It means that the labelled count is the actual count of the product. This compares with peeled-from counts, which are produced from shell-on tails of the quoted size. See Shrimp.

FINNANS: Also called finnan haddock and finnan haddie. Strictly, finnans are medium sized haddock split down the back with the backbone left on, then brined and cold smoked. The name has extended from this delicacy to all smoked haddock and even to other smoked fish. In the U.S.A., most finnans are fillets in deference to market dislike of bones. See also Smoked fish.

FISH BLOCKS: Frozen compressed slabs of fish fillets, usually without skin and bone, used as raw material for fish sticks, portions and other breaded and battered items. Most of the huge consumption in the U.S. is imported for manufacturing use but small quantities are used by some institutional caterers, who thaw blocks as a source of cheap fillets. Only small quantities of blocks are produced domestically.

Fish blocks are almost always 16½lbs each, packed four to a master carton. A small proportion is packed 3/18½lbs. The precise specifications for the manufacture of blocks that meet Grade A standards are spelled out in Title 50 of the U.S. Code of Federal Regulations, Paragraph 264.111. Contact the National Seafood Quality and Inspection Laboratory, Pascagoula, MS 39567 to obtain a copy of the standard. The Code defines a fish block as follows:

"Rectangular-shaped masses of cohering frozen fish flesh of a single species. They consist of adequately drained whole, wholesome fillets or pieces of whole, wholesome fillets cut into small portions but not ground or comminuted; and they are frozen and maintained at temperatures necessary for the preservation of the product."

Fish blocks may be skinless or skin-on, though the market is largely for skinless product.

To meet Grade A standards, blocks have to be very accurately shaped, have almost no bones at all, few voids (small gaps between the surface fillets) and of course be completely fresh and clean. Many blocks that do not quite meet these stringent standards are still entirely wholesome and produce wholesome portions from them.

Blocks may be made of almost any kind of fish. Pollock, cod, haddock, flounder, turbot and whiting are the most often used.

FISHERIES MANAGEMENT: Profits for the seafood business depend quite heavily on fisheries management. It is a complex and not very exciting subject, but worth learning.

Fisheries management theory followed in the U.S.A. is controlling the catch of a species to maintain the resource and so, in the long run, provide more of that species. This also ensures that a species does not become extinct. There are numerous flaws in the theory. One is that the risk of extinction, in practice, is limited to species which are caught so thoroughly that the population is reduced below the level at which it can regenerate. This certainly applies to whales; several species already have been efficiently hunted to extinction. This theory is also probably true for salmon, since they return to spawn in rivers and each river could be netted so that no fish escape. It is still far from true of most for our ocean-caught fish like cod, halibut or flounder. Catching techniques for such species simply do not yet have the power to eliminate a stock of fish.

The other major flaw in fisheries management theory is that it is based on the assumption that managers actually have the accurate data they need. In fact, assessment of fish stocks is far from an exact science. There are very few, if any, circumstances, where anyone has enough knowledge to state that he knows exactly how many fish there are and what is happening to them.

In practice, fisheries management in the U.S.A. is based on political and bureaucratic considerations much more than on practical considerations. The halibut fishery in the north Pacific, perhaps the most studied and regulated of all deep-sea fisheries, is subjected to a regime of short fishing openings of days or even hours. This results in far too many boats having far too little to do. All these boats have to be purchased and paid for. The price of halibut would surely decrease under a rational system. Further, this complex management scheme does not appear to have succeeded in preserving the resource.

At one time, flounder in the northeast was controlled by catch quotas, which regulated how much could be caught during a three month period. When the entire industry had caught the quota, the boats returned to port and were not allowed to catch any more for the rest of the quarter. This played havoc with the price of flounder causing violent short-term price fluctuations.

Many species are controlled by minimum size regulations. The idea is that if fishermen use larger nets, the small fish will escape to grow into bigger fish. In practice, a lot of small fish are still caught. Nobody has yet satisfactorily explained to a fisherman how throwing back a dead, small fish is going to help preserve the resource.

The political clout of sport-fishing interests has a great deal to do with fisheries management programs. Estimates of anglers in the U.S.A. range from 27 million up to 65 million. Either way, they have more votes than the entire seafood and restaurant industries combined. Regulators are often sympathetic to proposals to reserve pressured stocks for the sportsman. Gulf redfish is a prime example of this.

The end result is that fishing costs more than it would if market forces were left alone. Fish stocks that are reduced through heavy fishing often recover. Why? Because if the fisherman cannot make money fishing it, he will move to some other target species. The first one will then recover. Of course, this assumes that he has a boat able to switch to other resources. The technique does not work in primitive areas with small-scale equipment. A clam-digger's skiff cannot be used for much else. But a modern shrimp trawler can certainly be re-rigged for many other fisheries.

Management within three miles of the shore is reserved for the coastal state. Beyond that, the Federal jurisdiction ranges out to 200 miles. There are regional fisheries management councils around the coastline. All their proposals are open to public discussion, comment and review. The industry needs to pay more attention to what is going on. Currently, fishermen make sour jokes about needing law degrees before they can fish. The complexities of licensing systems, especially in the northwest, make the jokes far from funny.

FISH FARMING: See Aquaculture.

FISHLIST: See Names.

FISH MEAL AND FISH BY-PRODUCTS: Fish meal is cooked, dried fish, ground for use as animal feed. In large-scale production, such as the U.S. industry based on menhaden, whole fish are specifically caught for reduction to fish meal. In smaller scale operations, fish meal used to be produced from filleting waste and offal at the major fishing ports, where there is sufficient volume of such waste to justify the installation of fish meal plant. However, fish meal plants are not popular as neighbors and in recent years processing waste has become a problem to be solved rather than a source of additional revenue.

Fish meal is a vital part of animal feed, especially for pigs and poultry. About one third of the world's fish catch goes to fish meal production rather than for direct human consumption.

Fish oil is separated from the fish meal during production and used separately for various chemical, industrial and agricultural purposes.

Fish protein concentrate (FPC) is fish meal produced in a way suitable for human consumption. In general, this means that the intestines of the fish are removed and the fat in the meal is dissolved out to make the product palatable. It should be a light brown, tasteless and odorless powder, useful as a high-protein additive in processed foodstuffs. FPC has not caught the popular imagination and is little used.

Hydrolized fish proteins are liquid versions of fish meal, produced by dissolving fish to make a slurry suitable for mixing with silage in animal feeds.

There are numerous other fish by-products, including phar-maceuticals (such as fish-oil pills) and leather (from sharkskin, for example). They are important to the frozen seafood business because when they are produced strictly as a by-product, they help to keep down the cost of the frozen seafood you are buying by giving the processor a saleable outlet for what would other-wise be waste.

FISH STICKS: Also called fish fingers. Rectangular sticks of fish, breaded or battered, raw or precooked, usually weighing three-quarters to one ounce each.

FLAKE: Flake meat is the body meat from the blue crab. It consists of the smaller pieces of body meat. See Crabs.
• Flake is a name given to dogfish in Britain. It is not approved for use in the U.S.A.
• Many fish fillets are composed of flakes of flesh, joined together with connective tissues which run through each flake and join the membranes that are between each flake. A cod fillet has about fifty flakes down the full length of the fish. Fish like cod and haddock have large flakes. Flounder and sole have very small flakes. The differences in structure affect the appearance and the texture of the fish.
In certain circumstances, the flakes separate and the fillet "gapes." This may be sign of deterioration. See Gaping.

FLATFISH: This section covers the main flounder and sole spe-cies in alphabetical order. Flounder, fluke, sole, halibut and tur-bot are all flatfish, which are fish that live on the sea floor and have both eyes on the same side of the head. If you hold a flatfish with its belly towards you and the eyes on top, some species have the head at the left-hand end (these are left-eyed fish) and others have the head at the right-hand end (right-eyed fish). The dis-tinction is important for identification. If you have both a bottom and a top fillet, you can reconstruct the fish sufficiently to be able to tell whether it was a right-eyed or left-eyed type.
Flounder (and sole) are usually frozen as skinless fillets. Because of the bone structure of these fish, fillets are always boneless, unless careless cutting has left some of the bony "frill" which surrounds the whole body of the fish and is part of the fin

structure – this fault is uncommon. Flounder and sole fillets are usually skinned. Some packs are sold with white skin on, black skin removed. The skin of most species is very thin and is not a problem to eat. Nevertheless, the market generally prefers skinless product for the sake of appearance. Flounder or sole fillets are packed in cellos, layer packs, I.Q.F. and in blocks. Cellos are ungraded, with 3/5 count fillets the usual. Layer pack and I.Q.F. product is variously graded, but 3/5, 5/8, 8/10 ounce are the most frequent. Married fillets are also produced, usually for breading.

Canada is the largest supplier of flounder and sole, domestic supplies are the second largest. Many European countries ship flounder to the U.S., especially Holland, Denmark and Belgium. These countries produce top quality fish; their boats make very short trips, so the fish is extremely fresh when frozen.

Frozen flounder is available headless and dressed or pan-ready from domestic, Canadian and European packers. Grading is in two-ounce steps from 6/8 through 14/16 ounces. Boxes may be 10, 25, or 50lbs. Each fish should be polywrapped. This is usually low quality, high problem product. Flounder is only frozen in this form if it is too small or too soft for economical filleting, or if too much arrives at the plant at one time and filleters cannot handle it all. Often the fish is caught in shallow water when spawning: look for sand in the belly cavity and for remains of roe. Cook the fish to see if it is edible. Iceland produces some better product at a higher price but check this carefully as well.

Substitution is commonplace with flounder and sole, especially with the more expensive varieties of the fish, such as gray sole, which may cost 50 percent more than regular flounder. A frequent substitution is to pack turbot. If the turbot was previously replaced with arrowtooth, you can get a particularly bad deal. The only good defense is to know your fish and what it looks like and check both fish and cartons carefully for signs of switches. For example, Holland sole is not packed in boxes marked "printed in U.S.A." Such simple and obvious inconsistencies do occur. At one time, a large Canadian packer was using cartons printed with a list of the different flatfish that might be packed in it, giving distributors an easy opportunity to move the check mark indicating the product to show a more expensive variety. Be aware of the problem and look at your fish carefully. Experience is the best defense.

Flounder or sole?: The distinction is important for marketing, but quite unclear in practice. If the fish is labelled flounder or sole, it has to be one of the species listed below, according to Federal regulations listed in Paragraph 263.201 of Title 50 of the U.S. Code of Federal Regulations or it cannot be approved for U.S. Grading. This means it could not be sold to the military or other Federal purchasing programs. It would also be strong evidence for other purposes, including labelling and mislabelling disputes.

The following list shows the common name, the Latin name and the coast of habitat of all fish which may be labelled flounder or sole under the N.M.F.S. rules.

Sole

English name	Scientific name	Coast
Dover Sole	*Microstomus pacificus*	Pacific
English sole	*Parophrys vetulus*	Pacific
Gray sole	*Glyptocephalus cynoglossus*	Atlantic
Petrale sole	*Eopsetta jordani*	Pacific
Lemon sole	*Pseudopleuronectes americanus* over 3½lbs	Atlantic
Rock sole	*Lepidopsetta bilineata*	Pacific
Sand sole	*Psettichthys melanostictus*	Atlantic

Flounder

Blackback	*Pseudopleuronectes americanus* under 3½lbs	Atlantic
Yellowtail fldr	*Limanda ferruginea*	Atlantic
Dab, plaice	*Hippoglossoides platessoides*	Atlantic
Fluke	*Paralichthys dentatus*	Atlantic
Starry flounder	*Platichthys stellatus*	Pacific

The distinctions are not as scientific as they look. The difference between a 3¼lb blackback and a lemon sole half a pound larger, both of which are the same species (*Pseudopleuronectes americanus*,) is not detectable in terms of taste or appearance. The definitions are based on usage, and as such should perhaps be less rigid, since in practice there is no difference between sole and flounder.

The Fishlist newly prepared by the F.D.A. and N.M.F.S. takes a broader view. Eighty species of flatfish are included. The flounders and soles are all listed as such. Forty species have the market name "Flounder" and another twenty-five are called "Sole." The *Pseudopleuronectes americanus* mentioned above is called both winter flounder and lemon sole in the Fishlist (but the name blackback flounder appears to be out). Common and market names are legal to use on product in interstate commerce (see Names). The flatfish common names, market names and species are listed below:

Flatfish: Market Names and Common Names

Market name	Common name	Scientific name	Location
Flounder	Brill	*Colistium nudipinnis*	P
Flounder	Brill	*Scophthalmus rhombus*	A
Flounder	Brill, New Zealand	*Colistium guntheri*	P
Flounder	Flounder	*Arnoglossus scapha*	P
Flounder	Flounder	*Samariscus triocellatus*	P
Flounder	Flounder, Arctic	*Liopsetta glacialis*	P
Flounder	Flounder, Bering	*Hippoglossoides robustus*	P
Flounder	Flounder, Gulf	*Paralichthys albigutta*	A
Flounder	Flounder, Indian Ocean	*Psettodes erumei*	P
Flounder	Flounder, Patagonian	*Paralichthys patagonicus*	A
Flounder	Flounder, black	*Rhombosolea retiaria*	F
Flounder	Flounder, broad	*Paralichthys squamilentus*	A
Flounder	Flounder, eyed	*Bothus ocellatus*	A
Flounder	Flounder, fivespot	*Pseudorhombus pentophthalmus*	P
Flounder	Flounder, fourspot	*Paralichthys oblongus*	A
Flounder	Flounder, greenback	*Rhombosolea tapirina*	P
Flounder	Flounder, kamchatka	*Atheresthes evermanni*	P
Flounder	Flounder, largetoothed	*Pseudorhombus arsius*	P
Flounder	Flounder, longjawed	*Pelecanichthys crumenalis*	P
Flounder	Flounder, olive	*Paralichthys olivaceus*	A
Flounder	Flounder, panther	*Bothus pantherinus*	A
Flounder	Flounder, peacock	*Bothus lunatus*	A
Flounder	Flounder, sand	*Rhombosolea plebeia*	P
Flounder	Flounder, small-toothed	*Pseudorhombus jenynsii*	A-P

Market name	Common name	Scientific name	Location
Flounder	Flounder, starry	*Platichthys stellatus*	P-F
Flounder	Flounder, three-eye	*Ancylopsetta dilecta*	A
Flounder	Flounder, tropical	*Bothus mancus*	A
Flounder	Flounder, yellowbelly	*Rhombosolea leporina*	P
Flounder	Flounder, yellowtail	*Limanda ferruginea*	A
Flounder	Sole, New Zealand	*Peltorhampus novaezeelandiae*	P
Flounder	Sole, New Zealand lemon	*Pelotretis flavilatus*	P
Flounder	Windowpane	*Scophthalmus aquosus*	A
Flounder arrowtooth	Flounder, arrowtooth	*Atheresthes stomias*	P
Flounder/dab	Dab, common	*Limanda limanda*	A
Flounder/dab	Dab, longhead	*Limanda proboscidea*	A-P
Flounder/fluke	Flounder, European	*Platichthys flesus*	A
Flounder/fluke	Flounder, southern	*Paralichthys lethostigma*	A-F
Flounder/fluke	Flounder, summer	*Paralichthys dentatus*	A
Flounder/sole	Flounder, winter/lemon sole	*Pseudopleuronectes americanus*	A
Flounder/whiff	Megrim	*Lepidorhombus whiffiagonis*	A
Flounder/whiff	Scaldfish, fourspot	*Lepidorhombus boscii*	A
Halibut	Halibut, Atlantic	*Hippoglossus hippoglossus*	A
Halibut	Halibut, Pacific	*Hippoglossus stenolepis*	P
Halibut/California halibut	Halibut, California	*Paralichthys californicus*	P
Plaice	Plaice, Alaska	*Pleuronectes quadrituberculatus*	P
Plaice	Plaice, European	*Plueuronectes platessa*	A
Plaice/dab	Plaice, American	*Hippoglossoides platessoides*	A
Sanddab	Sanddab, Pacific	*Citharichthys sordidus*	P
Sole	Sole	*Austroglossus microlepis*	A
Sole	Sole	*Austroglossus pectoralis*	A
Sole	Sole, English	*Parophrys vetulus*	P
Sole	Sole, European	*Solea vulgaris*	A
Sole	Sole, kobe	*Aseraggodes kobensis*	P
Sole	Sole, lemon	*Microstomus kitt*	A
Sole	Sole, narrowbanded	*Aseraggodes macleayanus*	P
Sole	Sole, oriental black	*Synaptura orientalis*	A

Market name	Common name	Scientific name	Location
Sole	Sole, slender	*Lyopsetta exilis*	P
Sole	Sole, thickback	*Microchirus variegatus*	A
Sole dover	Sole, dover	*Microstomus pacificus*	P
Sole/flounder	Flounder, witch/gray sole	*Glyptocephalus cynoglossus*	A
Sole/flounder	Sole, C-O	*Pleuronichthys coenosus*	P
Sole/flounder	Sole, bigmouth	*Hippoglossina stomata*	P
Sole/flounder	Sole, butter	*Isopsetta isolepis*	P
Sole/flounder	Sole, curlfin	*Pleuronichthys decurrens*	P
Sole/flounder	Sole, deepsea	*Embassichthys bathybius*	P
Sole/flounder	Sole, fantail	*Xystreurys liolepis*	P
Sole/flounder	Sole, flathead	*Hippoglossoides elassodon*	P
Sole/flounder	Sole, petrale	*Eopsetta jordani*	P
Sole/flounder	Sole, rex	*Glyptocephalus zachirus*	P
Sole/flounder	Sole, rock	*Lepidopsetta bilineata*	P
Sole/flounder	Sole, roughscale	*Clidoderma asperrimum*	P
Sole/flounder	Sole, sand	*Psettichthys melanostictus*	P
Sole/flounder	Sole, yellowfin	*Limanda aspera*	P
Tonguesole	Tonguesole	*Cynoglossus spp.*	P
Turbot	Turbot	*Scophthalmus maximus*	A
Turbot	Turbot, diamond	*Hypsopsetta guttulata*	P
Turbot	Turbot, hornyhead	*Pleuronichthys verticalis*	P
Turbot	Turbot, spotted	*Pleuronichthys ritteri*	P
Turbot	Turbot, spottedtail	*Psettodes belcheni*	A
Turbot	Turbot, spring	*Psettodes bennetti*	P
Turbot, Greenland	Halibut, Greenland	*Reinhardtius hippoglossoides*	A-P

Locations: A = Atlantic P = Indo-Pacific F = Freshwater
Source: F.D.A.

This broader definition of flounder and sole should enable importers to experiment with flatfish from other parts of the world. There are good fish from west Africa and parts of Asia which might be marketed in the U.S.A.

There is, of course, a definite market distinction between flounder and sole and this is important. Sole and flounder are the most widely used and requested flatfish in the U.S. For most practical purposes, the two are interchangeable and all packing and other specifications are exactly the same for one as for the other. There are many buyers who will insist on sole, many others who will insist on flounder. There are cookery writers who praise the virtues of one fish over the other. As a supplier, all you can do is have available what your customers ask for.

There is also a market distinction between west and east coast fish. Although the Atlantic products are known and used throughout the country, they are generally more expensive than the Pacific items, and are not much used in the west. The Pacific products, which are accepted through the west, are regarded as inferior in the northeast. Alaskan efforts to handle and process some of these species better are beginning to show results. It is possible that Alaska will supply substantial quantities of flounder and sole products to the U.S. market in the future.

There are infrequent shipments of lemon sole (which is probably Pacific English sole) and other flounders from Japan and Korea, mostly packed I.Q.F. in the same way as Greenland turbot. Generally these are fairly soft fish and the price differential is rarely sufficient to make them worth even experimental use. For flatfish not listed below (halibut, turbot, dover sole etc.), see separate entries.

Alaska plaice *Scientific name: Pleuronectes quadrituberculatus:* Also called plaice. Do not confuse with American plaice, which is usually called dab (see below). This is a reasonable quality north Pacific right-eyed flatfish caught by Japanese and other factory vessels. Some fillet production from domestic sources is also predicted.

Arrowtooth flounder, arrowtooth sole *Scientific name: Atheresthes stomias:* A large Pacific flatfish similar in appearance to greenland turbot when filleted and skinned. Flounder and sole are used interchangeably in the name. The quality of the fish resembles neither flounder nor sole.

The flesh is very soft and breaks up when cooked. Although arrowtooth is cheap, it is basically unsatisfactory for most uses and its market is restricted. You may often persuade customers to try the fish on the basis of the cheap price, but few of them return for further supplies.

Most of the arrowtooth sold in the U.S.A. comes from Japan,

some from Korea; there is a resource available off British Columbia and Alaska which may provide further supplies in the future. The standard packing for the Asian products is 1/25lb IQF, individually wrapped, skinless and boneless fillets, graded 2/4, 4/8, 8/16 and 16/32 ounces, exactly as Greenland turbot from the same origins. Arrowtooth may also be packed in 10/5lb cellos and labelled Japanese flounder or Japanese sole.

Problems arise if arrowtooth is substituted for turbot or, as sometimes happens, is mixed with turbot and the whole pack labelled turbot. Although the two fish look much the same, the arrowtooth is very much softer and altogether less desirable in use than the turbot.

Arrowtooth packed in western Canada is known locally as turbot and may be labelled legally as such in Canada. This product should be avoided.

An indication of the quality of this fish is that it is used for pet food and fish meal.

Blackback flounder/lemon sole *Scientific name: Pseudopleuronectes americanus:* A right-eyed flatfish from the northeast Atlantic. It seems that "blackback," its most common name, is being dropped: it does not appear in the first published version of the Fishlist. The species still retains the distinction of being either a flounder or a sole, according to size (see above). The preferred flounder name is winter flounder. As a sole, it is lemon sole. There are numerous local names for the fish, which is one of the staple flatfish from the northeast. Most frozen flounder is imported from Canada.

This species gives an acceptable fillet with a bland taste. Fillets from the side with black skin tend to be grayish. The fish looks whiter and more attractive after it is cooked. It is the darkest flounder from the region, but like all fish the color varies widely. Like some other flounders, they change color slightly according to their surroundings. The species grows to as much as 8lbs but most of the fish caught are under 5lbs.

The fish is caught inshore from Massachusetts to New York in the winter when it is preparing to spawn, which explains the name winter flounder.

Dab *Scientific name: Hippoglossoides platessoides:* This right-eyed species is also called plaice and American plaice. In international trade statistics it is called long rough dab, but this

101

is not a term used commercially. The European common dab, *Limanda limanda*, is more like yellowtail flounder and is imported from time to time as flounder. The sanddab (*Lophopsetta maculata*) is a different fish, always small, reaching only about 1lb.

Dabs have good, firm flesh with a mild flounder flavor. They grow to about 6lbs. It is a good quality fish with a wide market, although when frozen it is unlikely to be distinguished from other Atlantic flounders.

Dover sole, Pacific *Scientific name: Microstomus pacificus:* A right-eyed Pacific flatfish, known to fishermen as slime sole because of the large quantity of skin slime on the fish when it is caught which makes it difficult to handle. This species can provide an acceptable fillet but it is nothing like genuine Dover sole from Europe, *Solea vulgaris*. (See separate entry on Dover sole). Dover sole is one of the few flatfish which cannot be called "sole" or "flounder" generically. The Dover should always be included.

According to some experimental processing work, Alaskan dover sole has better texture and eating qualities than the Californian variety, which is often very soft, with jelly-like flesh. The jellying is probably caused by feed and environmental factors, not by a parasite. The quality of the flesh is a significant problem. All Dover sole is delicate and must be processed and frozen very soon after catching to produce a good fillet. It is important to find a reliable source and stick with it. This is not a species to buy as a commodity on general description.

Dover sole, Genuine: See separate entry on Dover sole.

English sole *Scientific name: Parophrys vetulus:* A right-eyed flatfish found the full length of the Pacific coast. It is called lemon sole in Canada, apparently because it has a lemony flavor. It does not resemble the Atlantic lemon sole (blackback flounder – see above) or the fish imported as lemon sole from Asian factory vessels. The flesh is delicate and well regarded.

Fluke *Scientific name: Paralichthys dentatus:* Also frequently called summer flounder. This is a left-eyed flounder, one of the larger North Atlantic species. Fish of 8lbs to 10lbs are quite common. The flesh is firm and white. The market for fluke is particularly strong in the mid-Atlantic region. It is caught from southern Cape Cod to the Carolinas. Fisheries management plans control access to the species, which is also prized by sport fishermen.

Gray sole *Scientific name: Glyptocephalus cynoglossus:* A right-eyed fish also called witch and witch flounder. N.M.F.S. (Title 50, U.S. Code) says it must be called gray sole. The F.D.A. in the Fishlist says it may be called sole or flounder. Under either name, it is usually the most expensive Atlantic flounder/sole. The fillets are long and thin and have an excellent flavor. The species is found both sides of the Atlantic and frozen fillets are imported from Europe as well as Canada, which supplies most of the market for the frozen fish. Gray sole grow to about 4lbs and produce fillets around 8 ounces.

Halibut: See separate entry, Halibut.

Petrale sole *Scientific name: Eopsetta jordani:* This is a Pacific right-eyed flatfish, commercially the most important sole/flounder from the west coast and has the best eating quality. It is found from southern California to northern Alaska, grows to about seven pounds and has good, fairly firm flesh.

Rex sole *Scientific name: Glyptocephalus zachirus:* This is another right-eyed fish which can be called either sole or flounder. It is found the full length of the west coast. The fish is generally small and is often sold whole, because of low fillet yield. However, some Alaskan resources yield much larger fish which are filleted successfully. The meat is white and firm and some experts claim that it is similar to gray sole (it is a member of the same genus).

Rock sole *Scientific name: Lepidopsetta bilineata:* This is a right-eyed flatfish found from California to the Bering Sea. It is also caught on the Asian side of the Pacific. It is a fairly small fish, seldom exceeding five pounds and is the most important flounder/sole species for British Columbia fishermen. The flesh is firm and creamy-colored and strong enough to withstand recipes which call for rolling and stuffing.

Sand sole *Scientific name: Psettichthys melanostictus:* A right-eyed flatfish similar to petrale, found the length of the Pacific coast. It may be called sole or flounder.

Southern flounder *Scientific name: Paralichthys lethostigma:* This is an Atlantic left-eyed species similar to the fluke and sometimes called fluke. It is a comparatively small fish, usually reaching less than three pounds. The similar Gulf flounder

(*Paralichthys albigutta*) is caught with it and not distinguished in practice. These fish are available year-round and are at their peak in the winter months when the better northern species are scarce. The flesh is similar to fluke, though the fillets are generally smaller.

Starry flounder *Scientific name: Platichthys stellatus:* A right-eyed species found throughout the north Pacific from California to Japan. It is sometimes called a roughjacket because of its abrasive skin. It is an important commercial species and grows quite large, though most of the commercially caught fish are around three pounds. It has firm flesh with a larger flake than most soles and flounders, with a good flavor.

Yellowfin sole *Scientific name: Limanda aspera:* A right-eyed species caught in large quantities in the Bering Sea and north Pacific by factory trawlers. The fish is small and the flesh disintegrates when cooked. Frozen blocks and fillets are processed into prepared meals but the small, thin fillets are not generally suitable for either retail or institutional use.

Yellowtail flounder *Scientific name: Limanda ferruginea:* The yellowtail, also called rusty dab, is a right-eyed flatfish growing to about three pounds and is commercially the most important Atlantic flounder/sole. The fillets are sweet and firm and the fish is regarded as the standard to which other flounders are compared. It is caught from Rhode Island northwards to Labrador. The year-round fishery peaks in spring and fall, but frozen product is always available. There are state and Federal limits on catches. These change from time to time.

Other flounders and soles: There are many species from around the world that can be offered. There is no way of telling in advance what these might be or which ones will be worth using. The only way to find out is to try them. West Africa, in particular, has a number of fine soles which are used fresh (imported by air through New York's Fulton Fish Market). These other species could become the basis for expanding flatfish supply sources.

FLETCH: A boneless fillet of halibut. See Fillet.

FLOUNDER: See Flatfish.

FLUKE: See Flatfish.

F.O.B.: See Delivery terms.

FORMED FILLETS: Portions cut from blocks in such a way that they appear to be natural fillets, although all are exactly the same size and shape. This allows perfect portion control together with the appearance of serving a natural product. Technically, it is not easy to do, since the block must be handled and cut in such a way that the formed piece will not break into its constituent fillet parts when cooked.

FREEZE-DRYING: A drying process which is unlikely to replace the frozen food business. Product is frozen and then the moisture is removed by sublimation in a vacuum chamber. It gives excellent preservation, but the product has to be reconstituted before use. Product is also very fragile while freeze-dried and adequate, protective packaging is difficult to produce.

FREEZER BURN: Dehydration of frozen product. Freezer burn is caused by the evaporation loss of moisture from product. It is recognized by a whitish, cottony appearance of the flesh, especially at the cut edges or thinner places. This dehydration also encourages rancidity.

Fish slightly burned may be trimmed, if you have the time and facilities; the texture of even slightly burned areas is too bad for the fish to be edible without trimming.

Glaze is used to prevent freezer burn. Since the glaze itself evaporates, it may have to be renewed if the product is stored for long periods. Salmon, for example, should be reglazed every three months to maintain quality. Good packaging is most important in the prevention of freezer burn. Good bags or inner boxes and strong, well-sealed outer cartons can save a lot of product.

FREEZING AT SEA: An umbrella term covering several possible processes. Fish might be frozen whole (or dressed) for thawing and further processing on shore later, or it might be filleted and packed for distribution. It might be frozen on board the catching vessel, or it might be transferred to a mother ship for processing.

In general, it is better to freeze seafood products as soon as they are caught. Freezing at sea makes this possible. However, there are problems: do not assume that because a product is made "at sea" it is necessarily top quality.

Fishing vessels are small and the weather is often bad on fishing grounds. Boats make uncomfortable processing plants and it can be extremely difficult to operate machinery in moving, cramped conditions. Also, fish can be landed on deck in hugely varying quantities so that at times the processing areas cannot keep up with the supply while at other times there is nothing to do. Species that have to pass through rigor before processing may be frozen too soon and species that need fast handling may be left on deck for too long.

Despite all the difficulties, a great deal of frozen-at-sea product is excellent. The point is that buyers should not assume that it always will be. Check every time you buy until you are confident of the supplier.

FREEZING PROCESSES: The basic freezing methods used in the seafood industry affect the nature and quality of the product. The most important factor is to reduce the temperature in the center of the product to 0°F. or less as fast as possible. Generally, the freezing process selected should be the one which will best achieve this for the product in question.

All seafood, like all flesh, contains water. Seafoods contain 60 percent to 80 percent water depending on species and season. Water expands as its temperature drops from 39°F. to 32°F., and in expanding can damage the protein wall of the cell in which it is contained. For a simple demonstration of this effect, put a firm, ripe tomato in your freezer for two days, then defrost it and see what a soft mushy object you have. The expansion of the moisture in the cells breaks the cell structure and destroys the texture of the tomato.

If water freezes very quickly, it literally does not have time to expand fully and the damage done minimizes. So, the faster you freeze, the better. Many factors affect the speed of freezing, including the thickness of the material being frozen (the cold takes longer to penetrate a thicker slab, which can be frozen hard on the outside but still be soft in the center), and the temperature of the refrigerant used.

Modern technology achieves excellent results with all the usual methods, but it is still necessary to use the right method for each particular product and pack.

Plate Freezing: Also known as contact freezing. Product is placed on a metal plate, another plate is brought down on top and the product compresses slightly between the plates. This ensures good contact between the plates and the product. Refrigerant then pumps through the plates until the product freezes.

Plate freezing is the major technique used in the industry. It is used for blocks of shrimp, for fish blocks, layer pack products, blocks of scallops and for cello wraps – for most of the product handled by the industry. It is not suitable for product over five inches thick, or for very delicate items.

There are also vertical plate freezers, which work in a similar way. The vertical type are not much used anymore. They were suitable for bulk freezing of product that did not require too much care. Horizontal plate freezers allow the operator to pack product into end-user boxes and to add water to glaze it. Horizontal plate freezers produce better quality product.

Blast Freezing: Very cold air blows over the product, which is usually on trays set in racks in the freezer chamber to permit good circulation of the cold air.

Blast freezing is used for I.Q.F. products (except for very light items which might blow around) and is particularly useful for products of irregular shapes and varied sizes. Larger fish such as salmon, sablefish, halibut and turbot are normally blast frozen. From time to time you may find items which are normally block frozen, such as scallops, with bulging tops to the boxes. This may signify that the blocks were frozen in a blast freezer instead of under the compressing effect of a plate freezer. The product should be acceptable, but may cause problems in storage because the boxes will not stack properly.

The same symptom may indicate that the boxes were simply placed in a storage chamber to freeze. This is totally unsatisfactory since the time taken to freeze the center of the block will be so excessive that the product will certainly be poorly textured, and may actually decompose in the center. Blast freezers operate at much colder temperatures than storage freezers, which are not designed for the initial freezing of product. The use of storage freezers produces a product apparently in good shape, but which may be bad on the inside.

107

Blast freezing used to dehydrate some product, but modern equipment, if properly used, causes almost no loss of moisture and a highly satisfactory product for almost every use.

Cryogenic Freezing: This is an advanced application of blast freezing. The product moves on a belt, or is pushed, through a tunnel where it is exposed to very cold air, or to sprays of nitrogen or carbon dioxide at very low temperatures. Liquid cooled to as low as $-150°F$. may be used. Product less than two inches thick will freeze much more quickly than it would in a blast freezer, giving excellent quality product for I.Q.F. fillets, shrimp, shellfish and small packages of many products. As an example of the speed of cryogenic tunnels, nitrogen freezes small peeled shrimp at $-110°F$. ($-80°C$.) in about five minutes. By contrast, a 10lb salmon in a blast freezer at $-30°F$. ($-35°C$.) takes over five hours to freeze.

Brine freezing: Water saturated with salt is an excellent freezing medium for certain irregularly shaped and large products. It stays liquid at very low temperatures and the heat transference is good, so product freezes rapidly. Tuna is often frozen this way and swordfish should be. King crab sections are often brine frozen – this adds a certain amount of salt to the product but gives a moister meat than blast freezing used to do. Because of increasing consumer resistance to salt, brine frozen products may eventually prove less popular than blast frozen alternatives.

Whichever method is used, the most important thing is to ensure that the center of the product reaches zero Fahrenheit as quickly as possible.

The following rules are taken from the FAO/WHO "Recommended International Code of Practice for Frozen Fish." They are basic common sense:

Guidelines for Freezing Fish:

 1. Freeze only good-quality fresh fish. Freezing and frozen storage cannot improve quality. At best, freezing maintains fish and shellfish as they were before freezing.

 2. Freezing should be fast enough to prevent adverse quality changes. Slow freezing and incomplete freezing adversely affects texture, flavor and shelf-life.

 3. In vertical plate freezers, pack fish between plates with as few gaps as possible. Voids in the blocks slow down heat transfer and weaken the frozen block. Do not load fish

above the top of the freezer plates.

4. Defrost contact plate freeezers only long enough for easy unloading of the blocks. Otherwise, the blocks warm up and thaw, compromising quality.

5. Load a blast freezer to allow for sufficient flow of cold air around the product. Inadequate air circulation results in poor freezing rates and variable product quality.

6. In brine freezing, there should be rapid circulation of the cooling medium and the ratio of fish to brine should be carefully controlled.

7. Freezing processes should run their full allotted time to ensure their completion. Reducing the freezing time or overfilling freezers during heavy production periods results in incomplete freezing and subsequent breakage and quality problems.

8. Unless fish is packaged or wrapped, it should be glazed to prevent dehydration and oxidation during storage and distribution. Glaze fish uniformly, as quickly as possible after freezing.

FRIGATE MACKEREL *Scientific name: Auxis thazard:* For practical purposes, this is very similar to and is treated as bonito.

FROG LEGS: The large rear legs of the edible frog, (family Ranidae) with skin removed, attached at the top or single, poly-bagged and frozen, are considered a delicacy in many parts of the world. U.S. domestic production is very small and legs are sold fresh. The major origins for the substantial imports of frozen frogs are Bangladesh and Japan. Small quantities come also from Indonesia and other parts of southern Asia. India was the major supplier but now protects its frogs on the grounds that they help agriculture by eating vast numbers of insects.

Japanese frogs are whiter and considered superior to the rest. Japanese packers do a better job than most in trimming and packing their product.

Frogs sell throughout the U.S.A., especially in the big cities and in areas with French influence such as upper Michigan and Louisiana. Canada, especially Quebec province, is a large frog market.

Bangladesh and Japanese frogs are packed in 5lb units, 10 per master (10/5lbs).

Because of the prevalence of salmonella contamination on frogs from southern Asia, inspection by the F.D.A. at ports of entry is rigorous. At some periods, as much as 90 percent of shipments imported have been rejected. A business developed selling rejected frogs to European buyers, who irradiate the product to kill the salmonella and other bacteria and then ship the frogs back to the U.S.A. This is, or course, illegal, as the re-importation of rejected product is not permitted. See also Irradiation.

Frogs are graded by number of pairs per pound:

Pairs per lb	Designation
2/4	jumbo
4/6	large
6/8	medium
8/12	small
12/15	extra small
16/20	tiny

In general, the larger frogs (2/4 is the largest) are cheaper. Medium sizes are preferred but the relative prices fluctuate widely from time to time as the supplies of different sizes vary. The large French market will not use jumbos at all and the disproportionate amount of jumbos shipped to the U.S.A. helps to keep that size cheap.

As with all size grades, use counts instead of name descriptions to avoid disputes over definitions.

FRYER LEGS: The meat from the merus section of the Dungeness crab. See Crabs.

GAPING: The separation of the individual flakes which make up the fillet, so that slits or holes appear. In the worst cases the fillet may fall apart if the skin is removed.

Each flake on a fillet is separated from the next by a thin membrane, which looks like a shiny surface on the flake, where it parts from its neighbor. The flesh of the flake joins the membrane by connective tissues which run through the flake to the next membrane. If these threads are unduly strained they may break and the flesh will gape.

Gaping affects the usefulness of the fish and is caused by factors related to the fish itself and to the handling of the fish immediately after catching. Certain fish are more likely to gape than others. Haddock, cod, pollock and whiting probably suffer most. Soles and ocean catfish seem to suffer least. Some fish have weak connective tissues and almost always gape, like bluefish. Larger bluefish can gape very badly.

The condition of the fish when caught affects gaping, as it affects many other aspects of quality. Not every fish caught is in prime condition. It may be weak from a long migration, or from lack of food, or it may have struggled for a long time in the net or on a line, producing adrenalin and using up energy. It may be about to spawn, so that its energy reserves are concentrated into the reproductive organs instead of the muscle or it may have just spawned, leaving it weak, with watery flesh. All these factors may make a difference to how much a fillet may gape naturally.

The way the fish is handled after capture is also important. Fish pass through rigor mortis after they die. Rigor is the stiffening of the muscles of an animal shortly after death. In pre-rigor, a fish is soft and limp and bends easily. Once the muscles stiffen, the flesh is hard. If the fish is bent or strained during this period, connective tissue will tear and the fillets will gape.

When a fish goes into rigor and how long it stays there depends on the species, the temperature and the condition of the fish. Some fish are best processed immediately after they are killed, so that the fillets are produced before rigor sets in. However, most fish are better left in ice until they pass through rigor. This avoids any risk of the fillet tearing when the muscles stiffen, which will happen even though the fish is processed. Fish frozen pre-rigor tend to have a higher drip loss when thawing than fish frozen after rigor. Fillets cut pre-rigor may warp and distort.

Fillets may also gape simply because of poor handling. Fish that is not well-iced immediately after catching gapes more than fish that is properly handled. Fish that recently spawned and resumed feeding need particular care to avoid gaping.

Anything that tends to reduce the freshness and quality of fish can increase the possibility of gaping. Although it is sometimes a natural feature of a fish, it is most often a symptom of handling errors. Examine gaping fillets carefully before accepting them.

GASPAREAU: See Alewife.

GEFILTE FISH: A fish-ball product made from minced pike and whitefish, popular in Jewish cuisine. There are numerous recipes but freshwater fish are almost always used.

GEMFISH *Scientific name: Rexea solandri:* Valued in Japan, this species comes from southern Australia and New Zealand. It provides a white, delicate fillet with high fat which smokes well and stands up to most cooking methods. It used to be mistakenly called hake in Australia. Since the name change, a strong local market developed for the fish. Because of good local and Japanese markets, it is unlikely that much gemfish will be imported into the U.S.A.

GEODUCK: See Clams.

GIBBED: The gills, guts and stomach are removed through the gill flaps. The milt or roe is left in. This process is sometimes used for herring.

GILLNET: See Salmon.

GLAZE: Protective coating of ice on frozen product to prevent the flesh from dehydration. Product frozen in blocks should have a glaze covering the block. I.Q.F. product needs glaze all over. This is usually achieved either by spraying frozen product with very cold water, which freezes instantly into a protective film, or by dipping the frozen item in a bath of ice-cold water for the same effect.

Product that is stored for long periods may need to be re-glazed to restore the protection. Some product is glazed with water mixed with a small amount of corn syrup. This is thought to give better protection than water alone.

Glaze should not be included in the net weight of the product. The F.D.A. considers excess water an adulterant and will seize product that offends.

Determining the net weight of a product under its glaze is tricky. There are a number of procedures for determining net weights. See the description in the item Defrosting methods.

G.M.P.: See Good manufacturing practice.

GOATFISH: This family of fish includes the mullets known in the Mediterranean area. American mullets are true mullets and are rather different. Goatfish are good, small panfish with firm, white flesh. They can be caught along the Atlantic coast and in California, but are not eaten much in the U.S.A.

GONADS: Sex organs and parts. In fish, the female gonad is the roe, which contains the eggs. Male gonads are called milts and contain sperm. Some sea creatures have male and female gonads together (scallops are an example). See also Roe.

GOOD MANUFACTURING PRACTICE: G.M.P. for short. This is a section of the Food, Drug and Cosmetic Act defined in Part 110 of Title 21 of the U.S. Code. The regulations comprise a basic outline of how to set up and run a food processing plant. The rules cover personnel, buildings, equipment, production, warehousing and distribution.

GOOSEFISH: See Monkfish.

GRADE A: See U.S. Grade Standards.

G.R.A.S.: Means substances Generally Recognized As Safe. The concept is an important part of food safety law. Additives, chemicals and other substances that over many years have been accepted as part of our food are given this designation. Other substances may not be used in food unless specifically approved by the Food and Drug Administration. Salt, pepper and monosodium glutamate are G.R.A.S. substances.

This does not mean that any G.R.A.S. substance can be used at will. The regulations require that no more of it be used than is necessary for its intended purpose (which may be technical, physical or nutritional). It must also be clean and wholesome for use as food and be used in an appropriate and safe way.

G.R.A.S. substances are used for flavoring, for nutritional for-tification, as anti-caking agents, as preservatives and as flavor-ings. There are neutralizers, emulsifying agents, sequestrants and stabilizers. The lists are long and change from time to time. Current lists are available in the Code of Federal Regulations, Title 21, Part 182.

GRAVLAX: Also called gravadlax, dill salmon or marinated salmon. Gravlax is sides (fillets) of salmon dry-marinated in a mixture of salt, sugar and dill weed. It is a Scandinavian product finding increasing acceptance at retail and in restaurants in the U.S.A. It is similar to smoked salmon in taste and usage. Frozen gravlax is available sliced and portioned or in sides.

GRAYFISH: Name sometimes given to dogfish.

GREEN HEADLESS: Raw shell-on shrimp tails. Raw lobster tails are also sometimes called "green".

GREENLAND TURBOT *Scientific name: Reinhardtius hippoglossoides:* This is a large flatfish with moderate to inferior flesh which is sometimes passed off as the more expensive floun-der. F.D.A. (see Names) gives it the common name of Greenland halibut and the market name of Greenland turbot. Either is legal. The fish is neither a halibut nor a turbot and only small quantities come from Greenland. See Turbot for further discussion.

GREENLING: See Lingcod and Atka Mackerel.

GREEN SHEET: The name by which most people refer to the Market News Reports issued by the National Marine Fisheries Service (N.M.F.S.) from New York. The weekly summary lists first receiver selling prices of fresh and frozen seafood commod-ities in New York. It also gives fresh seafood receipts at Fulton Fish Market in New York and prices from New England and Mid-Atlantic ports. News and information items, including details of cold storage holdings of major seafood items, are published regularly.

A fuller service is published three times weekly, giving more data on fresh prices and movements than the weekly summary.

The prices given in the Green Sheet are for the most part pretty accurate. In any case they are the best available. The sheet is used all over the world as a source document for information on seafood prices in the U.S.A. Since it is devoutly followed by packers in many supplying countries it has a substantial influence on the market. You do not have to agree with it or believe it; but it is very useful to read it.

If you find that waiting for the weekly sheet is too much for your patience, you can call and listen to a recording of the prices, updated on Thursday afternoons. The number is 212/620-3244. You can also get fresh prices updated daily on 212/620-3577.

N.M.F.S. publishes four other similar reports, each in a different color to identify it, and each including particular regional items. If you buy fish blocks and fillets, the Boston Blue Sheet is important for you. If salmon is vital, add Seattle. New Orleans will give you the scoop on shrimp news and Los Angeles (Terminal Island) gives lots of space to the tuna industry.

For subscription information, write to any N.M.F.S. Market News Office. There are also telephone numbers for recorded information on various port prices and statistics. Market News will also supply you with these.

GREEN TICKET: If F.D.A. does not wish to sample a particular import, they issue a "May Proceed" notice on green paper. This is called a Green Ticket and means that the product is approved for domestic sale without sampling by F.D.A. It does not mean that the shipment is clean, perfect or anything else, just that it is permitted entry without further examination. If it is later suspected of causing problems, it can still be recalled and inspected.

GRENADIER: Also called rattail. These names are given to over 300 deep-water species found in most of the world's oceans. Attempts to commercialize them have not been very successful. Most species are small and they are not easy to process. Rattail is also not an attractive name for a consumer product. The flesh is white and mild tasting. Some New Zealand grenadier found markets for a while, although the flesh is soft and the fillet yield is very low.

The west coast species (*Coryphaenoides acrolepsis*), Pacific grenadier, is thought to be a very large resource. It is a small fish and lives in deep water. Small quantities are landed as by-catch with other species. Catches could expand if markets develop.

Hoki is sometimes referred to as "blue grenadier" but hoki is actually related to hake (whiting) and is not a grenadier biologically.

GROUPER: Also called jewfish, sea bass, sea perch, hind, scamp, warsaw and gag. There are many different groupers, most of which are very large fish. Smaller groupers reach three feet and fifty pounds. Large jewfish (*Epinephelus itajara*) have been recorded at nearly 700lbs. Groupers are in the Seabass family. The next table details the seabass, recorded by the Fishlist, with their market and common names.

Sea Bass: Market Names and Common Names

Market name	Common name	Scientific name	Location
Bass sea	Bass, black sea	*Epinephelus tauvina*	P
Bass, sea	Bass, Peruvian Sea	*Paralabrax callaensis*	P
Bass, sea	Bass, barred sand	*Paralabrax nebulifer*	P
Bass, sea	Bass, kelp	*Paralabrax clathratus*	P
Bass, sea	Bass, spotted sand	*Paralabrax maculatofasciatus*	P
Bass, sea	Creole-fish	*Paranthias furcifer*	A
Bass, sea	Grouper, speckled dwarf	*Epinephelus merra*	P
Bass, sea	Sea bass, bank	*Centropristis ocyurus*	A
Bass, sea	Sea bass, black	*Centropristis striata*	A
Bass, sea	Sea bass, rock	*Centropristis philadelphica*	A
Cabrilla	Cabrilla, spotted	*Epinephelus analogus*	P
Grouper	Coney	*Epinephelus fulva*	A
Grouper	Coney, gulf	*Cephalopholis acanthistius*	P
Grouper	Graysby	*Epinephelus cruentatus*	A
Grouper	Grouper	*Caprodon schlegelii*	P
Grouper	Grouper, black	*Mycteroperca bonaci*	A
Grouper	Grouper, blacktip	*Epinephelus fasciatus*	P

Market name	Common name	Scientific name	Location
Grouper	Grouper, broomtail	*Mycteroperca xenarcha*	P
Grouper	Grouper, chevron tailed	*Cephalopholis urodelus*	P
Grouper	Grouper, comb	*Mycteroperca rubra*	A-P
Grouper	Grouper, dusky	*Epinephelus guaza*	A
Grouper	Grouper, gulf	*Mycteroperca jordani*	P
Grouper	Grouper, marbled	*Epinephelus inermis*	A
Grouper	Grouper, misty	*Epinephelus mystacinus*	A
Grouper	Grouper, mottled	*Epinephelus fuscoguttatus*	P
Grouper	Grouper, nassau	*Epinephelus striatus*	A
Grouper	Grouper, purplespotted	*Cephalopholis argus*	P
Grouper	Grouper, red	*Epinephelus morio*	A
Grouper	Grouper, snowy	*Epinephelus niveatus*	A-P
Grouper	Grouper, spotted	*Cephalopholis taeniops*	A
Grouper	Grouper, tiger	*Mycteroperca tigris*	A
Grouper	Grouper, warsaw	*Epinephelus nigritus*	A
Grouper	Grouper, white	*Epinephelus aeneus*	A
Grouper	Grouper, yellowedge	*Epinephelus flavolimbatus*	A
Grouper	Grouper, yellowfin	*Mycteroperca venenosa*	A
Grouper	Grouper, yellowmouth	*Mycteroperca interstitialis*	A
Grouper	Perch, sand	*Diplectrum formosum*	A
Grouper	Rockcod, brownspotted	*Epinephelus chlorostigma*	A-P
Grouper	Rockcod, yellowspotted	*Epinephelus areolatus*	A-P
Grouper/gag	Gag	*Mycteroperca microlepis*	A
Grouper/hind	Hind, red	*Epinephelus guttatus*	A
Grouper/jewfish	Jewfish	*Epinephelus itajara*	A
Hamlet	Hamlet, mutton	*Epinephelus afer*	A
Hind	Hind, rock	*Epinephelus adscensionis*	A
Hind	Hind, speckled	*Epinephelus drummondhayi*	A
Scamp	Scamp	*Mycteroperca phenax*	A

Locations: A = Atlantic   P = Indo-Pacific   F = Freshwater
Source: F.D.A.

Imported grouper is increasingly popular, much of it as frozen product. There are groupers and seabass all over the world. This is a large and far-flung family. Market preferences are for skinless and boneless fillets. Individually polywrapping is a good idea. Fishermen should also bleed these fish when they catch them to lighten the flesh and delay oxidation.

Commercially frozen grouper comes historically from Mexico, in the form of skinless fillets or fingers, cut into portions in ounce grades from 1/2 ounces upwards, packed in 10lb boxes. It is a popular item for retail and institutional use and is excellent eating, providing firm flesh and good flavor. Grouper from South America is also imported with increasing frequency. The quality can vary.

Domestic grouper is mostly sold fresh and comes from the south Atlantic states and the Gulf of Mexico. Yellowfin grouper and misty grouper are both associated with ciguatera poisoning in the West Indies.

GURRY: Waste (guts, heads, skin, bones) from filleting fish. It may be turned into fish meal or used for mink food or lobster bait.

H.A.C.C.P.: See Inspection.

HADDOCK *Scientific name: Melanogrammus aeglefinus:* An important commercial species, haddock is a close relative of Atlantic cod distinguished from cod by a thumbprint mark on the skin and by its black lateral line. It has a slightly more pronounced flavor than cod. It is caught in the North Atlantic and there is no equivalent Pacific species.

Haddock is smaller than cod. Although the species reaches 20lbs, few fish over 5lbs are landed now. Head-on gutted fresh fish are graded under 1½lbs (snappers), 1½lbs to 2½lbs (scrod) and 2½lbs up (large).

In order to preserve its identity, much haddock sells with the skin on. Skinless haddock is not a real item: it is very likely another fish. Packs are virtually the same as for Atlantic cod. Haddock is smaller and the size range is less, but otherwise the same cellos, layer packs and blocks are produced.

Domestic and Canadian products supply the bulk of the market, with Canadian product usually earning a small price premium. Imports from Iceland, Norway and Denmark normally sell at higher prices for their presumed freshness and higher quality.

Cod and haddock are similarly priced; the relationship between them alters frequently due to supply and demand changes, but in general – and this is a very broad generalization – haddock is slightly more expensive than cod.

Haddock blanks are unlikely to be haddock. See Cellos.

HAGFISH *Scientific name: Eptatretus stouti:* Hagfish are also known as slime eels. There appears to be a moderate resource off central California. The skin is used in Asia for making leather. The leather products are often exported to the U.S.A.

HAKE: The scientific distinctions between hake and whiting are complex but largely irrelevant to commercial usage. Pacific hake (*Merluccius productus*) is now called whiting and marketed as whiting. The important commercial distinction is how the customer regards the fish. There is an added complication that a lot of whiting and hake comes from Spanish speaking countries and the Spanish name for both whiting and hake is "merluza".

For most purposes in the U.S.A., hake is regarded as a large cod-like fish with very soft flesh. Whiting is preferred in the marketplace and is perceived as a smaller, firmer product. Fish that are sold as hake include the following:

• red hake (*Urophycis chuss*) from the northeast
• Gulf hake (*Urophycis cirrata*) from the Gulf
• white hake (*Urophycis tenuis*) from the northeast.
The European hake, *Merluccius merluccius*, is not normally imported into the U.S.A., although there are substantial resources in the central Atlantic off the African coast which are widely traded internationally.

Hake is sold frozen headless and dressed, or filleted in 10/5lb cellos, layer packs and blocks. It is one of the cheapest white fish, selling for less than pollock.

HALIBUT: The largest flatfish and one of the largest of all fish. Atlantic halibut of 700lbs and Pacific halibut of nearly 500lbs have been recorded.

The following species are called halibut:

> *Hippoglossus hippoglossus* is the Atlantic halibut
> *Hippoglossus stenolepis* is the Pacific halibut
> *Paralychthys californicus* is California halibut.

California halibut is a much smaller fish, seldom growing larger than 50lbs. The meat is less firm than Pacific or Atlantic halibut. You are allowed to call Greenland turbot (*Reinhardtius hippoglossoides*) by the name of Greenland halibut, but not to call it "halibut" on its own. This is a totally different fish, anyway. See Turbot.

Halibut has rich, firm flesh and is a major Pacific coast fishery from Washington to Alaska. Catches have been limited since 1924 by the International Fisheries Commission. If you are concerned with halibut supplies, you need to keep track of quotas and other limits as well as catches and market data. Fishing is restricted to very short seasons, which attract a lot of fishing in a remarkably short time. The system seems inefficient (see Fishery Management). It encourages wide fluctuations in market prices and excludes any sort of reasonable market for fresh fish, which is only available occasionally and then in large quantities.

Atlantic halibut is a less important fishery in the U.S.A. The fish has been reduced in numbers to almost a rarity. It is caught more frequently in Canada and shipped fresh to U.S. markets. Eastern halibut is mainly sold fresh. The frozen halibut that fills most market needs is west coast product.

Frozen halibut is sold in a number of forms:

• Headless and dressed halibut graded in pounds 10/20, 20/40, 40/60, 60/80, 80/100 and 100-up are the usual form shipped out of Seattle and Vancouver. The smaller two sizes may be packed in 100lb boxes, larger fish in 200lb boxes. Often, the biggest fish are shipped individually in muslin wraps, without boxes, or in totes of 600lbs each. All halibut is eventually cut into portions suitable for serving and the yields from larger fish are higher. Nevertheless, the difficulty of handling larger fish and the risk of higher mercury concentrations in it, make the 20/40lb size the usually preferred grading.

• Steaks are prepared from frozen headless and dressed fish and are usually packed 6/5lbs, sometimes 10/5 lbs. Steaks should be layered with sheets of paper or poly between the layers. There is a U.S. Grade Standard for frozen halibut steaks. Size grades are either two ounce steps, 4/6, 6/8, 8/10 and 10/12 ounces, or are exact weight ounce grades, 4 ounces through 12 ounces. The smaller and larger size steaks are always harder to sell than the middle ranges. Halibut steaks often come from Japan. The fish is identical to the domestic and Canadian west coast fish and is usually well graded and packed.

• Boneless steaks are prepared from fillets, otherwise packed and graded as regular steaks. Boneless steaks are of course more expensive. They are sometimes called loin steaks.

• Fletches or loins are boneless fillets of halibut, used for preparing boneless steaks. They are generally individually wrapped and packed in 50lb or 100lb boxes. Fletches are mainly sold in the west. California halibut is usually filleted into fletches.

H AND G: Also called H and D. These are abbreviations for headed and gutted fish or headless, dressed fish.

HARD CURED: Dry salted and dried fish with moisture content less than 40 percent. See Curing

HARD SMOKED: Fish smoked in cold smoke for long periods until hard. West coast Indian smoked salmon is an example. The product is hard like beef jerky and will keep for long periods without refrigeration.

HATCHERY SALMON: Also called spent salmon. It is salmon which has spawned. The flesh is very soft and is fit only for animal food or the manufacture of fish paste, spreads or similar non-textured product. See Salmon.

HAZARD ANALYSIS CRITICAL CONTROL POINT: H.A.C.C.P. See Inspection.

HEAD MEAT: Meat from the body of the spiny lobster. Product is sometimes available from parts of Central America, packed 10/5lb or 10/5/1lb. The meat from the larger legs and shoulders is used, sometimes carefully cleaned but more often packed with tendons, shell fragments and even pieces of seaweed. Head meat has remarkably little flavor and is useful mainly to provide the "lobster" listed on an ingredient panel.

HEALTH AND NUTRITION: Seafood marketers are increasingly stressing the health benefits of fish and shellfish. Low in fat and calories compared with meat and poultry, seafoods also provide the only source of omega-3 fatty acids. (Despite claims that some plants have omega-3s, plant versions of the omega-3 molecules do not appear to have the same dietary effects as those from seafoods – it is still safe to claim seafood as the unique source). Omega-3s are believed to help reduce heart attacks and are linked with positive benefits in many areas of human health.

The term "n-3" is used by some scientists. It means exactly the same as omega-3, but adds to confusion among laypeople.

It is believed that the substantial increase in seafood consumption recorded in the second half of the 1980s is largely due to consumer concern with health and the benefits of eating seafood. While this appears to be a long-term trend in American habits, the industry would be more comfortable if consumers were buying seafood because it tastes good rather than because it does them good. Hopefully, more people will get hooked on seafood, whatever their reasons for eating it in the first place.

Knowledge of seafood's health benefits derives from a number of studies around the world, starting with the famous examination of the Greenland Eskimo diet. Cautious scientists, however, would still affirm that the case is not fully proven.

Nutrition information – knowing exactly what is in the fish and shellfish we eat – is also far from complete. The best source is still *Seafood Nutrition – Facts, Issues and Marketing of Nutrition in Fish and Shellfish* by Joyce A. Nettleton, D.Sc., R.D. The U.S. Department of Agriculture has more recently revised its *Agriculture Handbook Number 8-15 – Composition of Foods: Finfish and Shellfish Products*, which is a compilation of all the available nutrition data about seafoods.

Nutrition scientists seldom understand fish and shellfish. Unless the researcher is positive about the species he is testing, the reports of the test are not much use. Because some data suffers from this flaw, it is not possible for the seafood expert to be sure that the data is in fact about the right species.

Another problem is that far too little work has been done on the whole subject. Fish vary through the seasons, through their breeding cycles and because of variations in their diet. A particular species may be high in fat at one time of the year but very low in fat at other times. Without detailed knowledge of these variations, you really cannot define the true nutritional characteristics of the item. An example is the seasonal variation in the fat content of spot (*Leiostomus xanthurus*) which, according to an article by M.E. Waters in *Marine Fisheries Review* in 1982, varied from 0.6 percent in February to 8.96 percent in July.

The publicity about the health benefits of omega-3 fatty acids is being exploited by drug companies selling fish oil capsules. This is of no benefit to the seafood industry (other than those producing the small quantities of oily fish or fish livers which are processed into huge numbers of pills). There is no evidence that the large amounts of fish oil consumed in capsule form are any more beneficial to the average person than the very small amounts consumed when eating fish. Early in 1988, the F.D.A. stopped the use of health claims in fish-oil advertising on the grounds that there was insufficient evidence to support the claims being made.

One nutritional point which is greatly misunderstood is that shrimp is not a high-cholesterol item. The original research on shrimp was unable to distinguish between cholesterol and certain plant sterols. Current techniques can now discern the differences. Consumers can stop worrying about cholesterol in shrimp and concentrate on enjoying it.

HERRING *Scientific name: Clupea harengus:* A small oily fish, weighing about 1-1½lbs, found in large shoals in the north Atlantic and north Pacific. Similar fish are found in most seas around the world. North Atlantic herring was a staple food in northern Europe and though greatly reduced in numbers it is still a major commercial species. The Atlantic and Pacific herrings are subspecies of the same fish. The Atlantic herring is, in full scientific glory, *Clupea harengus harengus*. The Pacific herring in full is *Clupea harengus pallasi*.

Herrings are of less importance in the U.S.A. than in Europe. On the Atlantic coast, small herrings are canned as "Maine sardines" and larger fish are sold fresh or frozen for curing or for bait. Much larger quantities are landed in Canada, which also exports thousands of tons yearly to Europe. Quantities caught by U.S. fishermen are insufficient for development of a regular export trade.

On the Pacific coast, and especially in Alaska, herrings are now caught and frozen on a large scale for export to Japan, mainly for the roe. The roe is extracted and salted and the processed product also exported in many cases. A similar business based on exporting roe to Asia exists on the east coast, but is much less important.

In the U.S.A., most herring is eaten cured or pickled. Salted, Bismarck, dill, kippered and rollmops are among the popular forms.

Frozen herrings are used as raw material for curing and smoking. Lesser quality fish is widely used for bait and for animal feed. For these latter purposes, herring is frozen whole in 50lb blocks, often in trays without lids for cheapness.

Curers have very stringent quality requirements for their herring. Most prefer I.Q.F. or small blocks. Fish should meet the following criteria:

• The fish must be largely undamaged. Torn and bruised flesh detracts from the product and may make it unusable. Most buyers look at the bellies, the thinnest part, to check for tears.

• The fat content of the flesh must be high for virtually all smoking and curing. 10 percent is the lowest most buyers will accept and 18 percent is much preferred. Pacific herrings are generally less fat than Atlantic herrings. Some similar fish from tropical and Southern Hemisphere waters can be extraordinarily low in oil.

• Since the fat content is highest before the fish starts to develop roe or milt, the presence of maturing gonads will usually make the fish unacceptable to curers.

• At the stage when the flesh is fat, the fish is eating voraciously. Any delay in freezing the fish allows undigested food to ferment and form gas. Buyers will therefore check that the bellies are flat, not distended, as an indication that the fish was well handled and fresh.

• All the usual signs of freshness are necessary, such as bright eyes and fresh smell. Herring goes rancid and develops "off" odors at amazing speed.

There is little market for herring for direct consumer use, which is a pity since it is a tasty and nutritious fish and inexpensive. A few supermarkets will traypack I.Q.F. herring. Some fish is processed into fillets, usually butterfly fillets and layer packed, mostly for export to Europe.

Herring roe and milt are both prized in Europe. Roe is sought by the Japanese, but there is effectively no market for these items in the U.S.A.

There are many other herrings around the world. The U.S. has substantial resources of thread herring (*Opisthonema oglinum*) in the southeast and Gulf. This is smaller than the Atlantic herring but at certain times of year has plenty of fat and can be used much like its larger cousin. For river herring, see Alewife. See also Sardine, Pilchard and Anchovy.

HISTAMINES: Chemicals produced by decomposition in some species under certain conditions. Histamine poisoning is also called scombroid poisoning because it is often associated with the scombroid fish such as tunas and mackerels. Although rarely fatal, it is nasty. The problem first surfaced in imported mahi-mahi. Fish left in warm conditions, on the deck or on the beach, before processing were apt to produce histamines. Mahi and other species known to be a risk, such as tuna, are regularly monitored when imported. The problem can be avoided altogether by proper handling of the fish. There is no way the user can tell if a fish is affected – testing is quite complex. But good fresh fish is unlikely to be a problem. See also Seafood safety.

HOKI *Scientific name: Macruronus novaezelandiae:* Also called New Zealand whiting and New Zealand whiptail. The fish is distantly related to the hakes and looks similar to grenadier. It reaches about 3lbs and is found in large quantities around New Zealand, southern Australia and the southern tip of South America. It has whiting-like flesh – fairly soft but moist and white when cooked. The lateral fat line must be removed in fillets or for fish blocks.

Layer-packed frozen product is finding increasing markets. New Zealand processors pack loins (the center cut of the fillet after removing the lateral line) and found good acceptance for this premium product. The rest of the fillet is used for fish blocks.

Hoki with the lateral line has a fairly short shelf life. It is cheaper, but watch for it.

HOOLIHANS: See Smelts.

HORSE MACKEREL: Also called jack mackerel or scad. The name is sometimes given to bluefin tuna. Pacific jack mackerel is an important species, but for canning rather than for frozen use. Technically, the fish is a jack, but it is treated as a mackerel. See Mackerel.

HUMPBACK SALMON: Pink salmon. The smallest Pacific species. See Salmon.

HUSS: A name used for dogfish in Britain. The name is not approved for use in the U.S.A. See Dogfish.

IDENTIFICATION: See Economic fraud in the seafood business.

I.E.F.: See Iso-electric focusing.

ILLEX: See Squid.

INCONNU *Scientific name: Stenodus leucichthys:* This is the largest member of the freshwater whitefish group. The fish grow to over 20lbs. There is a seagoing strain which is even larger. Inconnu are excellent, trout-like fish, occasionally imported from Canada frozen and dressed.

INK: Squid, cuttlefish and octopus expel a black ink as a "smokescreen" to help them escape from predators. Squid and cuttlefish are sometimes cooked in their ink, which means that the ink sac must be removed carefully without breaking it.

INKFISH: Cuttlefish. Squid are sometimes incorrectly called inkfish.

INSPECTION: Mandatory inspection of seafood is a political issue. Voluntary inspection is available for a fee from the Department of Commerce (see U.S. Grade Standards). But unlike meat and poultry, seafood is not required to be inspected by the Federal government. Indeed, a General Accounting Office report in 1988 said that seafood was not often associated with health problems and that inspection was not necessary. In case mandatory inspection should become a reality, the following outlines the main technical aspects that seafood processors and purveyors will have to understand and implement.

THE HAZARD ANALYSIS CRITICAL CONTROL POINT (HACCP) system is the inspection, evaluation and quality control system of all procedures during processing, handling, distribution and storage where contamination or mishandling may affect the quality of the food product. Monitoring these areas regularly with the HACCP system avoids potential health hazards and insures top quality food product.

The principles of HACCP: The HACCP approach is to assess hazards, determine critical control points and establish procedures to monitor these points in food handling and processing. This assures food safety and prevents spoilage. Using HACCP system helps prevent health hazards from developing along the processing line and during distribution and food preparations.

Hazard Analysis: The evaluation of all procedures during production, processing, distribution and use of raw materials or food products including:

- identifying potentially hazardous raw materials and foods that may contain poisonous substances, pathogens, bacteria or conditions which may invite the growth of bacteria.
- observing each step of the processing operation to determine specific points and sources of chemical and bacterial contamination.
- determining the potential for bacteria or toxic substances to remain during handling and processing.
- determining the potential for bacteria to multiply.

Hazards are the unacceptable growth, survival or contamination by microorganisms which may affect the safety of food. The hazard analysis is conducted with all existing products, with new products and when any changes are made in raw materials, product formulation, processing, packaging or distribution.

Key questions to answer during hazard analysis:
Product formulation and packaging:
• What are the ingredients?
• What is the pH?
• Are toxic substances added? If so, what is the concentration?
• What type and numbers of bacteria are likely to be present?
• Are preservatives used? If so, what kind?
• What type of packaging is used and is it important for product stability?

Processing:
• Are live animals or raw products possibly contaminated with pathogens?
• Can pathogens spread to other products during processing?
• Will bacteria or pathogens be killed during processing?
• Can bacteria multiply or contaminate the product during or after processing or storage?

Conditions of distribution and use:
• Is the product distributed in warm or cold storage temperatures?
• What is its expected shelf life during distribution, storage and use?
• How will the product be prepared for consumption?
• Will it be cooked and held for a period before eating?
• If so, will it be held in hot, cold or warm temperatures?
• What mishandling could possibly occur during marketing or when the consumer handles it?

Answers to these questions provide valuable leads to potential hazards, including the effects of mishandling on product safety and stability.

An expert food microbiologist or toxicologist should check the analysis:
• test for bacteria or chemical substances.
• inoculate the product with appropriate food-borne pathogens and potential spoilage organisms.
• evaluate the effects of mishandling, simulate storage conditions, distribution, routine processing, marketing and any other expected conditions the product may encounter.

Critical control points are the potentially hazardous processing procedures and locations which are patrolled carefully to ensure that spoilage and contamination do not occur. These include:

- incoming raw materials, especially if they host heat-resistant bacteria
- the time and temperature of heat processing
- the temperature before, during and after freezing the product
- the amount of time the product is held in storage
- cleaning the equipment used for processing the product
- the way workers handle the product

Although many control points are obvious through hazard analysis, intensive research is sometimes needed to establish the best control points.

Monitoring: Critical points must be checked regularly to ensure that they are under full control. Appropriate tests should be determined for each critical control point. Tests must be carried out on a planned schedule. All results must be recorded. Checklists of locations and procedures of critical control points should always be used during testing.

HACCP techniques assure the highest degree of food safety when monitored properly. The difference between currently implemented meat and poultry inspection and HACCP is that the present system relies on finding problems after they have occurred rather than preventing them.

IMPORT INSPECTION: F.D.A. inspects imported foods for conformity with U.S. laws. Bacteria, contamination, filth and decomposition are the main reasons for finding foods unwholesome. For bacterial standards, see Bacteria. Contamination by metals and chemicals is covered in the entry Seafood safety. Filth and decomposition are covered below.

Filth action levels: Current Food and Drug Administration standards and definitions for filth on shrimp are quoted below. Filth standards for other seafood products are similar.

Interim Action Levels for Filth on Imported Fresh or Frozen Raw Shrimp: Samples of imported fresh or frozen raw shrimp may be detained when analyses of six 2 to 3 pound subsamples show filth at or above the following levels:

- Flies (whole or equivalent) 1. Filth flies – 2 in a sample.   2. Incidental flies – 10 in a sample.
- Filth Fly Fragments 1. Three fragments (excluding setae) in 5 of 6 sub-samples (these fragments are clearly identified as parts of a filth fly). 2. Large body parts (i.e.: thorax, abdomen) 1 in 3 of 6 sub-samples.
- Cockroaches 1. One whole or equivalent in the sample.   2. Excreta – 1 in 2 of 6 sub-samples.
- Hairs 1. Rat or mouse – 3 of any size in a sample.   2. Striated but not rat or mouse – 4 of any size in a sample.

Filth Flies Definition: Houseflies (Muscidae), humpbacked flies (Phoridae), moth flies (Psychodidae), black scavenger flies (Sepsidae), small dung flies (Sphaeroceridae), Chloropoid flies (Chloropidae), Anthoymiid flies (Anthoymiidae), blow flies (Calliphoridae), and flowe flies (Syrphidae). This is not necessarily a complete list of filth flies which might be found in shrimp.

Incidental Flies Definition: Dance flies (Empidiidae), beach flies (Canaccidae), shore flies (Ephydridae), (Natichiidae), tachinid flies (Tachinidae). This is not necessarily a complete list of incidental flies which might be found in shrimp.

Decomposition: The following is taken from Title 50 of the Code of Federal Regulations. This paragraph defines standard cooking procedures for shrimp which are necessary to judge decomposition, flavor and odor. A.O.A.C. methods are basically used. Decomposition of other seafoods is assessed in a similar way.

Procedures for cooking samples in sensory evaluation of cooked flavor and odor: "Cooked in a suitable manner" (Cooked style excepted) means that a portion of the thawed product has been cooked as follows:

Place two to four ounces of shrimp in a sauce pan with 1 pint of water and 1 teaspoon of salt (Salt optional). Cook until internal temperature reaches 160°F. (70°C.). Drain and cool without rinsing and check for flavor, odor and texture.

Defect Action Levels: These defect action levels apply to sample units of fresh or frozen shrimp. A defect action level occurs if the shrimp in a sample unit show Class 3 decomposition or if the percentage of shrimp showing

Class 2 decomposition plus four times the percentage of those showing Class 3 decomposition equals at least 20 percent of the shrimp in a sample unit. The classes are defined as follows:

- Class 1 – Passable
  This category includes fishery products that range from very fresh to those that contain fishy odors or other odors characteristic of the commercial product, not definitely identifiable as decomposition.
- Class 2 – Decomposed (Slight but Definite)
  The first stage of definitely identifiable decomposition. An odor is present that, while not really intense, is persistent and as readily perceptible to the experienced examiner as that of decomposition.
- Class 3 – Decomposed (Advanced)
  The product possesses a strong odor of decomposition which is persistent, distinct and unmistakable.

INTERLEAVED: Layer pack with polywrap separating each piece or layer of fish. See Packing styles.

I.P.W.: Individually polywrapped.

I.Q.F.: Individually quick frozen. Each piece of product is separate from every other. See Freezing processes.

IRRADIATION: Also called picowaving or ionizing irradiation. Irradiation is the treatment of food with low doses of radiation to kill surface bacteria. This extends the shelf life of the food, because the spoilage bacteria are no longer present. Experiments with fish indicate that good quality, fresh fillets could keep two to three times longer after irradiating. Irradiation is subject to complex political pressures. At least eight Federal bodies are involved. The Food and Drug Administration (F.D.A.) is responsible for deciding whether and how irradiated foods may be processed and marketed. F.D.A.'s initial approach is that irradiation is an additive and must be listed on the label of any irradiated food. Approval of irradiation has come very slowly, being permitted mainly for experimental purposes and for spices, which are not consumed in significant quantities by individuals. It is now permitted for pork products to reduce incidents of the trichinosis parasite. Scientific evidence of the effects of irradiation is unclear. The process appears to change some molecules of the flesh. Manchester University in England is developing a test for irradiated foods based on a distinctive form of carbon dioxide molecule produced by irradiation. There are concerns that irradiation reduces the nutritional value of foods. New substances, known as unique radiolytic products (URPs for short) are produced in foods by the irradiation process. We are told these are safe, but so far they have been neither identified nor tested. "Irradiation" usually means treatment with a low level of gamma radiation. However, there is a range of possible techniques, each with its own name.

Radurization is the use of "low" doses (below 100,000 rad) of ionizing irradiation.

Radicidation is the use of "medium" doses (100,000 – 1 million rad) of ionizing irradiation. This pasteurizes the product. Radicidized products should be packaged prior to irradiation and the dose of radiation depends on the nature of the product (ex: the size of its container and whether it is raw, dried, or frozen).

Raddapertization is the use of higher doses (above 1 million rad) of ionizing irradiation. With raddapertization, the radiation dosage must be high enough to sterilize the product (equivalent to a botulism cook). Because cooling is not necessary, post-radappertizing contamination is unlikely unless a package breaks. But the big concerns are outside the scientific area.

Safety: The nuclear industry insists that irradiation is safe. Very low dosages of radiation are used. The radiation certainly does not remain in the food. However, opponents point to other safety issues. Irradiation plants are supplied with radioactive materials and produce significant quantities of radioactive waste. Both supplies and wastes must be transported. Any plant using radioactive materials presents a hazard to its neighbors. The industry's case was not helped when managers of one of the pioneering companies were convicted of hiding safety defects from inspectors.

Marketing: Many leading retailers are understandably nervous about offering food that is labelled as "irradiated." The processing industry attempted to persuade F.D.A. that the label does not have to mention irradiation. Failing this, other words such as "picowaved" are offered, presumably to avoid the use of anything that sounds like radiation. Consumer groups are almost universally hostile to irradiation ("killer tomatoes" was a popular phrase not long ago when the subject was discussed) though most consumers are probably unaware of the controversy.

Recontamination: The surface of irradiated foods is almost entirely free of bacteria. If the food is then contaminated with a new bacteria – for example if the packaging is less than perfect, or simply from handling – there is no existing bacteria to compete with the new one and prevent it from multiplying. In fact, irradiated surfaces are prime, virgin real estate for bugs. Botulinus in particular is not killed by irradiation, which leaves the food's surface clear for the bug to spread without competition from other bacteria.

Re-irradiation: The nuclear industry is keen to avoid labelling irradiated products. Lack of comprehensive labelling could mean that product might be re-irradiated, since a secondary processor would not know that the product he was using was already treated. The risks from the additional dosage of gamma rays are unknown. For the seafood industry there is one separate problem. Some seafoods have for many years been irradiated and illegally imported into the country. Irradiation is used in several European countries to process shrimp, frog legs and other seafood items that are rejected for salmonella contamination. The bacteria is killed by the process and the product is then re-imported. This procedure is against the law, but has been difficult to detect and enforce. F.D.A. inspectors look for unusually clean product as an indication that it was irradiated. Irradiation is a very complex subject, which we have space only to present in bare outline. It may become an important issue or it may become a non-issue as better, less controversial ways of preserving food are developed. Freezing technology already does the job and is improving all the time.

ISO-ELECTRIC FOCUSING: The full term is "thin layer polyacrylamide gel iso-electric focusing"; IEF for short. This is a technique for making positive identification of species by analyzing the pattern of proteins in the flesh. The proteins in the flesh of every species, when charged with an electric current, form a unique pattern which is like a "fingerprint" of the species. No two species are the same: even some sub-species show different patterns. The IEF technique has been approved for raw seafoods by the A.O.A.C – the Association for Official Analytical Chemists. This means that properly conducted IEF tests will stand up in court as proof of the species identity of raw seafood products. The technique is useful in two ways. One is to make a positive identification of what you have. The other, possibly more important, is to determine that what you have is NOT what you ordered. There are two drawbacks to IEF. The minor one is that it cannot, as yet, be used for cooked seafoods. For example, it cannot determine accurately whether there is real crabmeat in a surimi product. The major problem, however, is that the data base of proved samples is not nearly big enough. To demonstrate the species, you have to be able to compare the pattern with that from a definitively identified sample of the species. The N.M.F.S. laboratory in Gloucester, Massachusetts has a fairly large library of authenticated samples. But there is a need for many more samples. Nevertheless, in any given situation it is possible to obtain an authenticated sample of the correct species, then compare your own sample's pattern with this. The technique allows clear and accurate decision in disputes over what a seafood product actually is. IEF is not the ultimate technique. Monoclonal antibodies developed from different fish species can be used to make better, positive identifications. However, this work has not advanced far. In the meantime, IEF offers the industry sufficient assurance for everyday business needs.

JACK MACKEREL: See Mackerel.

JACKS: Also called trevally, crevalle jack, bumber, blue runner and green runner. The names cover a wide variety of tropical and subtropical fish, some of which are also good game fish. Some may be frozen and sold pan-ready, but most when traded are used as bait fish and zoo food. Pompano and amberjack are also jacks, though not usually so regarded commercially. The following is from the Fishlist (see Names) and covers the 56 species of the jack family recognized for sale in the U.S.A.

Jacks: Market Names and Common Names

Market name	Common name	Scientific name	Location
Amberjack	Amberjack, greater	*Seriola dumerili*	A
Amberjack	Amberjack, lesser	*Seriola fasciata*	A
Amberjack	Rudderfish, banded	*Seriola zonata*	A
Amberjack/ yellowtail	Amberjack, king	*Seriola quinqueradiata*	P
Amberjack/ yellowtail	Yellowtail	*Seriola lalandei*	P
Bumper	Bumper, Atlantic	*Chloroscombrus chrysurus*	A
Bumper	Bumper, Pacific	*Chloroscombrus orqueta*	P
Jack	Jack crevalle	*Caranx hippos*	A
Jack	Jack, almaco	*Seriola rivoliana*	A
Jack	Jack, bar	*Caranx ruber*	A
Jack	Jack, black	*Caranx lugubris*	A
Jack	Jack, cottonmouth	*Uraspis secunda*	A-P
Jack	Jack, green	*Caranx caballus*	P
Jack	Jack, horse-eye	*Caranx latus*	A
Jack	Jack, mazatlan/striped	*Caranx vinctus*	P
Jack	Jack, whitemouth	*Caranx helvolus*	P
Jack	Jack, yellow	*Caranx bartholomaei*	A
Jack	Leatherjacket	*Oligoplites saurus*	A
Jack	Lookdown	*Selene vomer*	A
Jack	Moonfish, Atlantic	*Selene setapinnis*	A
Jack	Moonfish, Pacific	*Selene peruviana*	P
Jack mackerel	Mackerel, jack	*Trachurus declivis*	A
Jack mackerel	Mackerel, jack	*Trachurus symmetricus*	P
Jack mackerel	Scad, Japanese	*Trachurus japonicus*	P
Jack mackerel	Scad, inca	*Trachurus murphyi*	P
Jack mackerel	Scad, rough	*Trachurus lathami*	A
Jack/blue runner	Runner, blue	*Caranx crysos*	A
Jack/rainbow runner	Runner, rainbow	*Elegatis bipinnulata*	A-P
Jack/roosterfish	Roosterfish	*Nematistius pectoralis*	P
Jack/trevally	Jack, spotted	*Caranx melampygus*	P
Jack/trevally	Trevally, giant	*Caranx ignobilis*	P
Jack/trevally	Trevally, white	*Caranx georgianus*	P
Jackfish/crevalle	Jack, threadfin	*Alectis indicus*	P

Locations: A = Atlantic   P = Indo-Pacific   F = Freshwater
Source: F.D.A.

Market name	Common name	Scientific name	Location
Mackerel/scad	Mackerel, jack	*Trachurus novaeze-landiae*	P
Pompano	Pompano, African	*Alectis ciliaris*	A
Pompano	Pompano, Florida	*Trachinotus carolinus*	A
Pompano	Pompano, paloma	*Trachinotus paitensis*	P
Pompano	Pompano, tropical	*Trachinotus blochi*	P
Pompano/palometa	Palometa	*Trachinotus goodei*	A
Pompano/permit	Permit	*Trachinotus falcatus*	A
Pompano/permit	Permit, palometta	*Trachinotus kennedyi*	P
Pompano/pompanito	Pompano, gafftopsail	*Trachinotus rhodopus*	P
Scad	Horse mackerel, Atlantic	*Trachurus trachurus*	A-P
Scad	Koheru	*Decapterus koheru*	P
Scad	Scad, Mexican	*Decapterus scombrinus*	P
Scad	Scad, amberstripe	*Decapterus muroadsi*	P
Scad	Scad, bigeye	*Selar crumenophthalmus*	A
Scad	Scad, blue	*Trachurus picturatus*	A
Scad	Scad, mackerel	*Decapterus macarellus*	A
Scad	Scad, northern mackerel	*Decapterus russelli*	P
Scad	Scad, redtail	*Decapterus tabl*	A
Scad	Scad, round	*Decapterus punctatus*	A
Scad	Scad, yellowtail	*Caranx mate*	P
Trevally	Trevally, bigeye	*Caranx sexfasciatus*	P
Trevally	Trevally, white	*Caranx dentex*	P

Locations: A = Atlantic   P = Indo-Pacific   F = Freshwater
Source: F.D.A.

JAPANESE FLOUNDER AND SOLE: Deceptive labels for arrowtooth. See Flatfish.

JAPANESE TURBOT: Greenland turbot. See Turbot.

JEWFISH: See Grouper.

JUMBO COD: Large fresh cod 25lbs and over; fillets from cod of this size. In current practice, almost any cod fillet over 16 ounces may be misdescribed as a "jumbo." The use of such descriptive terms should be avoided. Size definitions are much more precise.

JUMBO LUMP: Large pieces of meat from the body of the blue crab. See Crabs.

JUMBO SHRIMP: In everyday use, a jumbo shrimp means almost any large shrimp. Under all circumstances use numerical counts to define shrimp and never use descriptive names, which are open to differing interpretations.

KAMABOKO: See Surimi.

KG or KILOGRAM: A metric weight equivalent to 2.2046lbs. In the U.S.A. it is usually calculated as 2.2lbs, so if you buy shrimp packed in 2 kilo blocks, you will normally be billed for 4.4lbs, not 4.4092lbs. Because a 2kg block of shrimp is similar in size and shape to a 5lb block, some distributors will resell the 2kg block as a 5lb block, effectively overcharging by 12 percent. You should be aware of which origins pack in kilos and also, of course, check the weights on the product you receive.

KING CRAB: See Crabs.

KINGFISH *Scientific name: Scomberomorus cavalla:* Also called king mackerel. Unapproved names include cavalla, cero and sierra. A large mackerel, fairly common in southern Florida, reaching 25lbs with sportfishermen occasionally landing fish as large as 100lbs. It is sold frozen headless and dressed in 25lb and 50lb boxes. It is frequently filleted or steaked and packed 10/5lbs or 5/10lbs. It is an oily fish with a good pronounced flavor.

KINGFISH, SOUTHERN *Scientific names: Menticirrhus americanus, Menticirrhus saxatilis, Menticirrhus littoralis.* These fish are also called king whiting, although the name is not approved by the F.D A. and is confusing. These species are members of the drum tribe. They are found from Maine southwards into the Gulf of Mexico. The fish has white to pink flesh and is usually between 12 ounces and 3 pounds.

Southern kingfish is an inexpensive and palatable seafood. There are substantial resources which could be caught and used as frozen pan-dressed product.

KINGKLIP *Scientific name: Genypterus spp.:* These fish are known as cusk-eels in Europe but not in North America. South Africa was the first fishing country to harvest kinglip. The species *Genypterus capensis*, has been sold in frozen fillet form for many years in Europe. The very similar *Genypterus blacodes* has been marketed from Chile and New Zealand since the middle 1980s. Red kingklip (*Genypterus chilensis*) and black kingklip (*Genypterus maculatus*) are also harvested in the southern oceans. New Zealanders may call their product ling, a name that is not appropriate in the U.S.A.

Kingklip flesh is dense, white and firm and has gained some market share as an alternative to orange roughy. Skinless and boneless fillets are the usual product form, usually size graded and I.Q.F. or layer packed.

There appear to be large resources of kingklip, which is a comparatively inexpensive and acceptable fish.

KING SALMON: Also called chinook or spring salmon. The largest of the Pacific salmon, averaging 20lbs when mature. See Salmon.

KING WHITING: A confusing name applied to many different fish, including large whiting or hake, corvina (drum) and even kingfish. This is a term to avoid using.

KIPPER: A smoked herring product. The precise definition from the Torry Research Laboratory in Aberdeen, Scotland – Aberdeen is where kippers originated – is "fat herring with guts and gills removed, split down the back from head to tail, lightly brined, dyed if desired, and cold smoked at air temperatures not higher than 30°C. (86°F.)."

The U.S. market prefers kipper fillets and most smoked herring is called kipper. Freezing smoked products accentuates the salty taste, so product intended to be frozen should be specifically cured for freezing.

Domestic, Canadian and Scottish kippers and kipper fillets are widely available. Packs vary, but all should be well wrapped and sealed to protect the fish and to prevent the odor from affecting other product stored nearby.

KIPPERED FISH: Hot smoked fish, especially salmon, is sometimes called "kippered."

KLIPFISH: See Curing.

KOSHER: Food approved under the dietary laws of the Jewish religion. For seafood, only fish that have fins and scales may be consumed, excluding all shellfish, shrimp, lobster and creatures such as shark which do not have regular scales. Preparation of the food must also conform to certain rules and take place under the supervision of a rabbi. It is not possible for an already packed product to be approved. The supervision must be performed throughout the production process.

The supervisor authorizes the imprint of his organization's symbol, such as the widely known u in a circle. There are a number of supervisory services and each has its own symbol. If you need further assistance, contact a local rabbi. New York Sea Grant has a useful publication *Old Laws in a New Market* by Joe and Carrie Regenstein. Contact your local Sea Grant to get a copy.

Non-kosher fishes include:
- Billfishes (Family Istiophoridae) including: Sailfishes (*Istiophorus spp.*), Marlins and Spearfishes (*Tetrapturus spp.*, *Makaiara spp.*)
- Catfishes (Order Siluriformes) including: Channel catfish (*Ictalurus punctatus*), Bullheads (*Ictalurus spp.*), Sea catfish (*Arius felis* which is also known as *Ariopsis felis*)
- Cutlassfishes (Family Trichjuridae) including: cutlassfishes (*Trichiurus spp.*), Scabbardfishes (*Lepidopus spp.*)
- Eels (Order Anguilliformes) including: American and European eel (*Anguilla rostrata* and *Anguilla anguilla*) and Conger eel (*Conger oceanicus*)
- Gars (Order Semionotiformes) Freshwater gars (*Lepisosteus spp.*)
- Goosefishes, anglers or monkfish (*Lophius spp.*)

- Lampreys (Family Petromyzontidae)
- Leatherjacket (*Oligoplites saurus*)
- Lumpsuckers (Family Cyclopteridae) including: Lumpfish (*Cyclopterus lumpus*), Snailfishes (*Liparis spp.*)
- Ocean pout or eelpout (*Macrozoarces americanus*)
- Oilfish (*Ruvettus pretiosus*)
- Puffers (Family Tetraodontidae) Puffers, blowfishes, swell-fishes, sea-squab (*Sphoeroides spp.*)
- Rock prickleback or rockeel (*Xiphister mucosus*)
- Sculpins (Family Cottidae) including: Sculpins (*Myoxocephalus spp.*, *Cottus spp.*, *Leptocottus spp.*, etc.), Cabezon (*Scorpaenichtys marmoratus*), Searaven (*Hemitripterus americanus*)
- Sharks, rays, and their relatives (Class Chondrichthyes) including: Grayfishes or dogfishes (*Mustelus spp.*, *Squalus spp.*), Soupfin shark (*Galeorhinus zyopterus*), Sawfishes (*Pristis species*), Skates (*Raja spp.*), Chimaeras or ratfishes (Order Chimaeriformes)
- Snake mackerels (*Gempylus spp.*)
- Sturgeons (Order Acipenseriformes) including: Sturgeons (*Acipenser spp.*, *Scaphirhynchus spp.*), Beluga (*Huso huso*) and Paddlefish or spoonbill cat (*Polydon spathula*)
- Swordfish (*Xiphias gladius*)
- Toadfishes (Family Batrachoididae) including: Toadfishes (*Opsanus spp.*), Midshipmen (*Porichthys spp.*)
- Triggerfishes and filefishes (Family Balistidae) including: Triggerfishes (*Balistes spp.*, *Canthidermis spp.*)
- Trunkfishes (Family Ostraciidae) including: Trunkfishes and cowfishes (*Lactophrys spp.*)
- Wolffishes (Family Anarhichadidae) including: Wolffishes or ocean catfishes (*Anarhichas spp.*).

Packing seafoods according to kosher rules is not particularly difficult and this is a growing area of the market which is worth attention. Even kosher surimi is now available, made entirely from pollock, without any crabmeat or crab essence.

KRILL: Species of plankton, which look and taste rather like shrimp. Although plankton is usually microscopic, krill may be several inches long. There is a lot of krill in the North Pacific and hundreds of millions of tons are estimated in the Antarctic, where they used to be eaten by the whales. Now that the whales are almost extinct, man is working on ways to harvest and utilize the krill. The Antarctic species is *Euphausia superba*. It is the largest of the 85 known species of krill, reaching 4.6 inches in length. It also forages actively for food, making it much more like a shrimp than like any other animal plankton.

Factory vessels from a number of countries have caught the animal and experimented with different processing techniques. Krill is difficult to remove from the hard, thick shell and has a low yield of meat. There is so far no way to make krill into a product familiar to consumers.

However, there is a lot of krill to harvest and much interest in utilizing the resource, which in the Antarctic alone is greater than the present world catch of all existing marine foods.

Meanwhile, very small quantities of frozen or freeze-dried krill are being used as treats for pet fish in home aquaria and as special food for farmed fish. Japan and the U.S.S.R. have developed small markets for human consumption. You may expect to see "krillburgers" or similar product on offer at some time in the future.

LABELLING: The U.S. Food and Drug Administration regulates the labelling of all foods, including fish and shellfish. In 1973, the F.D.A. began enforcing a final set of regulations which state what kinds of information are required on labels and what claims are prohibited.

The following must be included on labels: product name; net contents or weight (including packing liquid); name and address of the manufacturer, packer, or distributor; and the ingredients listed in descending order by weight. Including the ingredients is not mandatory, however, if the product conforms to "standards of identity."

Standards of identity are products conforming to an established recipe. There are established standards of identity for canned tuna and salmon.

The Fair Packaging Act of 1966 requires that all information be written in simple English and placed conspicuously on the label. F.D.A. may decide a product is misbranded if statements, designs, or pictures on the label are false or misleading or if the label fails to provide required information.

Information which the manufacturer may include if he chooses, but are not mandatory, are open dating, preparation instructions, nutrition information, grading symbols, recipes, code dating for shelf life, universal product code and other defined symbols.

The F.D.A. may also regulate product description if the product is called something misleading or confusing. Surimi is a prime example because the consumer does not know what the description means. The F.D.A. also insists that the common names of fish originate from the zoological name of their species (For more information see Names).

The net weight, volume or count of a product (excluding the weight of the box, can or jar) must be included on the label in bold face or some other noticeable type. Net weight includes the liquid in which the food is packed. Terms that may exaggerate the amount of product (such as "full" gallon or "jumbo" quart) are not allowed.

The name of the country of origin of imported product is required on all labels by the U.S. Customs Service. Fish imported from country "A" must indicate that it is produced in that country. The same rule applies to electronic equipment or anything that comes from overseas. Imported product that is processed in the U.S.A. becomes domestic product if it undergoes a substantial transformation. For many years, the National Marine Fisheries Service was advising its inspection service clients that peeling and deveining imported shrimp was sufficient change in the product to justify its domestication. Customs has decided that in fact peeling and deveining is not sufficient and that such product must continue to be labelled with its country of origin.

At this time, it is not entirely clear how much processing is necessary for a seafood to be substantially transformed. If in doubt, consult the proper experts.

This is only a brief summary: labelling regulations are detailed and complex. It pays to consult experts. For a summary of rules on nutrition claims on labels, see Nutrition and labelling.

LABORATORY TESTS: See A.O.A.C.

LACEY ACT: Laws which make it a Federal felony to break any state, Indian tribal or foreign law relating to taking, possessing, transporting, trading or selling any fish. Shipping fish into a state which bans the species is an offence under the Lacey Act. So is buying fish from a foreign country knowing that the fish was taken in violation of conservation laws. The Lacey Act is comprehensive and tough. Copies are available from U.S. Fish and Wildlife Service or National Marine Fisheries Service.

LADYFISH *Scientific name: Elops saurus:* Tarpon. A soft, bony fish prized by game fishermen (who sometimes call it tenpounder). Dressed fish are sometimes sold commercially in California and may be labelled skipjack.

LAKE HERRING: See Cisco.

LAKE PERCH *Scientific name: Perca flavescens:* A small northern freshwater fish widely available frozen. It is also called yellow perch, striped perch, jack perch and many other names that are not approved for trading. It is usually pan-fried. Fillets, skin-on, I.Q.F., are a popular item throughout the mid-west. The available supply is limited since most of the fish caught are too small to fillet. Ocean perch and west coast rockfish are frequently used as substitutes. Perch has a distinctive reddish skin, as do the products that are substituted for it.

LAKE WHITEFISH: See Whitefish.

LANGOSTINOS *Scientific name: Cervimunida johni:* Squat lobster. The other, very similar, commercial species is *Pleuroncodes monodon*. Both are fished off Chile in large quantities. A related species, *Pleuroncodes planipes*, is found from Baja California southwards through Central America. Although the name langostino is specific enough for this product in the U.S.A. it can be a source of much confusion with overseas suppliers. Langostino means shrimp in Spanish. In some countries it is the official name for particular species of shrimp.

The product widely known and marketed in the U.S.A. as langostino is the cooked and peeled tail meat of these small crustaceans which are between shrimp and small lobster in appearance. Large quantities are imported from Chile and parts of Central America. The frozen product is a tasteless, soft-textured item, usable mainly as a substitute for lobster meat in recipes that contain more strongly flavored ingredients, such as salads for sandwiches where the mayonnaise and vegetables mask the lack of flavor of the langostino.

Langostinos are usually packed in 12 ounce bars, polywrapped and then put into printed cartons for retail sale. Retail business on this item used to be huge when the product was cheap. Usual mastering is one dozen bars in a box, four boxes per carton, expressed as 4/12/12oz. To overcome poor plant hygiene and F.D.A. rejections, most langostinos are pasteurized to destroy bacteria. This process requires a thinner bar, so pasteurized langos have two 6oz bars wrapped as a 12oz, giving the complicated packing description of 4/12/twin 6oz.

I.Q.F. langos are also available packed in 6/5lbs bulk for institutional use and 8oz and 16oz retail bags. I.Q.F. lango prices are usually quoted per pound, while the bars are frequently quoted per 12oz bar. Make sure the price structure is clear when you buy or sell this item. Also check whether the bars are in printed cartons, or in polywraps without cartons. Preferences vary.

The Chilean langostino is regarded as the market leader. Generally those from other origins sell at a substantially lower price, since the flavor and texture are thought to be inferior. It is worth trying these products and making your own judgement.

LANGOUSTINE: Not to be confused with langostino, this is the French name for *Nephrops spp*. See Lobsterette.

LATIN NAMES: See Scientific names.

LAYER PACK: See Packing styles.

L/C: See Letter of credit.

LEAN FISH: Species where most of the fat is contained in the liver rather than in the muscle. Cod, flounder, sole and pollock are lean fish. For more information, see Health and nutrition.

LEGS AND CLAWS: King crab product. See Crabs.

LEMON SOLE: In the U.S. this name is given to blackback flounder over 3½lbs. In Europe it is a different flatfish, *Microstomus kitt*. Frozen Japanese lemon sole is sometimes available, I.Q.F. packed 1/25lbs. This is neither of the lemon soles. See Flatfish.

LETTER OF CREDIT: A banking document allowing a supplier to exchange documentary evidence of shipment for his payment. A bank is usually designated to handle the transfer and ensure documents are in order. Letters of credit make international trade possible and are also used domestically, especially where large sums are involved.

The buyer instructs his bank to pay the seller when the seller gives the bank certain specified documents. These include a commercial invoice and proof that the goods have been shipped into control of the buyer – a warehouse transfer or a Bill of Lading from a trucker or ship, for example. Documents may also include inspection service reports to prove that the goods are actually those ordered and any papers needed in handling the goods, such as Certificates of Origin in international trade. When the seller ships the goods, he is then able to assemble all the documents, present them to the bank and receive payment because the bank has already made sure that it has the money available from the buyer (under a "confirmed" L/C).

By this system, the buyer knows that the goods are correct and available to him; and the seller knows that he will be paid by a bank, not by a fish buyer, when he ships according to the contract. Both sides are protected and the bank takes a small fee. It is a thoroughly developed, tested and effective commercial tool and could be much more utilized in the domestic seafood business.

LING *Scientific name: Molva molva:* A North Atlantic relative of the cod, often used for salting. It is a large fish with firm, sweet flesh, but not very common. Frozen fillets are packed in cellos and layer packs. The fish is sometimes substituted for ocean catfish.

Kingklip (cusk-eel) is called ling in New Zealand. Cobia is sometimes incorrectly called ling.

LINGCOD *Scientific name: Ophiodon elongatus:* A Pacific greenling, neither a cod nor a ling, with fairly soft flesh which may sometimes have a naturally greenish tint. This is normal and cooks out, but deters some buyers.

Skinless I.Q.F fillets are usually packed in 10lb or 25lb boxes and may or may not be graded. Boneless fillets are also available at extra expense. Lingcod is an adequate cheap fillet favored for fish and chip meals in the Pacific northwest but must not be confused with either cod or ling, as it is definitely neither, and resembles neither.

Frozen-at-sea lingcod, headless and dressed, is sometimes available from Alaska. Lingcod steaks are sometimes substituted for halibut steaks. The skin is spotted, whereas halibut has white skin on one side and black skin on the other. The appearance of the skin is an easy way to distinguish the two fish.

Lingcod meat cooks up white and mild. It will stand up to most cooking methods. The large pinbones in the fillets are best removed with pliers by the end-user.

LISTERIA: A common, food-borne bacteria, *Listeria monocytogenes*, once thought to be restricted to dairy products. It causes listeriosis, which is a fairly dangerous form of food poisoning. Some seafoods may be affected by it. Keeping processing areas clean and sanitized and separating raw from cooked product help greatly to reduce the risks of listeria contamination. Although it is destroyed by heat, the bug can survive freezer temperatures. There is particular cause for concern with cooked product since this is often not fully heated before it is eaten. Health officials are extremely concerned about listeria, which seems to be spreading rapidly.

LITTLENECK: Small hard clam. See Clams.

LOBSTER: This section covers lobsters, spiny or rock lobsters and slipper lobsters. For lobsterettes (*Nephrops spp.*) see Lobsterette. For squat lobsters see Langostino. For freshwater crayfish (crawfish) see Crayfish.
Lobster *Scientific name: Homarus americanus:* Also called Maine lobster, Canadian lobster and American lobster. This is the true lobster, with two large claws.

Genuine lobster is the animal with two claws which is found only in the North Atlantic. The species *Homarus americanus* is caught from Labrador south to Maryland. The virtually identical species *Homarus gammarus* lives on the eastern side of the north Atlantic from Norway south to Portugal. These are the only animals that should be called lobster. In some New England states, the description of anything else as lobster is illegal.

Nearly all lobsters are sold live. Frozen lobsters are available and are a second-rate substitute in taste and texture. Lobster is one of the few seafoods that does not freeze well. The flavor deteriorates and the flesh toughens in the freezing process. Freezing lobster in the shell also makes the animal brittle, so that claws and legs fall off. However, a live lobster, cooked and immediately brine frozen, then packed in a sealed plastic "bubble" with water to keep it moist can be an acceptable product. Alternative packing, using parchment or polywraps, or polystyrene tubes, does not protect the lobster as well so breakage is high and shelf life short.

"Bubble" packs are so far the best way of utilizing lobsters in frozen form. They and other frozen whole cooked lobsters are usually graded the same way as live lobsters:

Chix or chickens	1lb or less
Eighths	over 1lb to 1lb 2oz
Quarters	over 1lb 2oz to 1lb 4oz
X-halves	over 1lb 4 oz to 1lb 6oz
Halves	over 1lb 6oz to 1lb 8oz
Three quarters	over 1½ to 1lb 12oz
Deuces	over 1lb 12oz to 2 lb
2½lb	over 2 to 2½lb
2-3lb	over 2 to 3lb
3-4lb	over 3 to 4lb
Jumbos	4lb and up

Quarters to deuces are known as selects. Jumbos are seldom frozen, except for special order for buffet display or similar use. Lobsters up to 30lb used to be available, but the number of lobsters over three pounds is small now.

Lobsters with one claw are called culls and are usually graded as chicken, select and large culls. Minimum sizes for lobsters are based on the length of the carapace of the body and not on the weight. Minimum sizes are increasing on the following schedule:

1/1/83	3³⁄₁₆inch
1/1/88	3⁷⁄₃₂inch
1/1/89	3¼inch
1/1/90	escape vent size to be compatible with a minimum carapace length of 3⁵⁄₁₆inch. (Escape vent must be large enough to allow lobsters 3⁵⁄₁₆ and smaller to escape.)
1/1/91	3⁹⁄₃₂inch
1/1/92	3⁵⁄₁₆inch

Lobster meat is produced in Canada. It is cooked, picked, packed into cans and frozen without heat-treating. This process is called cold-canning. This product comes only from Canada and is not made in the U.S.A. because the conservation laws differ.

In the U.S. conservation of lobster resources depends on regulating the minimum size of lobster that may be taken, so that the animals are permitted to grow to breeding size before capture. Any undersize lobsters caught must be put back in the sea alive. In Canada, conservation has taken the approach of limiting seasons in fishing areas, so that although during the season any size lobster may be fished, the seasons are short and sufficient breeding stock is left in the water. Whatever the relative merits may be, the effect of the Canadian rules is that large quantities of small lobsters are landed in Canada and these cannot be exported to the main markets in the U.S.A. and Europe because of minimum size rules.

The Canadians therefore cook the small lobsters, known as "canners" and pick the meat for cold canning as described above. Freezing instead of autoclaving the cans retards bacteria growth without spoiling the texture of the meat.

The cans are mostly color lithographed and come in three sizes:

- 11.3 ounces, sold on a price per can basis, packed 12 or 24 per case. The size used to be sold as 12 ounces and is still generally known as 12oz can, but weights and measures rules have required greater honesty in the labelling, which is now 11.3oz.
- 2lb cans, 6 or 12 per case, sold on a per pound basis.
- 5lb cans, 6 per case, sold on a per pound basis.

Five different grades of meat are packed:

Tail and claw (T & C) meat is the most expensive, and the highest quality pack. This contains only meat from the tails and claws of the lobster. All pieces should be unbroken.

Tail, knuckle and claw (TCK) meat additionally contains meat from the knuckles, that is the joints between the claw and the body.

Regular meat contains claw, tail and body meat in natural proportions as it comes from the lobster. Tails should be whole, but may be slightly broken. Regular meat is the bulk of the pack and is entirely satisfactory for most uses.

New Hampshire pack is regular meat made from larger lobsters (lobsters that are over the minimum size required for live lobsters in the U.S.A.). This pack is seldom seen now.

Broken meat is usually the cheapest. It is sometimes made from jumbo lobsters, which are difficult to ship alive. Broken jumbo meat is an excellent buy, since it contains large pieces and very few shreds.

Lobster meat naturally varies greatly in texture and taste according to the moulting stage of the lobster. It is produced all along the immense coastlines of the Atlantic Provinces, sometimes in large modern factories, but more often in small seasonal packing sheds and even in fishermen's kitchens.

It is therefore inevitable that quality should vary and brands are inconsistent. Mostly the product is good, but for those times when it is not, protect yourself by purchasing from major label packers, their U.S. brokers, or from major distributors. Production seasons are short, and speculation is customary, but you must have a supplier capable of replacing inferior product. A single shipment with the same label on the cans may have originated in a number of different packing places, so sampling your shipment is not always an adequate precaution.

A few lobster tails, usually cooked, are frozen and may be available from time to time. Like whole frozen lobsters, they also are a poor product compared to fresh, live lobster.

Spiny lobster or Rock lobster: Mostly sold as frozen lobster tails, there is a wide variety of species from most of the world's marine coastal waters. For full information on the major commercial species, how to identify them and much more, see *Lobsters of the World, an Illustrated Guide* by Austin B. Williams published in 1988 by Osprey Books.

The terms spiny lobster and rock lobster are interchangeable. We have been unable to find any consistent distinction between the two terms. Some people prefer one, some the other.

In market terms, there are two distinct types of spiny lobster tails; cold water and warm water. Even so, the distinction is partly one of perception. The temperature of the water in which the various species live is less important than the market's ideas of the climate of the supplying countries. Scientists generally avoid defining lobsters in these two categories only, preferring to classify the animals in three groups: tropical, subtropical and temperate. Tropical lobsters are warmwater and temperate lobsters are cold water. The subtropical ones may be in the market as either. The following table lists the more common species in these three categories. This table also shows which species come from the major supplying regions.

All lobster tails should show clean white meat at the end which is broken from the body. This meat should be well glazed for protection. Most producers also remove the vein (digestive tract). The shell should be lightly glazed overall. Each tail should be well wrapped or polybagged for protection. Size grading varies but is obviously vital for such expensive items.

Cold water tails are the more expensive. Most used to be imported into the U.S.A. from South Africa, but this product was banned as part of trade sanctions against South Africa. New Zealand and Australia are currently the most important suppliers. Cold water tails are good, firm, tasty product. The major origins pack carefully and well. There are minor differences in appearance and taste between the different tails, but all offer a superior product and consistency. South African tails, not cur-

Common species of spiny lobsters, their areas of significant fishery, and approximate catch

in millions of pounds, 1976 (adapted from Morgan, 1980).

Species	Areas of significant fishery	Catch
Tropical		
Panulirus argus	Florida, Bahamas, Caribbean, Brazil	50.25
Panulirus echinatus	None	
Panulirus gracilis	Ecuador, Panama	0.60
Panulirus guttatus	None	
Panulirus homarus[1]	East Africa, Indonesia	0.88
Panulirus laevicauda	Brazil	6.61
Panulirus longipes[2]	None	
Panulirus ornatus	New Guinea, East Africa	1.19
Panulirus penicillatus	Reunion, Pacific Islands, Galapagos	0.88
Panulirus polyphagus	Pakistan, India, Southeast Asia	8.16
Panulirus regius	West Africa	0.99
Panulirus versicolor	None	
Subtotal		69.58
Subtropical		
Jasus verreauxi	Eastern Australia, New Zealand	0.28
Palinurus charlestoni	Cape Verde Islands	0.01
Palinurus delagoae	Southeast Africa	0.13
Palinurus mauritanicus	Mauritania, West Africa	0.33
Panulirus cygnus	Western Australia	19.62
Panulirus inflatus	West Mexico, Guatemala	3.31
Panulirus interruptus	California	0.27
Panulirus japonicus	Japan, South China Sea	2.65
Panulirus marginatus	Hawaii	0.02
Panulirus pascuensis	Easter Island	0.01
Panulirus stimpsoni	Hong Kong	0.02
Subtotal		26.65
Temperate		
Jasus edwardsii	New Zealand	8.16
Jasus frontalis	Juan Fernandez Island	0.11
Jasus lalandii	Southwest Africa	13.67
Jasus novaehollandiae	South and southeast Australia	7.72
Jasus paulensis	St. Paul and New Amsterdam Islands	1.98
Jasus tristani	Tristan da Cunha	0.01
Palinurus elephas	U.K., France, Spain, Italy	3.31
Palinurus gilchristi	South Africa	2.14
Subtotal		37.10
World total		133.33

[1] Three subspecies.

[2] Two subspecies.

rently available in the U.S., are size-graded by letter grades. See the next table for details.

Code	Ounces
K	2
KZ	2½
M	3½
J	4 to 4½
H	4½ to 5½
G	5½ to 6½
F	6½ to 7½
E	7½ to to 8
D	8 to 9
C	9½ to 11
B	11½ to 12
A	12 to 16
AA	16 to 20
AAA	20 to 40

These grades are used by some other origins so are still relevant in the marketplace.

Australian and New Zealand packers sometimes use letter codes for size designations, but the grading varies from packer to packer and it is preferable to use gradings in ounces. Grades may be in one ounce or two ounce steps, or straight sizes, like those used for Brazil tails (see below). Australian and New Zealand tails are normally packed in 20lb or 25lb boxes, though occasionally a metric pack of 10kg will appear. These were intended for the Japanese market when packed. Because of the various packs, it is especially advisable to check weights before accepting shipments. A few cold water tails are offered from unusual origins, such as France or Spain. Although cold water tails are harvested in these places, the quantities are small and the local markets strong. It is important to examine any such offered product in case it is something masquerading as an expensive cold water tail.

Warm water tails are cheaper and generally less tasty and consistent. They come from a wider range of sources. Brazil and domestic packers in Florida supply the major quantities. Many warm water tails also come from the Bahamas, where the resource is shared with Florida fishermen and from many parts of the Caribbean including Cuba and Nicaragua, although imports from these two countries are not permitted. Most Central American countries supply some lobster tails. Quantities also come from Asia, especially from India and the Arabian Gulf.

Florida tails are usually packed 4/10lb and graded in 2 ounce steps from 4/6 through 10/12, larger sizes are graded in 4oz steps. Brazil grading is in straight sizes from 3oz to 14oz and this portion control grading has given the Brazilian packers an important edge in the market: because the buyer knows how many tails he will get in every box, he can plan and control more effectively. Brazil tails are always packed 4/10lbs and size definitions are based on counts per 10lb box as follows:

Size (ounces)	Count per 10lb box
3	over 50
3X	50
3XX	38-45
4	40
5	32
6	27
7	23
8	20
9	18
10	16
11	15
12	13
13	12
14	11

To clarify, 3oz Brazil tails are under 3 ounces; 3X tails are about 3¼oz; 3XX are about 3½oz; all sizes are graded by eye to look similar – these gradings do not imply that every tail in a box is identical in weight. Honduran tails are graded similarly to Brazilian without 3X and 3XX sizes. Indian tails are sometimes packed in one ounce steps. Otherwise, most warm water tails are packed like Florida tails in two ounce gradings and 4/10lb cartons.

Most buyers have firm opinions about the differences in tails, and about which they prefer. Many believe that Indian tails have too much sand in the vein and are too dark in color; however, Indian tails are frequently repacked and passed off as Florida tails, so the distinction is clearly not that great in practice.

Some of the most blatant cheating in seafoods applies to lobster tails. Less expensive species may be repacked as cold water tails, for example. Indian tails, which are comparatively cheap, may be repacked as Florida tails. As mentioned earlier, *Lobsters of the World – An Illustrated Guide* provides the information for you to determine the species from the tail alone. The knowledge can protect against substantial losses.

Apart from repacking tails from one source as those from another and more highly valued source, glazing is a popular activity in the lobster tail business. It is a practice which seems to be accepted by those most at risk: the restaurant buyers. Tails are glazed in order to sell less weight of product for the same money and also to increase the nominal size of a tail to a size that is generally more expensive.

Glazing may be done in two ways. The obvious way is to dip the tail in cold water and refreeze it until it has the required weight. It is possible to add considerable weight in this way, especially if the process is repeated. The more sophisticated method is to inject icy cold water between the shell and the meat and freeze it there, where it is not detectable until the tail defrosts. Glaze up to 30 percent is not uncommon and 20 percent is "normal" in some markets.

A simple technique for detecting under-shell glaze is being developed in California, based on certain size relationships of the tails. If the method proves to be accurate as well as simple it will be a great asset to all buyers and users of lobster tails. For information on valid defrosting techniques, see Defrosting methods.

One further lobster tail scam is to remove one or two tails from each ten-pound box. It is surprisingly easy to do this and still leave the box looking complete. The only defense is to check carefully, weigh the tails and defrost some to check the glaze. Always take extra care with any boxes that seem to have been opened, restrapped, cut, or look so good that they probably never suffered the knocks of shipping from overseas destinations.

Whichever way it is done, excessive glaze means that you are buying water instead of lobster – not a good bargain. The rationale seems to be that if the competition is doing it, then the only way to compete is to copy. If the competition is advertising an eight ounce tail at a price that demonstrates the use of heavily glazed product which would thaw out to, say, 6½oz each, then the only way to match the price is to offer the same bad deal to the customer. This thinking assumes that the consumer is unaware of what he is getting and is surely wrong. The consumer may not know what is wrong with the deal, but consumers have a well developed sense for bad value for money. In the long run, the widespread use of dishonest weights and sizes will simply nudge the consumer towards steak or other alternative foods.

It is unfortunate that enforcement of honest weights is sparse – buyers who deliberately use glazed tails often rely on this. But there are also many buyers who do not appreciate that they are being sold glaze instead of lobster – it is absolutely essential that you check the thawed weights of every shipment of tails you receive, no matter what boxes they are in. For information on general seafood scams, see Economic fraud in the seafood business.

Spiny/rock lobsters are sometimes sold whole frozen, individually wrapped in 25lb boxes. This product is usually cooked before being frozen. Spiny lobsters stand freezing better than true lobsters and this product can be very good.

Lobster tail meat: Peeled spiny lobster tails. Rock lobster tail meat is packed in small quantities, often as a way of handling inferior product. Taiwan, Hong Kong and similar Asian origins are the usual sources.

A high quality lobster tail meat comes from Japan and the east coast of China and is known as red rock meat (species is mainly *Linuparus trigonus*). This has a particularly deep color, both in the shell and when peeled and is favored by Chinese restaurant buyers and others. The meat is usually graded in 2oz steps and packed 10/5lbs. It is prone to black spot (melanosis) and should be carefully inspected.

Slipper lobsters: Also called flat, locust, Spanish, shovel-nosed and bulldozer. Australians call some of them "bugs." These species are distributed through many of the world's warmer coastal waters, but nowhere in large quantities. They are distinctly different from spiny lobsters and are always worth much less. The major commercial species is probably *Thenus orientalis*, which is found from northern Australia throughout southeast and southern Asia, around the east coast of Africa and into the eastern half of the Mediterranean. Harvested mainly in Asia, the tails are small and tasteless. Sales depend a great deal on the name "lobster" which is attached to them.

Slipper tails are sold with shell, or as peeled and deveined meats. Both products are usually size graded under-1oz, 1/2oz, 2/3oz (or 1/3oz), 2/4oz and 4/6oz. Normal packing is 24/1lb bags for small tails and retail sale, 5lb bags and 10lb boxes for institutional use. Hawaii produces a very large slipper lobster, with tails as large as 20 ounces.

Slipper lobster products are not renowned for high quality and need to be checked carefully each time.

LOBSTERETTE: *Scientific names: Nephrops spp.* and *Metanephrops spp.* Also called scampi, Dublin Bay prawn, Norway lobster, langoustine, baby lobster, dainty tails, lobster dainties, Aden tails and Somali tails.

The "original" seafood is *Nephrops norvegicus*, which is the Mediterranean scampi, the French langoustine and the British Dublin Bay prawn. This is a relative of the true (clawed) lobster (see Lobsters). In the U.S.A. "scampi" usually refers to shrimp cooked in butter and garlic, but in their native Italy, these animals rightly hold that name for themselves, not for the recipe.

The species is found from Iceland and western Norway to Morocco, and in the western and central Mediterranean, including the Adriatic.

Whole tails are usually carefully graded by count (7/9, 9/12, 12/15, 15/18, 18/24 per lb) packed in 2kg boxes and heavily glazed for protection. There is little standardization in the size grading or the pack size, however. Peeled meats are available I.Q.F. or breaded, but this product, while very popular in the United Kingdom, has never caught on here. When available, it is usually described as scampi meat.

There are other, very similar, species, such as *Nephrops andamanicus*, which is found off southeastern Africa, in the East Indies and Andaman Sea and also off northern Australia. There are two species, *Metanephrops binghami* and *Metanephrops rubellus* which are found in the western Atlantic. The first of these ranges from Florida, through the Gulf to northern Brazil. The second is found off central and southern Brazil. New Zealand and Australia have *Metanephrops challengeri*, which is a close relative.

There are similar animals, which look much like Nephrops. Aden and Somalia ship a rather dark colored tail with sharp points on the underside of the shell. India exports a similarly shaped tail, but the color is closer to that of scampi. Some Indian packers clip the points to improve the acceptability. These are packed in 5lb blocks just like shrimp. All of these tails are good to eat, although perhaps less good than genuine Norway lobster. Importers might be more successful selling tails for their own qualities instead of for substitutes.

There is no reason not to use deep sea tails, so long as you and your customers know which product is being shipped.

Canadian demand for lobsterette tails is much stronger than U.S. demand. Much of the product imported into the U.S.A. is reshipped to Canadian customers.

LOLIGO: See Squid.

LOTTE: French name for monkfish.

LOX: Smoked salmon. The name comes from the German word for salmon, "Lachse" (or from the similar Scandinavian "Laks") and is used for lightly salted and smoked salmon. Lox originally meant salted salmon.

LUMPFISH *Scientific name: Cyclopterus lumpus:* Also called lump sucker and henfish. The North Atlantic species is eaten smoked in Scandinavia and the U.S.S.R. The unfertilized eggs are colored and salted and used as a substitute for caviar. This product is available in the U.S.A.

The North Pacific (Bering Sea) lumpfish is caught by Japanese vessels. Neither this nor the Atlantic lumpfish is used in the U.S.A. The fish lives in far northern waters and is caught mainly for its eggs. If meat is offered, make sure it does not come from a ripe or spent female fish.

LUMP MEAT: The two large pieces of body meat from the blue crab's back fin. See Crabs.

MACKEREL: Fish of the mackerel family are listed in the following table.

Atlantic Mackerel *Scientific name: Scomber scombrus:* Mackerel is a small oily fish growing to about 2lbs and found in large shoals. It is sometimes called Boston mackerel. It has a distinctive brightly colored skin with blue, silver and green flashes. Mackerel is not highly regarded as a food fish in the U.S.A. although salted mackerel was once an important item of trade for New England. The flesh is brownish, cooking up to a creamy color. Much of the catch is now frozen whole and packed into 25lb and 50lb blocks for bait and for animal food.

For human consumption, I.Q.F. whole or headless dressed mackerel, skin-on fillets in 10/5lb cellos and 10lb and 15lb layer packs are all available.

Mackerel is used for curing and smoking. Good quality fish with high oil content is required for these purposes. Mackerel turns rancid very quickly, therefore fast, clean handling of the fish is essential. Look for bright skins, bright eyes and undamaged fish especially undamaged belly walls. If the fish is gutted, look for belly burn. Look for the same qualities described under herring for fish that are cured.

Hot smoked mackerel can be very close in taste and texture to smoked trout and is gaining in popularity.

Pacific mackerel *Scientific name: Scomber japonicus:* Pacific mackerel is very similar to Atlantic mackerel although it is a little

Mackerel: Market Names and Common Names

Market name	Common name	Scientific name	Location
Bonito	Bonito, Atlantic	*Sarda sarda*	A
Bonito	Bonito, Pacific	*Sarda chiliensis*	P
Bonito	Bonito, striped	*Sarda orientalis (& S. velox)*	A-P
Mackerel	Cero	*Scomberomorus regalis*	A
Mackerel	Mackerel, Atlantic	*Scomber scombrus*	A
Mackerel	Mackerel, Indian	*Rastrelliger kanagurta*	P
Mackerel	Mackerel, Spanish	*Scomberomorus maculatus*	A
Mackerel	Mackerel, Spanish	*Scomberomorus tritor*	A
Mackerel	Mackerel, chub	*Scomber japonicus*	A-P
Mackerel	Mackerel, double-lined	*Grammatorcynus bicaneatus*	P
Mackerel	Mackerel, frigate	*Auxis thazard*	A-P
Mackerel	Mackerel, narrow-barred	*Scomberomorus commerson*	P
Mackerel	Sierra, Pacific	*Scomberomorus sierra*	P
Mackerel	Sierra, gulf	*Scomberomorus concolor*	P
Mackerel chub	Mackerel, spotted chub	*Scomber australasicus*	P
Mackerel king	Mackerel, king	*Scomberomorus cavalla*	A
Tuna	Albacore	*Thunnus alalunga*	A-P
Tuna	Kawakawa	*Euthynnus affinis*	P
Tuna	Skipjack, black	*Euthynnus lineatus*	P
Tuna	Tuna, bigeye	*Thunnus obesus*	A-P
Tuna	Tuna, blackfin	*Thunnus atlanticus*	A
Tuna	Tuna, bluefin	*Thunnus thynnus*	A-P
Tuna	Tuna, bullet	*Auxis rochei*	A-P
Tuna	Tuna, longtail	*Thunnus tonggol*	P
Tuna	Tuna, skipjack	*Euthynnus pelamis*	A-P
Tuna	Tuna, southern bluefin	*Thunnus maccoyii*	A-P
Tuna	Tuna, yellowfin	*Thunnus albacares*	A-P
Tuna	Tunny, little	*Euthynnus alletteratus*	A
Wahoo	Wahoo	*Acanthocybium solanderi*	A-P

Locations: A = Atlantic   P = Indo-Pacific   F = Freshwater
Source: F.D.A.

smaller and may have a lower oil content. It is a large and potentially important resource found mostly as canned product. The species is found in the Atlantic also, where it is generally known as chub mackerel.

Jack mackerel *Scientific name: Trachurus symmetricus:* Also called scad. Technically, this fish is a jack, not a mackerel. It is an important Pacific species, growing to about one pound and used mainly for canning. It looks much like a Pacific mackerel and is used like it. Jack mackerel are highly regarded for swordfish bait. Horse mackerel, *Trachurus trachurus*, is a similar Atlantic species.

Spanish mackerel and frigate mackerel are covered in separate entries in this book. Atka mackerel is a greenling, not a mackerel. See Atka mackerel for more details.

MAHI-MAHI *Scientific name: Coryphaena hippurus:* Also legally called dolphin-fish. Smart marketers avoid the name. Mahi-mahi, the Hawaiian name, is legal, well-known and easy to sell. The Spanish name is dorado. This is not the mammal porpoise or dolphin, but a large (up to six feet) colorful fish unfortunately named dolphin and found in most of the world's oceans. It is common around Hawaii and is a popular sport fish off both the Atlantic and Pacific coasts. The fish is found throughout tropical and subtropical oceans. It is imported as frozen fillets from South and Central America, Taiwan, Japan and other countries.

Fillets are always packed with the colorful skin on, partly because the skin is attractive and partly because without the skin the fish falls apart when cooked. Usual size grading is in pound steps, 1/2, 2/3, 3/4, 4/5 and 5lbs up, with fillets over 4lbs preferred in most markets. Asian packers may grade in 2lb increments. Fillets should be I.Q.F., individually wrapped. They are usually packed in 50lb boxes. Fillets are sometimes cut and sold as portions. Bellies should be trimmed to remove the oily strip at the bottom. Fish that is bled on capture has lighter flesh and better shelf life. Japanese product is usually frozen at sea and commands the highest prices for frozen product. Other origins are generally frozen on shore.

Mahi is excellent eating, with firm and well flavored flesh. When cooked, the meat is white with a large flake. Mahi is often found on cold buffets, Polynesian style and sells best in Hawaii,

California and Florida, as well as in parts of the mid-west. It is a comparatively cheap fillet and makes an attractive serving.

Yellowtail is occasionally substituted for mahi.

The one major problem with mahi is the possible presence of histamines in the flesh. Histamines cause severe food poisoning. They are difficult to detect because presence is far from uniform in batches of the fish. See Histamines and Seafood safety for full details.

MAINE LOBSTER: Canadian lobster; see Lobster.

MAKO: See Sharks.

MARINATED SALMON: See Gravlax.

MARKET NEW REPORTS: See Green Sheet.

MARRIED FILLETS: The two fillets from one fish frozen together, skin sides out, giving the appearance of a whole fish but without the bones. This technique is usually applied to flounder or sole. It is mainly used for very small fillets to give thicker meat for breading, or to make an attractively shaped product for serving.

MASU *Scientific name: Oncorhynchus masou:* Cherry salmon. A species of Pacific salmon found only on Asian coasts. It is not known or marketed in the U.S.A.

MELANOSIS: Also called black spot. Blackening of the shell in crustacea, especially shrimp and some crabs. Glands secreting the pigment melanin are present in the skin-like membrane beneath the shell of some crustacea. In time, the melanin causes spots and patches of blackening on the shell, which though harmless is aesthetically unpleasing.

Melanosis occurs particularly fast on the heads of whole shrimp, which is not much of a problem in the U.S.A. since shrimp with heads on is seldom used. Melanosis occurs also on the tails of shrimp and on crab. It is not prevented by freezing. It does not affect the eating quality of the meat, but severe cases can blacken parts of the meat also.

Melanosis always appears in time, but it happens much more quickly if product is not promptly handled before freezing. It is an indication either that product is old, or that it was not well processed in the first place. It is therefore a valid ground for refusing product.

Melanosis can be slowed or prevented by the use of acidic dips, most of which are not permitted for use in the U.S.A.

MENHADEN *Scientific name: Brevoortia tyrannus:* Also called pogy. A small Atlantic and Gulf herring-like fish of great economic importance for fish meal and oil. It is not regarded as edible, being very oily and bony. There are several similar species. Menhaden supports the largest volume in U.S.A. fishery.

The possibilities of using menhaden for surimi are under investigation.

MERCURY: A heavy metal occurring naturally in some seafood. It tends to accumulate and so is higher in creatures such as tuna and swordfish which live a long time.

The F.D.A. monitors imports and interstate shipments of items known for high mercury content. Some states also watch for mercury. The current F.D.A. standard permitting up to one part per million of mercury is about in line with most of the world. Higher levels are only likely in very large fish, such as swordfish weighing over 150lbs.

The problem of mercury in seafoods has been grossly overstated in the past. See also Seafood safety.

MERUS: The section of the leg of a king, snow or Dungeness crab which is closest to the shoulder. It is the largest and thickest segment and contains the choicest meat. See Crabs.

METRIC WEIGHTS AND MEASURES: The metric system is unfortunately spreading to the U.S.A. and increasing amounts of product packed in metric quantities are being imported. The basic unit of weight is the kilo, which is 2.2046lbs and is usually traded in the U.S.A. as 2.2lbs. A 2kg block of product therefore weighs 4.4lbs.

It is not uncommon for distributors to sell 2kg blocks of shrimp as 5lb blocks, giving themselves an additional 12 percent profit.

Since shrimp has to be heavily glazed for protection and since many 2kg packs are the same external dimensions as 5lb packs, it is impossible to tell by eye whether you are being cheated in this way. Insist on product in original packing, inspect boxes for signs of altered markings and check net weights. When you check, report the results to your supplier, who will be more careful if he knows that you check. The importance of this for high priced product cannot be overstated. At $6/lb, if you receive one case of 10/2kg (44lbs) instead of 10/5lb (50lbs), you are paying $36 for product that is not there. You also make yourself vulnerable to claims or prosecution for short weight sales if you pass along these packs, even in good faith, to your own customers. Know which origins pack in kilos, check your purchases and remain at all times vigilant for signs of cheating.

Approximate equivalent counts	
per lb	per kg
2	4.4
4	8.8
5	11
6	13
7	15.5
10	22
12	26.5
15	33
16	35
20	44
21	46
25	55
30	66
35	77
40	90
50	110
60	132
70	154
90	198
100	220
130	285
200	440

MILKFISH *Scientific name: Chanos chanos:* A large pink-fleshed fish widely used in south-east Asia where it has been farmed for centuries. Small quantities are also farmed in Hawaii. Frozen whole milkfish is available from specialist importers. The flesh is rather soft.

MILT: Male gonads. Sometimes called "soft roes." Herring milts are an important item in Europe and the milts of striped mullet are highly regarded in east Asia. Milts of other species are not much utilized anywhere else.

MOLLUSC: Frequently spelled mollusk. Shellfish are either molluscs or crustaceans. The shells are the equivalent of the skeletons in mammals and fish, so shellfish have no bones in the meat. The biological definition of a mollusc is too complex to be helpful in everyday use. Commonly eaten molluscs include clams, oysters, conch, whelks, scallops, abalone, mussels and snails. Squid, octopus and sepia are all molluscs and in these animals the shell is a piece of cartilage inside rather than a shell on the outside.

There are three groups of molluscs:

Bivalves have two shells that close around the animal. Clams, oysters and scallops are examples of bivalves.

Univalves have a single shell and the animal lives inside it. Snails and abalone are univalves.

Cephalopods, the word indicating feet growing out of the head, include octopus, cuttlefish and squid.

MONKFISH *Scientific names: Lophius americanus* (Atlantic) and *Lophius piscatorius* (Pacific). Also known as anglerfish, goosefish, frogfish, ocean blowfish, sea devil and bellyfish. F.D.A. seems willing to accept only monkfish and goosefish. The French name, lotte, is frequently used on menus. A large deep sea fish, reaching four feet in length and fifty pounds in weight. Only the tail section is used. The enormous head and the central belly section are discarded.

The tails provide good, white, meaty, firm flesh, versatile in use for a variety of fish recipes and as an extender for lobster and scallops. Monkfish tails are packed whole with skin, or skinless. Alternatively, fillets are prepared by cutting the skinless tail in half lengthwise and removing the central cartilage. Fillets are always totally boneless. Monkfish should be individually wrapped for protection.

Grading varies between different packers, but since the domestic market is small and monkfish is exported to Europe, grading tends to be in metric steps, such as under 1kg, 1/2kg and 2/4kg per piece.

There are similar species all over the world. It has been imported from New Zealand, for example, although the species there, *Kathetostoma giganteum*, is actually a totally different family. This species contains pinbones. The imported fish tends to be a darker color than domestic monkfish and less acceptable. However, it is generally substantially cheaper than domestic and is marketed on that basis.

Because of its firm, sweet flesh and the guaranteed absence of bones, monkfish is becoming more popular, especially in the mid-west. It is well worth examining the possibilities of using it. Although supplies are never abundant, it is usually obtainable most of the year, fresh or frozen.

MONOCLONAL ANTIBODIES: See Economic fraud in the seafood business.

MORWONG: See Painted sweet-lips and Tarakihi.

MULLET *Scientific name: Mugil cephalus:* Also called lisa and striped mullet. Outside Florida, lisa is not an approved name for this species. Although almost all of the U.S. catch comes from Florida, the species is found from North Carolina to Texas as well as off the Pacific coast. The same species is also found in Asia.

Frozen mullet is available whole, dressed, pan ready, or as fillets, usually packed in 25lb boxes. Frozen mullet has a short shelf life because of its high oil content. Most of the fish caught are about 1½lbs live weight, which is too small for economical filleting. The flavor is well liked by many, who describe it as "nutty" and disliked by some who think it tastes "muddy." It is an inexpensive fish and the large resource is capable of producing even larger quantities if markets develop. Users of frozen product should check for freshness because of the short storage life of this species.

Large quantities of mullet are processed for roe in the late fall and early winter. Either the roe or the fish containing it are exported to Taiwan and other Asian countries. The similar white mullet, *Mugil curema*, which ripens in the early spring, is also caught and processed for roe. Packers selling female fish for roe may offer male fish for bait and animal food.

There is a growing market for smoked mullet. The oiliness of the fish makes it a good raw material for smoking.

There are numerous other mullets available in the U.S.A. but these are not normally fished. The European mullet, one of the classic fishes of Mediterranean cuisine, is technically a goatfish. It is rather different from striped mullet.

Canadians sometimes call white sucker (*Catostomus commersoni*,) mullet. Although sucker is clearly a poor market name, the fish is a buffalofish related to catfish. It is totally unlike a mullet.

MUSKELLUNGE: See Pike.

MUSSEL *Scientific name: Mytilus edulis:* Also called blue mussel or common mussel. It is not spelled "mussell" – one "l" is sufficient. Mussels are abundant, nutritious, cheap bivalve molluscs which are underexploited in the U.S.A. The market is expanding.

Washed live mussels sell along the eastern seaboard and to a lesser extent along the Pacific coast. As market acceptance grows, a number of processors are offering a variety of frozen mussel products. Frozen mussels are imported from Ireland, Korea and other countries.

Among products currently available are I.Q.F. cooked mussel meats, usually in 5lb bags, sometimes also in 8oz or 1lb bags for retail sale. Cooked meats in block frozen packs are used by processors. Breaded mussels are sometimes used as a cheap constituent of fried platters. There is a wide variety of products based on mussels on the half shell with sauces or marinades. There is no standardization of packs.

Mussel meats should be plump. Color varies and is not significant. If shells are included they should be clean and free of barnacles, stones and other encrustations. Mussels are monitored under the Shellfish Sanitation Program.

Farmed mussels are increasingly important. They offer cleaner product since they are grown generally on ropes or stakes and so are clear of sea bottom mud. Farmed product tends to be more consistent in size and meat content than mussels harvested from the wild. Atlantic and Pacific coasts both offer cultured mussels. The prospects are good for greatly increasing supplies.

A larger and different species from New Zealand, *Perna canaliculus*, the green mussel or green-lipped mussel, has established itself in the U.S. market. Supplies should be augmented by increasing aquaculture of the species. This is a large mussel growing over five inches long and three ounces gross weight. It is offered in a variety of fresh and frozen packs and preparations, which are sold retail as well as in restaurants.

N-3: Alternative term for omega-3. See Health and nutrition.

NAMES: There are thousands of edible fish and shellfish species; perhaps as many as 500 are in regular use in the U.S.A. But most consumers (and quite a few people in the fish business, the restaurant business and in the retail fish trade) would be hard put to name more than a couple of dozen. Everyone knows shrimp, lobster, crab, flounder, sole, cod and salmon. Very few know painted sweet-lips, goosefish, hair crabs or arctic char.

Because so few of the varieties of fish and shellfish are known (and therefore trusted) by consumers, marketers often like to sell lesser-known species under the common English name of one that is familiar. Sometimes this is harmless. It really matters little whether you say "salmon" or "Atlantic salmon". But in other circumstances, it can be misleading and sometimes definitely fraudulent. Calling a pink-fleshed tilapia "red snapper" will fool the user into thinking that he is getting a well-known, well-liked and expensive fish. In fact, the tilapia is not often sold in the U.S.A. and is much less expensive than snapper.

The U.S. Food and Drug Administration (F.D.A.) is the agency responsible for determining and policing nomenclature of foodstuffs, including fish and shellfish. The National Marine Fisheries Service (N.M.F.S.) is obviously closely concerned, but it is the F.D.A. which has the final say and which makes the rules.

The book *A List of Common and Scientific Names of Fishes from the United States and Canada*, published by The American Fisheries Society (A.F.S.) is the prime source recognized by the F.D.A. and other Federal agencies for names of fish. This book gives only one common name for each scientific name. However, the book is not recognized everywhere as the source for common names. In California, for example, the Department of Fish and Game decides the common names for fish within its state borders (see Snapper for more information on this). The A.F.S. has a new publication *Common and Scientific Names of Aquatic Invertebrates from the United States and Canada: Mollusks* which presumably also will be authoritative.

The A.F.S. list covers only North American species. If it does not have the necessary information, the F.D.A. usually then refers to *Fishes of the World* (second edition) by Joseph S. Nelson, which covers fishes extensively, but not shellfish at all. After that, the next resource is *The Multilingual Dictionary of Fish and Fish Products* compiled by the Organization for Economic Cooperation and Development. This covers over 1,100 fish and shellfish species and products.

Nevertheless, there are still many items which are for sale in the U.S.A. with no common names given in any of these sources.

To confront and, hopefully, to solve this problem, N.M.F.S. and the F.D.A. together have drafted a document listing *Approved Market Names for Fish* or Fishlist for short. This covers over 1,000 fish species (a separate list is being started for molluscs and crustacea) and defines "market names" as well as common names. It is likely that both of these names will be accepted in interstate trade and other names will not be legal. The Fishlist is now being published for comments, before it becomes a regulation.

The problem in establishing acceptable common names in English for seafood items is that so many different names are given to the same species. There are a number of reasons, identified by the drafters of the FDA/NMFS document:

• Regional names given to the same species may differ. Striped bass in New York is called rockfish in Maryland.

• A small proportion of commercial sellers deliberately use the name of a more expensive variety in order to sell a lower-valued fish at a higher price by trading on the name of the more desirable one.

• The need to establish a name for underutilized or imported species which may carry names that would automatically deter consumers from trying them. The best-known example of this is the popular orange roughy, which might well have been called "slimehead" since it most closely resembles the Atlantic slimehead. It might never have become popular under that name.

The writers of the *Approved Market Names for Fish* established a list of seven criteria for selecting an acceptable common name. These are listed below in order of priority, which means that if a name from a higher priority exists, that is the name that will be ruled acceptable.

• A common or usual name established by Federal law or regulation.

• A common name selected and listed by the American Fisheries Society in its *List of Common and Scientific Names of Fishes from the United States and Canada* or in the updated version due for publication in 1990 or 1991 called *Worldwide Listing of Fishes and Invertebrates*. The 1988 publication listing names of molluscs – *Common and Scientific Names of Aquatic Invertebrates from the United States and Canada* – is also used.

• A common name most often cited in authoritative literature.

• For species from foreign waters being marketed in the U.S.A., a market name most often used in international marketing or a common name cited in the Food and Agriculture Organization's *Yearbook of Fishery Statistics* for the species, with preference given to an English name or the English translation of the foreign language name.

• A market name most often applied historically by the industry in marketing the species.

• If the species has not established a domestic market name or foreign common name, a market name which describes the species as long as it does not trade on the established market name of another species.

• The market name used for other species of the same genus, or other genera in the same scientific family.

In addition to scientific family names and scientific species names, *The Approved Market Names for Fish* also has common names and market names that are or will be acceptable in interstate trade. There are also (mainly unpublished) lists of regional names and other names found, most of which are not acceptable.

The acceptable common and market names are given throughout this book. For convenience and easy reference *The Approved Market Names for Fish* is reproduced here also.

The Fishlist helps standardize seafood names and to avoid a great deal of confusion. It will also ensure that you stay within the law. More attention is now paid to economic fraud in seafoods than ever before. A significant part of such fraud consists of labelling a cheap fish as an expensive one – substitution of a low-price product for one that the buyer thinks is worth more. The Fishlist provides a standard. Everyone in the seafood industry should know what their product should be called.

The other main advantage of the Fishlist: if you have a product that is not already known in the U.S.A., it gives the means and methods for arriving at a name that is acceptable for marketing purposes without misleading the customer. Not every fish can be called "red snapper" or "sole."

The Fishlist: Approved Market Names for Fish

Market name	Common name	Scientific name	Location
Aholehole	Aholehole, Hawaiian	*Kuhlia sandvicensis*	P
Aholehole	Flagtail, rock	*Kuhlia rupestris*	P
Aholehole	Flagtail, spotted	*Kuhlia marginata*	P
Alewife/river herring	Alewife	*Alosa pseudoharengus*	A-F
Alfonsin	Alfonsin	*Trachichthodes affinis*	P
Alfonsin	Alfonsin a casta	*Beryx splendens*	P
Alfonsin	Bream, red	*Beryx decadactylus*	A
Amberjack	Amberjack, greater	*Seriola dumerili*	A
Amberjack	Amberjack, lesser	*Seriola fasciata*	A
Amberjack	Rudderfish, banded	*Seriola zonata*	A
Amberjack/ yellowtail	Amberjack, king	*Seriola quinqueradiata*	P
Amberjack/ yellowtail	Yellowtail	*Seriola lalandei*	P
Anchovy	Anchoveta	*Cetengraulis mysticetus*	P
Anchovy	Anchoveta	*Engraulis ringens*	P
Anchovy	Anchovy	*Anchoviella letidentostole*	A
Anchovy	Anchovy	*Stolephorus purpureus*	P

Locations: A = Atlantic   P = Indo-Pacific   F = Freshwater
Source: F.D.A.

Market name	Common name	Scientific name	Location
Anchovy	Anchovy, European	*Engraulis encrasicolus*	A
Anchovy	Anchovy, Japanese	*Engraulis japonica*	P
Anchovy	Anchovy, New Jersey	*Anchoa duodecim*	A
Anchovy	Anchovy, bay	*Anchoa mitchilli*	A
Anchovy	Anchovy, camiguana	*Anchoviella estauqual*	A
Anchovy	Anchovy, deepbody	*Anchoa compressa*	P
Anchovy	Anchovy, dusky	*Anchoa lyolepis*	A
Anchovy	Anchovy, flat	*Anchoviella perfasciata*	A
Anchovy	Anchovy, key	*Anchoa cayorum*	A
Anchovy	Anchovy, longnose	*Anchoa nasuta*	A
Anchovy	Anchovy, northern	*Engraulis mordax*	P
Anchovy	Anchovy, round headed	*Stolephorus buccaneeri*	P
Anchovy	Anchovy, silver	*Engraulis eurystole*	A
Anchovy	Anchovy, slim	*Stolephorus miarcha*	A
Anchovy	Anchovy, slough	*Anchoa delicatissima*	P
Anchovy	Anchovy, southern	*Engraulis australis*	P
Anchovy	Anchovy, striped	*Anchoa hepsetus*	A
Angelfish	Angelfish, French	*Pomacanthus paru*	A
Angelfish	Angelfish, blue	*Holacanthus bermudensis*	A
Angelfish	Angelfish, gray	*Pomacanthus arcuatus*	A
Angelfish	Angelfish, queen	*Holacanthus ciliaris*	A
Angelfish	Rock beauty	*Holacanthus tricolor*	A
Argentine	Argentine, silverside	*Argentina elongata*	A-P
Armourhead	Armourhead, pelagic	*Pentaceros richardsoni*	P
Barracuda	Barracuda, Pacific	*Sphyraena argentea*	P
Barracuda	Barracuda, great	*Sphyraena barracuda*	A
Barracuda	Guaguanche	*Sphyraena guachancho*	A
Barracuda	Sennet, southern	*Sphyraena picudilla*	A
Barracuda	Vicuda	*Sphyraena ensis*	A
Bass	Bass, Guadalupe	*Micropterus treculi*	F
Bass	Bass, Ozark	*Ambloplites constellatus*	F
Bass	Bass, Roanoke	*Ambloplites cavifrons*	F
Bass	Bass, blackmouth	*Synagrops bellus*	A
Bass	Bass, largemouth	*Micropterus salmoides*	F
Bass	Bass, rock	*Ambloplites rupestris*	F
Bass	Bass, smallmouth	*Micropterus dolomieui*	F
Bass	Bass, spotted	*Micropterus punctulatus*	F
Bass	Bass, striped	*Morone saxatilis*	A-F-P

Market name	Common name	Scientific name	Location
Bass	Bass, sunshine	*Morone chrysops X saxatilis*	F
Bass	Bass, suwannee	*Micropterus notius*	F
Bass	Bass, white	*Morone chrysops*	F
Bass	Bass, yellow	*Morone mississippiensis*	F
Bass	Warmouth	*Lepomis gulosus*	F
Bass sea	Bass, European sea	*Dicentrarchus labrax*	A
Bass sea	Bass, Japan sea	*Lateolabrax japonicus*	P
Bass sea	Bass, black sea	*Epinephelus tauvina*	P
Bass sea	Wreckfish	*Polyprion americanus*	A
Bass sea	Wreckfish	*Polyprion moene*	P
Bass, sea	Bass, Argentine sea	*Acanthistius brasilianus*	A
Bass, sea	Bass, Peruvian Sea	*Paralabrax callaensis*	P
Bass, sea	Bass, barred sand	*Paralabrax nebulifer*	P
Bass, sea	Bass, kelp	*Paralabrax clathratus*	P
Bass, sea	Bass, spotted sand	*Paralabrax maculatofasciatus*	P
Bass, sea	Creole-fish	*Paranthias furcifer*	A
Bass, sea	Grouper, speckled dwarf	*Epinephelus merra*	P
Bass, sea	Sea bass, bank	*Centropristis ocyurus*	A
Bass, sea	Sea bass, black	*Centropristis striata*	A
Bass, sea	Sea bass, rock	*Centropristis philadelphica*	A
Bigeye	Bigeye	*Priacanthus arenatus*	A
Bigeye	Bigeye, short	*Pristigenys alta*	A
Bluefish	Bluefish	*Pomatomus saltatrix*	A
Bluegill	Bluegill	*Lepomis macrochirus*	F
Bluenose	Cutlerfish, Antarctic	*Hyperoglyphe antarctica*	P
Boarfish	Boarfish, deepbody	*Antigonia capros*	A
Boarfish	Boarfish, giant	*Paristiopterus labiosus*	P
Boarfish	Boarfish, shortspine	*Antigonia combatia*	A
Bonefish	Bonefish	*Albula vulpes*	A-P
Bonito	Bonito, Atlantic	*Sarda sarda*	A
Bonito	Bonito, Pacific	*Sarda chiliensis*	P
Bonito	Bonito, striped	*Sarda orientalis (& S. velox)*	A-P
Bonnetmouth	Bonnetmouth	*Emmelichthys nitidus*	P
Bonnetmouth	Bonnetmouth	*Plagiogenion rubiginosus*	P
Bowfin	Bowfin	*Amia calva*	F

Market name	Common name	Scientific name	Location
Bream	Bream, gilt-headed	*Sparus auratus*	A
Bream	Bream, long-spined red	*Argyrops spinifer*	A-P
Bream	Bream, threadfin	*Pentapodus macrurus*	P
Bream	Tai, Taiwan	*Argyrops bleekeri*	P
Bream, threadfin	Bream, Japanese threadfin	*Nemipterus japonicus*	P
Bream/bogue	Bogue	*Boops boops*	A
Brotula	Brotula, bearded	*Brotula barbarta*	A
Buffalo	Buffalo, bigmouth	*Ictiobus cyprinellus*	F
Buffalo	Buffalo, black	*Ictiobus niger*	F
Buffalo	Buffalo, smallmouth	*Ictiobus bubalus*	F
Bullhead	Bullhead, flat	*Ictalurus platycephalus*	F
Bullhead	Bullhead, yellow	*Ictalurus natalis*	F
Bullhead/catfish	Bullhead, black	*Ictalurus melas*	F
Bullhead/catfish	Bullhead, brown	*Ictalurus nebulosus*	F
Bumper	Bumper, Atlantic	*Chloroscombrus chrysurus*	A
Bumper	Bumper, Pacific	*Chloroscombrus orqueta*	P
Burbot	Burbot	*Lota lota*	F
Butterfish	Butterfish	*Peprilus triacanthus*	A
Butterfish	Butterfish, Gulf	*Peprilus burti*	A
Butterfish	Harvestfish	*Peprilus alepidotus*	A
Butterfish	Pompano, Pacific	*Peprilus simillimus*	P
Butterflyfish	Butterflyfish, banded	*Chaetodon striatus*	A
Butterflyfish	Butterflyfish, spotfin	*Chaetodon ocellatus*	A
Cabrilla	Cabrilla, spotted	*Epinephelus analogus*	P
Capelin	Capelin	*Mallotus villosus*	A-P
Cardinalfish	Cardinalfish, bigeye	*Epigonus telescopus*	P
Carp	Carp, common	*Cyprinus carpio*	F
Catfish	Caparari	*Pseudoplatystoma tigrinum*	F
Catfish	Catfish, Brazilian	*Brachyplatysoma vaillanti*	F
Catfish	Catfish, blue	*Ictalurus furcatus*	F
Catfish	Catfish, channel	*Ictalurus punctatus*	F
Catfish	Catfish, flathead	*Pylodictis olivaris*	F
Catfish	Catfish, flatwhiskered	*Pinirampus spp.*	F
Catfish	Catfish, white	*Ictalurus catus*	F
Catfish	Catfish, yaqui	*Ictalurus pricei*	F

Market name	Common name	Scientific name	Location
Catfish	Coroata	*Platynematichthys notatus*	F
Catfish sea	Catfish, gafftopsail	*Bagre marinus*	A
Catfish sea	Catfish, hardhead	*Arius felis*	A-F
Catfish, ocean	Wolffish, Atlantic	*Anarhichas lupus*	A
Catfish, ocean	Wolffish, Bering	*Anarhichas orientalis*	P
Catfish, ocean	Wolffish, northern	*Anarhichas denticulatus*	A
Catfish, ocean	Wolffish, spotted	*Anarhichas minor*	A
Char	Char, Arctic	*Salvelinus alpinus*	A-F-P
Chimaera	Chimaera, longnosed	*Harriotta raleighana*	P
Chimaera	Ratfish	*Hydrolagus novaezelandiae*	P
Chimaera	Ratfish	*Hydrolagus spp.*	A-P
Chub	Chub, Bermuda	*Kyphosus sectatrix*	A
Chub	Chub, yellow	*Kyphosus incisor*	A
Chub	Kiyi	*Coregonus kiyi*	F
Cisco	Cisco, shortnose	*Coregonus reighardi*	F
Cisco/chub	Cisco, longjaw	*Coregonus alpenae*	F
Cisco/chub	Cisco, shortjaw	*Coregonus zenithicus*	F
Cisco/tullibee	Cisco/lake herring	*Coregonus artedii*	F
Cobia	Cobia	*Rachycentron canadum*	A
Cod	Cod, Artic	*Boreogadus saida*	A-P
Cod	Cod, Greenland	*Gadus ogac*	A
Cod	Cod, polar	*Arctogadus glacialis*	A
Cod	Cod, saffron	*Eleginus gracilis*	P
Cod	Cod, toothed	*Arctogadus borisovi*	A
Cod morid	Cod, morid	*Pseudophycis breviusculus*	P
Cod, morid	Cod, morid	*Mora pacifica*	P
Cod, morid	Cod, rock	*Lotella rhacina*	P
Cod/Alaska cod	Cod, Pacific	*Gadus macrocephalus*	P
Cod/codfish	Cod, Atlantic	*Gadus morhua*	A
Conger eel	Conger eel	*Conger oceanicus*	A
Conger eel	Conger eel	*Conger oligoporus*	P
Conger eel	Conger eel	*Congrina aequoreus*	P
Conger eel	Conger, bandtooth	*Ariosoma balearicum*	A
Conger eel	Conger, catalina	*Gnathophis catalinensis*	P
Conger eel	Conger, eel gray	*Conger cinereus*	P
Conger eel	Conger, manytooth	*Conger triporiceps*	A

Market name	Common name	Scientific name	Location
Conger eel	Conger, margintail	*Paraconger caudilimbatus*	A
Conger eel	Conger, whiptail	*Hildebrandia gracilior*	A
Conger eel	Conger, yellow	*Hildebrandia flava*	A
Conger eel	Eel, conger	*Conger conger*	A
Conger eel	Eel, white	*Conger marginatus*	P
Corvina	Corvina, shortfin	*Cynoscion parvipinnis*	P
Cowfish	Cowfish, honeycomb	*Lactophrys polygonia*	A
Cowfish	Cowfish, scrawled	*Lactophrys quadricornis*	A
Crappie	Crappie, black	*Pomoxis nigromaculatus*	F
Crappie	Crappie, white	*Pomoxis annularis*	F
Croaker	Captainfish	*Pseudotolithes spp.*	A
Croaker	Cob	*Argyrosomus hololepidotus*	A-P
Croaker	Croaker	*Nibea spp.*	P
Croaker	Croaker	*Pachypops spp.*	A
Croaker	Croaker	*Pachyurus spp.*	A
Croaker	Croaker	*Paralonchurus spp.*	A-P
Croaker	Croaker	*Plagioscion spp.*	A
Croaker	Croaker	*Pterotolithus spp.*	P
Croaker	Croaker, Atlantic	*Micropogonias undulatus*	A-F
Croaker	Croaker, Japanese	*Argyrosomus japonicus*	P
Croaker	Croaker, black	*Argyrosomus nibe*	P
Croaker	Croaker, black	*Cheilotrema saturnum*	P
Croaker	Croaker, blue	*Bairdiella batabana*	A
Croaker	Croaker, reef	*Odontoscion dentex*	A
Croaker	Croaker, smalleye	*Nebris microps*	A-F
Croaker	Croaker, spotfin	*Roncador stearnsi*	P
Croaker	Croaker, striped	*Bairdiella sanctaeluciae*	A
Croaker	Croaker, white	*Argyrosomus argentatus*	A-P
Croaker	Croaker, white	*Argyrosomus macrophthalmus*	A-P
Croaker	Croaker, white	*Genyonemus lineatus*	P
Croaker	Croaker, yellowfin	*Umbrina roncador*	P
Croaker	Drummer, whitemouth	*Micropogonias furnieri*	A
Croaker	Jewfish, spotted	*Johnius spp.*	P
Croaker/corvina	Corvina	*Micropogonias opercularis*	A
Croaker/corvina	Corvina, bigtooth	*Isopisthus parvipinnis*	A
Croaker/corvina	Corvina, gulf	*Cynoscion orthonopterus*	P

Market name	Common name	Scientific name	Location
Croaker/shadefish	Shadefish, Atlantic	*Argyrosomus regius*	A
Croaker/yellowfish	Croaker, yellow	*Pseudosciaena spp.*	P
Cunner	Cunner	*Tautogolabrus adspersus*	A
Cusk	Cusk	*Brosme brosme*	A
Cusk-eel	Cusk-eel, blackedge	*Lepophidium graellsi*	A
Cusk-eel	Cusk-eel, fawn	*Lepophidium cervinum*	A
Cutlassfish	Cutlassfish, Atlantic	*Trichiurus lepturus*	A
Cutlassfish	Cutlassfish, Pacific	*Trichiurus nitens*	P
Cutlassfish	Hairtail, smallhead	*Trichiurus savaka*	P
Cutlassfish	Scabbardfish	*Lepidopus caudatus*	P
Cutlassfish	Scabbardfish, black	*Aphanopus carbo*	A
Cutlassfish	Scabbardfish, silver	*Lepidopus caudatus*	A-P
Dogfish	Catshark	*Centrophorus squamosus*	P
Dogfish	Dogfish	*Mustelus antarcticus*	P
Dogfish	Dogfish, black	*Centroscymnus fabricii*	A
Dogfish	Dogfish, large spotted	*Scyliorhinus stellaris*	A
Dogfish	Dogfish, lesser spotted	*Scyliorhinus canicula*	A
Dogfish	Dogfish, northern	*Squalus blainvillei*	A-P
Dogfish	Dogfish, smooth	*Mustelus canis*	A
Dogfish	Dogfish, spiny/spring	*Squalus acanthias*	A-P
Dogfish	Shark, dogfish	*Mustelus lenticulatus*	P
Dory	Dory, buckler	*Zenopsis conchifer*	A
Dory	Dory, mirror	*Zenopsis nebulosa*	P
Dory	Dory, silver	*Cyttus novae-zelandiae*	P
Dory	John Dory, European	*Zeus faber*	P
Driftfish	Barrelfish	*Hyperoglyphe perciformis*	A
Driftfish	Driftfish, black	*Hyperoglyphe bythites*	A
Drum	Drum	*Larimus spp.*	A
Drum	Drum	*Stellifer spp.*	A
Drum	Drum, black	*Pogonias cromis*	A
Drum	Drum, sand	*Umbrina corides*	A
Drum	Drum, spotted	*Equetus punctatus*	A
Drum, freshwater	Drum, freshwater	*Aplodinotus grunniens*	F
Drum/cubbyu	Cubbyu	*Equetus umbrosus*	A
Drum/lion fish	Lion fish	*Collichthys spp.*	P
Drum/meagre	Drum/meagre	*Sciaena spp.*	A
Drum/queenfish	Queenfish	*Seriphus politus*	P
Drum/redfish	Drum, red	*Sciaenops ocellatus*	A-F

Market name	Common name	Scientific name	Location
Drummer	Drummer, lowfinned	*Kyphosus vaigiensis*	P
Eel	Eel, European	*Anguilla anguilla*	A-F
Eel	Eel, Japanese	*Anguilla japonicus*	P-F
Eel	Eel, long-finned	*Anguilla dieffenbachii*	P-F
Eel	Eel, short-fin	*Anguilla australis*	P-F
Eel, freshwater	Eel, American	*Anguilla rostrata*	A-F
Eelpout	Eelpout	*Zoarces viviparus*	A
Eelpout/ocean pout	Pout, ocean	*Macrozoarces americanus*	A
Elephant fish	Fish, elephant	*Callorhynchus millii*	P
Emperor	Emperor	*Lethrinus spp.*	P
Fanfish	Fanfish, Pacific	*Pteraclis aesticola*	P
Filefish	Filefish, orange	*Aluterus schoepfi*	A
Filefish	Filefish, unicorn	*Aluterus monocers*	A
Flounder	Brill	*Colistium nudipinnis*	P
Flounder	Brill	*Scophthalmus rhombus*	A
Flounder	Brill, New Zealand	*Colistium guntheri*	P
Flounder	Flounder	*Arnoglossus scapha*	P
Flounder	Flounder	*Samariscus triocellatus*	P
Flounder	Flounder, Arctic	*Liopsetta glacialis*	P
Flounder	Flounder, Bering	*Hippoglossoides robustus*	P
Flounder	Flounder, Gulf	*Paralichthys albigutta*	A
Flounder	Flounder, Indian Ocean	*Psettodes erumei*	P
Flounder	Flounder, Patagonian	*Paralichthys patagonicus*	A
Flounder	Flounder, black	*Rhombosolea retiaria*	F
Flounder	Flounder, broad	*Paralichthys squamilentus*	A
Flounder	Flounder, eyed	*Bothus ocellatus*	A
Flounder	Flounder, fivespot	*Pseudorhombus pentophthalmus*	P
Flounder	Flounder, fourspot	*Paralichthys oblongus*	A
Flounder	Flounder, greenback	*Rhombosolea tapirina*	P
Flounder	Flounder, kamchatka	*Atheresthes evermanni*	P
Flounder	Flounder, largetoothed	*Pseudorhombus arsius*	P
Flounder	Flounder, longjawed	*Pelecanichthys crumenalis*	P
Flounder	Flounder, olive	*Paralichthys olivaceus*	A
Flounder	Flounder, panther	*Bothus pantherinus*	A
Flounder	Flounder, peacock	*Bothus lunatus*	A
Flounder	Flounder, sand	*Rhombosolea plebeia*	P

Market name	Common name	Scientific name	Location
Flounder	Flounder, small-toothed	*Pseudorhombus jenynsii*	A-P
Flounder	Flounder, starry	*Platichthys stellatus*	P-F
Flounder	Flounder, three-eye	*Ancylopsetta dilecta*	A
Flounder	Flounder, tropical	*Bothus mancus*	A
Flounder	Flounder, yellowbelly	*Rhombosolea leporina*	P
Flounder	Flounder, yellowtail	*Limanda ferruginea*	A
Flounder	Sole, New Zealand	*Peltorhampus novaezeelandiae*	P
Flounder	Sole, New Zealand lemon	*Pelotretis flavilatus*	P
Flounder	Windowpane	*Scophthalmus aquosus*	A
Flounder arrowtooth	Flounder, arrowtooth	*Atheresthes stomias*	P
Flounder/dab	Dab, common	*Limanda limanda*	A
Flounder/dab	Dab, longhead	*Limanda proboscidea*	A-P
Flounder/fluke	Flounder, European	*Platichthys flesus*	A
Flounder/fluke	Flounder, southern	*Paralichthys lethostigma*	A-F
Flounder/fluke	Flounder, summer	*Paralichthys dentatus*	A
Flounder/sole	Flounder, winter/lemon sole	*Pseudopleuronectes americanus*	A
Flounder/whiff	Megrim	*Lepidorhombus whiffiagonis*	A
Flounder/whiff	Scaldfish, fourspot	*Lepidorhombus boscii*	A
Flyingfish	Flyingfish, Atlantic	*Cypselurus melanurus*	A
Flyingfish	Flyingfish, California	*Cypselurus californicus*	P
Flyingfish	Flyingfish, bandwing	*Cypselurus exsiliens*	A
Flyingfish	Flyingfish, blackwing	*Hirundichthys rondeleti*	A-P
Flyingfish	Flyingfish, blotchwing	*Cypselurus hubbsi*	P
Flyingfish	Flyingfish, bluntnose	*Prognichthys gibbifrons*	A
Flyingfish	Flyingfish, clearwing	*Cyspelurus comatus*	A
Flyingfish	Flyingfish, cuvier's	*Cypselurus speculiger*	P
Flyingfish	Flyingfish, fourwing	*Hirundichthys affinis*	A
Flyingfish	Flyingfish, jenkins	*Cypselurus atrisignis*	P
Flyingfish	Flyingfish, margined	*Cypselurus cyanopterus*	A
Flyingfish	Flyingfish, ocean two-wing	*Exocoetus obtusirostris*	A
Flyingfish	Flyingfish, sailfin	*Parexocoetus brachypterus*	A
Flyingfish	Flyingfish, sharpchin	*Fodiator acutus*	P
Flyingfish	Flyingfish, shortnosed	*Cypselurus simus*	P

Market name	Common name	Scientific name	Location
Flyingfish	Flyingfish, smallwing	*Oxyporhamphus micropterus*	A
Flyingfish	Flyingfish, spotfin	*Cypselurus furcatus*	A
Flyingfish	Flyingfish, spotted wing	*Cypselurus spilonopterus*	P
Flyingfish	Flyingfish, trop. two-wing	*Exocoetus volitans*	A
Gar	Gar, alligator	*Lepisosteus spatula*	F
Gar	Gar, longnose	*Lepisosteus osseus*	F
Gemfish	Domine	*Epinnula magistralis*	A-P
Gemfish	Escolar	*Lepidocybium flavobrunneum*	A-P
Gemfish	Gemfish, black	*Nesiarchus nasutus*	A-P
Gemfish/barracouta	Gemfish, silver	*Rexea solandri*	P
Gemfish/barracouta	Mackerel, snake	*Thyrsites atun*	P
Gemfish/caballa	Mackerel, white snake	*Thyrsites lepidopoides*	A
Goatfish	Goatfish	*Mulloidichthys spp.*	A
Goatfish	Goatfish	*Parupeneus spp.*	P
Goatfish	Goatfish	*Upeneus spp.*	A
Goatfish	Goatfish, bluespotted	*Upeneichthys lineatus*	P
Goatfish	Goatfish, red	*Mullus auratus*	A
Goatfish	Goatfish, spotted	*Pseudupeneus spp.*	A
Goldeye	Goldeye	*Hiodon alosoides*	F
Goldfish	Goldfish	*Carassius auratus*	F
Grayling	Grayling, Arctic	*Thymallus arcticus*	F
Greenbone	Greenbone	*Coridodax pullus*	P
Greenling	Greenling, kelp	*Hexagrammos decagrammus*	P
Greenling	Greenling, masked	*Hexagrammos octogrammus*	P
Greenling	Greenling, rock	*Hexagrammos lagocephalus*	P
Greenling	Greenling, whitespotted	*Hexagrammos stelleri*	P
Grenadier	Grenadier	*Macrourus spp.*	P
Grenadier	Grenadier, rock	*Coryphaenoides rupestris*	A
Grenadier	Grenadier, roughnose	*Trachyrhynchus murrayi*	A
Grenadier	Marlin-spike	*Nezumia bairdi*	A

Locations: A = Atlantic   P = Indo-Pacific   F = Freshwater
Source: F.D.A.

Market name	Common name	Scientific name	Location
Grenadier	Rattail, giant	*Coryphaenoides pectoralis*	P
Grenadier	Whiptail, deepsea	*Lepidorhynchus denticulatus*	P
Grouper	Coney	*Epinephelus fulva*	A
Grouper	Coney, gulf	*Cephalopholis acanthistius*	P
Grouper	Graysby	*Epinephelus cruentatus*	A
Grouper	Grouper	*Caprodon schlegelii*	P
Grouper	Grouper, black	*Mycteroperca bonaci*	A
Grouper	Grouper, blacktip	*Epinephelus fasciatus*	P
Grouper	Grouper, broomtail	*Mycteroperca xenarcha*	P
Grouper	Grouper, chevron tailed	*Cephalopholis urodelus*	P
Grouper	Grouper, comb	*Mycteroperca rubra*	A-P
Grouper	Grouper, dusky	*Epinephelus guaza*	A
Grouper	Grouper, gulf	*Mycteroperca jordani*	P
Grouper	Grouper, marbled	*Epinephelus inermis*	A
Grouper	Grouper, misty	*Epinephelus mystacinus*	A
Grouper	Grouper, mottled	*Epinephelus fuscoguttatus*	P
Grouper	Grouper, nassau	*Epinephelus striatus*	A
Grouper	Grouper, purplespotted	*Cephalopholis argus*	P
Grouper	Grouper, red	*Epinephelus morio*	A
Grouper	Grouper, snowy	*Epinephelus niveatus*	A-P
Grouper	Grouper, spotted	*Cephalopholis taeniops*	A
Grouper	Grouper, tiger	*Mycteroperca tigris*	A
Grouper	Grouper, warsaw	*Epinephelus nigritus*	A
Grouper	Grouper, white	*Epinephelus aeneus*	A
Grouper	Grouper, yellowedge	*Epinephelus flavolimbatus*	A
Grouper	Grouper, yellowfin	*Mycteroperca venenosa*	A
Grouper	Grouper, yellowmouth	*Mycteroperca interstitialis*	A
Grouper	Perch, sand	*Diplectrum formosum*	A
Grouper	Rockcod, brownspotted	*Epinephelus chlorostigma*	A-P
Grouper	Rockcod, yellowspotted	*Epinephelus areolatus*	A-P
Grouper/gag	Gag	*Mycteroperca microlepis*	A
Grouper/hind	Hind, red	*Epinephelus guttatus*	A
Grouper/jewfish	Jewfish	*Epinephelus itajara*	A

Market name	Common name	Scientific name	Location
Grunion	Grunion, California	*Leuresthes tenuis*	P
Grunt	Grunt, French	*Haemulon flavolineatum*	A
Grunt	Grunt, Latin	*Haemulon steindachneri*	A-P
Grunt	Grunt, Spanish	*Haemulon macrostomum*	A
Grunt	Grunt, barred	*Conodon nobilis*	A-P
Grunt	Grunt, black	*Haemulon bonariense*	A
Grunt	Grunt, bluestriped	*Haemulon sciurus*	A
Grunt	Grunt, burrito	*Anisotremus interruptus*	A
Grunt	Grunt, burro	*Pomadasys crocro*	A
Grunt	Grunt, caesar	*Haemulon carbonarium*	A
Grunt	Grunt, smallmouth	*Haemulon chrysargyreum*	A
Grunt	Grunt, striped	*Haemulon striatum*	A
Grunt	Grunt, white	*Haemulon plumieri*	A
Grunt	Pigfish	*Orthopristis chrysoptera*	A-F
Grunt	Prieta mojarra	*Haemulon scudderii*	P
Grunt	Sailors choice	*Haemulon parrai*	A
Grunt/catalina	Catalina	*Anisotremus taeniatus*	A
Grunt/cottonwick	Cottonwick	*Haemulon melanurum*	A
Grunt/margate	Margate	*Haemulon album*	A
Grunt/margate	Margate, black	*Anisotremus surinamensis*	A
Grunt/porkfish	Porkfish	*Anisotremus virginicus*	A
Grunt/sargo	Sargo	*Anisotremus davidsoni*	P
Grunt/sweetlips	Sweetlips, Oriental	*Plectorhynchus orientalis*	P
Grunt/sweetlips	Sweetlips, brown	*Plectorhynchus nigrus*	P
Grunt/sweetlips	Sweetlips, harlequin	*Plectorhynchus chaetodonoides*	P
Grunt/sweetlips	Sweetlips, painted	*Plectorhynchus pictus*	P
Grunt/sweetlips	Sweetlips, yellowbanded	*Plectorhynchus lineatus*	P
Grunt/tomtate	Tomtate	*Haemulon aurolineatum*	A
Grunt/tomtate	Tomtate	*Haemulon rimator*	A
Guitarfish	Guitarfish, Atlantic	*Rhinobatos lentiginosus*	A
Guitarfish	Guitarfish, banded	*Zapteryx exasperata*	P
Guitarfish	Guitarfish, shovelnose	*Rhinobatos productus*	P
Guitarfish	Thornback	*Platyrhinoidis triseriata*	P
Haddock	Haddock	*Melanogrammus aeglefinus*	A

Market name	Common name	Scientific name	Location
Hake	Hake, Brazilian	*Urophycis brasiliensis*	A
Hake	Hake, Carolina	*Urophycis earlli*	A
Hake	Hake, Gulf	*Urophycis cirrata*	A
Hake	Hake, longfin	*Phycis chesteri*	A
Hake	Hake, red	*Urophycis chuss*	A
Hake	Hake, southern	*Urophycis floridana*	A
Hake	Hake, spotted	*Urophycis regia*	A
Hake	Hake, white	*Urophycis tenuis*	A
Halfmoon	Halfmoon	*Medialuna californiensis*	P
Halibut	Halibut, Atlantic	*Hippoglossus hippoglossus*	A
Halibut	Halibut, Pacific	*Hippoglossus stenolepis*	P
Halibut/California halibut	Halibut, California	*Paralichthys californicus*	P
Hamlet	Hamlet, mutton	*Epinephelus afer*	A
Herring	Herring, round	*Etrumeus teres*	A-P
Herring	Ilisha, African	*Ilisha africans*	A
Herring	Ilisha, Indian	*Ilisha melastoma*	P
Herring	Ilisha, Pacific	*Ilisha furthi*	P
Herring	Ilisha, bigeye	*Ilisha megaloptera*	P
Herring	Ilisha, javan	*Ilisha pristigastroides*	P
Herring	Ilisha, pugnose	*Ilisha elongata*	P
Herring	Pellona, Indian	*Pellona ditchela*	P
Herring	Tardoore	*Opisthopterus tardoore*	P
Herring, thread	Thread herring, Atlantic	*Opisthonema oglinum*	A-F
Herring/river herring	Herring, blueback	*Alosa aestivalis*	A-F
Herring/river herring	Herring, skipjack	*Alosa chrysochloris*	A-P
Herring/sea herring/ sild	Herring, Atlantic	*Clupea harengus harengus*	A
Herring/sea herring/ sild	Herring, Pacific	*Clupea harengus pallasi*	P
Hind	Hind, rock	*Epinephelus adscensionis*	A
Hind	Hind, speckled	*Epinephelus drummondhayi*	A
Hogfish	Hogfish	*Lachnolaimus maximus*	A
Hogfish	Hogfish, Spanish	*Bodianus rufus*	A
Hogfish	Hogfish, spotfin	*Bodianus pulchellus*	A
Houndfish	Houndfish	*Tylosurus crocodilus*	A
Icefish	Icefish	*Notothenia moariensis*	P

Market name	Common name	Scientific name	Location
Icefish	Icefish, Japanese	*Salangichthys spp.*	P
Icefish	Icefish, mackerel	*Champsocephalus gunnari*	A
Jack	Jack crevalle	*Caranx hippos*	A
Jack	Jack, almaco	*Seriola rivoliana*	A
Jack	Jack, bar	*Caranx ruber*	A
Jack	Jack, black	*Caranx lugubris*	A
Jack	Jack, cottonmouth	*Uraspis secunda*	A-P
Jack	Jack, green	*Caranx caballus*	P
Jack	Jack, horse-eye	*Caranx latus*	A
Jack	Jack, mazatlan/striped	*Caranx vinctus*	P
Jack	Jack, whitemouth	*Caranx helvolus*	P
Jack	Jack, yellow	*Caranx bartholomaei*	A
Jack	Leatherjacket	*Oligoplites saurus*	A
Jack	Lookdown	*Selene vomer*	A
Jack	Moonfish, Atlantic	*Selene setapinnis*	A
Jack	Moonfish, Pacific	*Selene peruviana*	P
Jack mackerel	Mackerel, jack	*Trachurus declivis*	A
Jack mackerel	Mackerel, jack	*Trachurus symmetricus*	P
Jack mackerel	Scad, Japanese	*Trachurus japonicus*	P
Jack mackerel	Scad, inca	*Trachurus murphyi*	P
Jack mackerel	Scad, rough	*Trachurus lathami*	A
Jack/blue runner	Runner, blue	*Caranx crysos*	A
Jack/rainbow runner	Runner, rainbow	*Elegatis bipinnulata*	A-P
Jack/roosterfish	Roosterfish	*Nematistius pectoralis*	P
Jack/trevally	Jack, spotted	*Caranx melampygus*	P
Jack/trevally	Trevally, giant	*Caranx ignobilis*	P
Jack/trevally	Trevally, white	*Caranx georgianus*	P
Jackfish/crevalle	Jack, threadfin	*Alectis indicus*	P
Jobfish	Jobfish, green	*Aprion virescens*	P
Jobfish	Jobfish, lavender	*Pristipomoides sieboldii*	P
Jobfish	Jobfish, rusty	*Aphareus rutilans*	P
Jobfish	Jobfish, smalltooth	*Aphareus furcatus*	P
Jobfish	Snapper/jobfish goldeneye	*Pristipomoides flavipinnis*	P
Kahawai	Kahawai	*Arripis trutta*	P
Kelpfish	Kelpfish	*Chironemus marmoratus*	P
Killifish	Killifish, marsh	*Fundulus confluentus*	A-F
Killifish	Killifish, striped	*Fundulus majalis*	A
Killifish	Mummichog	*Fundulus heteroclitus*	A-F

Market name	Common name	Scientific name	Location
Kingfish	Kingfish, Gulf	*Menticirrhus littoralis*	A
Kingfish	Kingfish, northern	*Menticirrhus saxatilis*	A
Kingfish	Kingfish, southern	*Menticirrhus americanus*	A
Kingfish/corbina	Corbina, California	*Menticirrhus undulatus*	P
Kingklip	Kingklip, South African	*Genypterus capensis*	A
Kingklip	Kingklip, black	*Genypterus maculatus*	P
Kingklip	Kingklip, golden	*Genypterus blacodes*	P
Kingklip	Kingklip, red	*Genypterus chilensis*	A
Ladyfish	Ladyfish	*Elops hawaiensis*	P-F
Ladyfish	Ladyfish	*Elops saurus*	A-F
Ladyfish	Machete	*Elops affinis*	P-F
Ling	Ling	*Molva molva*	A
Ling	Ling, blue	*Molva dypterygia*	A
Ling Mediterranean	Ling, Spanish	*Molva macrophthalus*	A
Lingcod	Lingcod	*Ophiodon elongatus*	P
Lizardfish	Lizardfish, inshore	*Synodus foetens*	A
Lizardfish	Sand diver	*Synodus intermedius*	A
Louvar	Louvar	*Luvarus imperialis*	A-P
Lumpfish	Lumpfish	*Cyclopterus lumpus*	A
Mackerel	Cero	*Scomberomorus regalis*	A
Mackerel	Mackerel, Atlantic	*Scomber scombrus*	A
Mackerel	Mackerel, Indian	*Rastrelliger kanagurta*	P
Mackerel	Mackerel, Spanish	*Scomberomorus maculatus*	A
Mackerel	Mackerel, Spanish	*Scomberomorus tritor*	A
Mackerel	Mackerel, chub	*Scomber japonicus*	A-P
Mackerel	Mackerel, double-lined	*Grammatorcynus bicaneatus*	P
Mackerel	Mackerel, frigate	*Auxis thazard*	A-P
Mackerel	Mackerel, narrow-barred	*Scomberomorus commerson*	P
Mackerel	Sierra, Pacific	*Scomberomorus sierra*	P
Mackerel	Sierra, gulf	*Scomberomorus concolor*	P
Mackerel chub	Mackerel, spotted chub	*Scomber australasicus*	P
Mackerel king	Mackerel, king	*Scomberomorus cavalla*	A
Mackerel, atka	Mackerel, atka	*Pleurogrammus monopterygius*	P
Mackerel, snake	Oilfish	*Ruvettus pretiosus*	A-P
Mackerel/scad	Mackerel, jack	*Trachurus novaeze-landiae*	P

Market name	Common name	Scientific name	Location
Mahi-mahi	Dolphin	*Coryphaena hippurus*	A-P
Mahi-mahi	Dolphin, pompano	*Coryphaena equisetis*	A
Manta	Manta, Atlantic	*Manta birostris*	A
Manta	Manta, Pacific	*Manta hamiltoni*	P
Manta	Mobula, smoothtail	*Mobula lucasana*	P
Manta	Mobula, spinetail	*Mobula japanica*	P
Manta	Ray, devil	*Mobula hypostoma*	A
Marlin	Marlin, black	*Makaira indica*	P
Marlin	Marlin, blue	*Makaira nigricans*	A-P
Marlin	Marlin, striped	*Tetrapturus audax*	P
Marlin	Marlin, white	*Tetrapturus albidus*	A
Menhaden	Menhaden, Atlantic	*Brevoortia tyrannus*	A
Menhaden	Menhaden, Gulf	*Brevoortia patronus*	A
Menhaden	Menhaden, finescale	*Brevoortia gunteri*	A
Menhaden	Menhaden, yellowfin	*Brevoortia smithi*	A
Milkfish	Milkfish	*Chanos chanos*	P
Mojarra	Mojarra, striped	*Diapterus plumieri*	A-F
Mojarra	Pompano, Irish	*Diapterus auratus*	A
Monkfish	Goosefish	*Lophius americanus*	A
Monkfish	Monkfish	*Lophius piscatorius*	P
Mooneye	Mooneye	*Hiodon tergisus*	F
Moray	Moray, recticulate	*Muraena retifera*	A
Morwong	Marblefish	*Aplodactylus meandratus*	P
Morwong	Morwong	*Nemadactylus douglasi*	P
Morwong	Morwong, blue	*Nemadactylus carponotatus*	P
Morwong	Morwong, brownband	*Cheilodactylus spectabilis*	P
Morwong	Morwong, magpie	*Cheilodactylus gibbosus*	P
Morwong	Tarakihi	*Cheilodactylus macropterus*	P
Mullet	Liza	*Mugil liza*	A
Mullet	Mullet	*Neomyxus chaptalii*	P
Mullet	Mullet, fantail	*Mugil trichodon*	A
Mullet	Mullet, mountain	*Agonostomus monticola*	A-F
Mullet	Mullet, red	*Mullus brabatus*	A
Mullet	Mullet, red	*Mullus surmuletus*	A
Mullet	Mullet, redeye	*Mugil gaimardianus*	A
Mullet	Mullet, striped	*Mugil cephalus*	A-P-F
Mullet	Mullet, wartynosed	*Crenimugil crenilabis*	A

185

Market name	Common name	Scientific name	Location
Mullet	Mullet, white	*Mugil curema*	A-F
Mullet	Mullet, yelloweye	*Aldrichetta forsteri*	P
Muskellunge	Muskellunge	*Esox masquinongy*	F
Nile perch	Perch, Nile	*Lates nilotica*	F
Opah	Opah	*Lampris guttatus*	A-P
Opaleye	Opaleye	*Girella nigricans*	P
Oreo dory	Oreo, dory black	*Allocyttus spp*	P
Oreo dory	Oreo, dory smooth	*Pseudocyttus maculatus*	P
Oscar	Oscar	*Astronotus ocellatus*	F
Paddlefish	Paddlefish	*Polyodon spathula*	F
Pargo	Pargo, striped	*Hoplopagrus guntheri*	A
Parrotfish	Parrotfish, midnight	*Scarus coelestinus*	A
Parrotfish	Parrotfish, stoplight	*Sparisoma viride*	A
Perch	Perch, silver	*Bairdiella chrysoura*	A-F
Perch	Perch, zebra	*Hermosilla azurea*	P
Perch yellow/lake perch	Perch, yellow	*Perca flavescens*	F
Perch, ocean	Deepwater, redfish	*Sebastes mentella*	A
Perch, ocean	Ocean perch, Pacific	*Sebastes alutus*	P
Perch, ocean	Redfish, Labrador	*Sebastes fasciatus*	A
Perch, ocean	Redfish, Norway	*Sebastes viviparus*	A
Perch, ocean	Redfish/ocean perch	*Sebastes marinus*	A
Perch, pile	Perch, pile	*Rhacochilus vacca*	P
Perch, white	Perch, white	*Morone americana*	A-F
Pickerel	Pickerel, chain	*Esox niger*	F
Pickerel	Pickerel, grass	*Esox americanus vermiculatus*	F
Pickerel	Pickerel, redfin	*Esox americanus americanus*	F
Pike	Pike, northern	*Esox lucius*	F
Pilchard/sardine	Pilchard, European	*Sardina pilchardus*	A
Pilchard/sardine	Pilchard, Japanese	*Sardinops sagax melanosticta*	P
Pilchard/sardine	Pilchard, South African	*Sardinops sagax ocellata*	A-P
Pilchard/sardine	Sardine, Australian	*Sardinops neopilchardus*	P
Pipefish	Pipefish, northern	*Syngnathus fuscus*	A
Plaice	Plaice, Alaska	*Pleuronectes quadrituberculatus*	P
Plaice	Plaice, European	*Plueuronectes platessa*	A

Market name	Common name	Scientific name	Location
Plaice/dab	Plaice, American	*Hippoglossoides platessoides*	A
Pollock	Pollock	*Pollachius pollachius*	A
Pollock	Pollock	*Pollachius virens*	A
Pollock/Alaska pollock	Pollock, walleye	*Theragra chalcogramma*	P
Pomfret	Pomfret	*Taractes rubescens*	P
Pomfret	Pomfret, Atlantic	*Brama brama*	A
Pomfret	Pomfret, Pacific	*Brama japonica*	P
Pompano	Pompano, African	*Alectis ciliaris*	A
Pompano	Pompano, Florida	*Trachinotus carolinus*	A
Pompano	Pompano, paloma	*Trachinotus paitensis*	P
Pompano	Pompano, tropical	*Trachinotus blochi*	P
Pompano/palometa	Palometa	*Trachinotus goodei*	A
Pompano/permit	Permit	*Trachinotus falcatus*	A
Pompano/permit	Permit, palometta	*Trachinotus kennedyi*	P
Pompano/pompanito	Pompano, gafftopsail	*Trachinotus rhodopus*	P
Porgy	Dentex	*Dentex gibbosus*	A
Porgy	Pinfish	*Lagodon rhomboides*	A-F
Porgy	Porgy	*Calamus spp.*	A-P
Porgy	Porgy	*Diplodus spp.*	A
Porgy	Porgy	*Pagrus pagrus*	A-P
Porgy	Porgy, longspine	*Stenotomus caprinus*	A
Porgy	Porgy, red Hawaiian	*Chrysophrys auratus*	P
Porgy/scup	Scup	*Stenotomus chrysops*	A
Puffer	Puffer, bandtail	*Sphoeroides spengleri*	A
Puffer	Puffer, blunthead	*Sphoeroides pachygaster*	A
Puffer	Puffer, checkerd	*Sphoeroides testudineus*	A
Puffer	Puffer, least	*Sphoeroides parvus*	A
Puffer	Puffer, longnose	*Sphoeroides lobatus*	P
Puffer	Puffer, northern	*Sphoeroides maculatus*	A
Puffer	Puffer, smooth	*Lagocephalus laevigatus*	A
Puffer	Puffer, southern	*Sphoeroides mephelus*	A
Puffer, bullseye	Puffer, bullseye	*Sphoeroides annulatus*	P
Puffer, marbled	Puffer, marbled	*Sphoeroides dorsalis*	P
Puffer, oceanic	Puffer, oceanic	*Lagocephalus lagocephalus*	A-P

Locations: A = Atlantic   P = Indo-Pacific   F = Freshwater
Source: F.D.A.

Market name	Common name	Scientific name	Location
Racehorse	Pigfish, southern	*Congiopodus leucopaecilus*	P
Ray, bat	Ray, bat	*Myliobatis californica*	P
Ray, bullnose	Ray, bullnose	*Myliobatis freminvillei*	A
Ray, cownose	Ray, cownose	*Rhinoptera bonasus*	A
Ray, eagle	Ray, southern eagle	*Myliobatis goodei*	A
Ray, eagle	Ray, spotted eagle	*Aetobatus narinari*	A
Ray, electric	Ray, Pacific electric	*Torpedo califonica*	P
Ray, electric	Ray, lesser electric	*Narcine brasiliensis*	A
Rockfish	Bocaccio	*Sebastes paucispinis*	P
Rockfish	Chilipepper	*Sebastes goodei*	P
Rockfish	Cowcod	*Sebastes levis*	P
Rockfish	Rockfish	*Helicolenus papillosus*	P
Rockfish	Rockfish, Mexican	*Sebastes macdonaldi*	P
Rockfish	Rockfish, Puget Sound	*Sebastes emphaeus*	P
Rockfish	Rockfish, aurora	*Sebastes aurora*	P
Rockfish	Rockfish, bank	*Sebastes rufus*	P
Rockfish	Rockfish, black	*Sebastes melanops*	P
Rockfish	Rockfish, black & yellow	*Sebastes chrysomelas*	P
Rockfish	Rockfish, blackgill	*Sebastes melanostomus*	P
Rockfish	Rockfish, blue	*Sebastes mystinus*	P
Rockfish	Rockfish, bronzespotted	*Sebastes gilli*	P
Rockfish	Rockfish, brown	*Sebastes auriculatus*	P
Rockfish	Rockfish, calico	*Sebastes dalli*	P
Rockfish	Rockfish, canary	*Sebastes pinniger*	P
Rockfish	Rockfish, chameleon	*Sebastes phillipsi*	P
Rockfish	Rockfish, china	*Sebastes nebulosus*	P
Rockfish	Rockfish, copper	*Sebastes caurinus*	P
Rockfish	Rockfish, darkblotched	*Sebastes crameri*	P
Rockfish	Rockfish, dusky	*Sebastes ciliatus*	P
Rockfish	Rockfish, dwarf-red	*Sebastes rufinanus*	P
Rockfish	Rockfish, flag	*Sebastes rubrivinctus*	P
Rockfish	Rockfish, freckled	*Sebastes lentiginosus*	P
Rockfish	Rockfish, gopher	*Sebastes carnatus*	P
Rockfish	Rockfish, grass	*Sebastes rastrelliger*	P
Rockfish	Rockfish, greenblotched	*Sebastes rosenblatti*	P
Rockfish	Rockfish, greenspotted	*Sebastes chlorostictus*	P

Market name	Common name	Scientific name	Location
Rockfish	Rockfish, greenstriped	*Sebastes elongatus*	P
Rockfish	Rockfish, halfbanded	*Sebastes semicinctus*	P
Rockfish	Rockfish, honeycomb	*Sebastes umbrosus*	P
Rockfish	Rockfish, kelp	*Sebastes atrovirens*	P
Rockfish	Rockfish, northern	*Sebastes polyspinis*	P
Rockfish	Rockfish, olive	*Sebastes serranoides*	P
Rockfish	Rockfish, pink	*Sebastes eos*	P
Rockfish	Rockfish, pinkrose	*Sebastes simulator*	P
Rockfish	Rockfish, pygmy	*Sebastes wilsoni*	P
Rockfish	Rockfish, quillback	*Sebastes maliger*	P
Rockfish	Rockfish, red	*Scorpaena cardinalis*	P
Rockfish	Rockfish, redbanded	*Sebastes babcocki*	P
Rockfish	Rockfish, redstripe	*Sebastes proriger*	P
Rockfish	Rockfish, rosethorn	*Sebastes helvomaculatus*	P
Rockfish	Rockfish, rosy	*Sebastes rosaceus*	P
Rockfish	Rockfish, rougheye	*Sebastes aleutianus*	P
Rockfish	Rockfish, semaphore	*Sebastes melanosema*	P
Rockfish	Rockfish, sharpchin	*Sebastes zacentrus*	P
Rockfish	Rockfish, shortbelly	*Sebastes jordani*	P
Rockfish	Rockfish, shortraker	*Sebastes borealis*	P
Rockfish	Rockfish, silvergray	*Sebastes brevispinis*	P
Rockfish	Rockfish, speckled	*Sebastes ovalis*	P
Rockfish	Rockfish, splitnose	*Sebastes diploproa*	P
Rockfish	Rockfish, squarespot	*Sebastes hopkinsi*	P
Rockfish	Rockfish, starry	*Sebastes constellatus*	P
Rockfish	Rockfish, stripetail	*Sebastes saxicola*	P
Rockfish	Rockfish, swordspine	*Sebastes ensifer*	P
Rockfish	Rockfish, tiger	*Sebastes nigrocinctus*	P
Rockfish	Rockfish, vermillion	*Sebastes miniatus*	P
Rockfish	Rockfish, widow	*Sebastes entomelas*	P
Rockfish	Rockfish, yelloweye	*Sebastes ruberrimus*	P
Rockfish	Rockfish, yellowmouth	*Sebastes reedi*	P
Rockfish	Rockfish, yellowtail	*Sebastes flavidus*	P
Rockfish	Treefish	*Sebastes serriceps*	P
Rockling	Rockling, fourbeard	*Enchelyopus cimbrius*	A
Rosefish	Rosefish, blackbelly	*Helicolenus dactylopterus*	A
Roughy	Roughy, pinkfinned	*Paratrachichthys trailli*	P
Roughy	Roughy, silver	*Hoplostethus mediterraneus*	A-P

Market name	Common name	Scientific name	Location
Roughy, orange	Roughy, orange	*Hoplostethus atlanticus*	A-P
Rudderfish	Rudderfish	*Kyphosus cinerascens*	P
Ruff black	Ruff, black	*Centrolophus niger*	P
Sablefish	Sablefish	*Anoplopoma fimbria*	P
Sailfish	Sailfish	*Istiophorus platypterus*	A-P
Sailfish	Sailfish, Indo-Pacific	*Istiophorus gladius*	A-P
Salmon sockeye/ blueback/red	Salmon, sockeye	*Oncorhynchus nerka*	P-F
Salmon, cherry	Salmon, cherry	*Oncorhynchus masou*	P-F
Salmon, chinook/ king/spring	Salmon, chinook	*Oncorhynchus tshawytscha*	P-F
Salmon, chum/keta	Salmon, chum	*Oncorhynchus keta*	P-F
Salmon, coho/silver/ med.red	Salmon, coho	*Oncorhynchus kisutch*	A-P-F
Salmon, pink/ humpback sal.	Salmon, pink	*Oncorhynchus gorbuscha*	A-F-P
Salmon/Atlantic salmon	Salmon, Atlantic	*Salmo salar*	A-F
Sanddab	Sanddab, Pacific	*Citharichthys sordidus*	P
Sandlance	Sandlance, Pacific	*Ammodytes hexapterus*	A-P
Sandperch	Weever	*Parapercis spp.*	A-P
Sardine	Pilchard, false	*Harengula clupeola*	A
Sardine	Sardine, Spanish	*Sardinella anchovia*	A
Sardine	Sardine, Spanish	*Sardinella aurita*	A
Sardine	Sardine, fringescale	*Sardinella fimbriata*	P
Sardine	Sardine, oil	*Sardinella longiceps*	P
Sardine	Sardine, orangespot	*Sardinella brasiliensis*	A
Sardine	Sardine, perforated-scale	*Sardinella perforata*	P
Sardine	Sardine, redear	*Harengula humeralis*	A
Sardine	Sardine, scaled	*Harengula jaguana*	A-F
Sardine/pilchard	Sardine, Pacific	*Sardinops sagax*	P
Sauger	Sauger	*Stizostedion canadense*	F
Saury	Saury, Atlantic	*Scomberesox saurus*	A
Saury	Saury, Pacific	*Cololabis saira*	P
Sawfish	Sawfish, largetooth	*Pristis perotteti*	A
Sawfish	Sawfish, smalltooth	*Pristis pectinata*	A
Scad	Horse mackerel, Atlantic	*Trachurus trachurus*	A-P
Scad	Koheru	*Decapterus koheru*	P
Scad	Scad, Mexican	*Decapterus scombrinus*	P

Market name	Common name	Scientific name	Location
Scad	Scad, amberstripe	*Decapterus muroadsi*	P
Scad	Scad, bigeye	*Selar crumenophthalmus*	A
Scad	Scad, blue	*Trachurus picturatus*	A
Scad	Scad, mackerel	*Decapterus macarellus*	A
Scad	Scad, northern mackerel	*Decapterus russelli*	P
Scad	Scad, redtail	*Decapterus tabl*	A
Scad	Scad, round	*Decapterus punctatus*	A
Scad	Scad, yellowtail	*Caranx mate*	P
Scamp	Scamp	*Mycteroperca phenax*	A
Schoolmaster	Schoolmaster	*Lutjanus apodus*	A
Scorpionfish	Scorpionfish, orange	*Scorpaena scrofa*	A
Sculpin	Sculpin, great	*Myoxocephalus polyacanthocephalus*	P
Sculpin	Sea raven, Atlantic	*Hemitripterus americanus*	A
Sculpin/cabezon	Cabezon	*Scorpaenichthys marmoratus*	P
Seabream	Bream, sea	*Archosargus rhomboidalis*	A
Seabream	Seabream	*Pagellus spp.*	A
Searobin	Gurnard, spotted	*Pterygotrigla picta*	P
Searobin	Gurnard, tub	*Chelidonichthys lucerna*	A
Searobin	Searobin, armored	*Peristedion miniatum*	A
Searobin	Searobin, bluefin	*Chelidonichthys kumu*	P
Searobin	Searobin, northern	*Prionotus carolinus*	A
Seatrout	Seabass, white	*Cynoscion nobilis*	P
Seatrout	Seatrout, sand	*Cynoscion arenarius*	A
Seatrout	Seatrout, silver	*Cynoscion nothus*	A
Seatrout	Seatrout, spotted	*Cynoscion nebulosus*	A-F
Shad	Shad, Alabama	*Alosa alabamae*	A-F
Shad	Shad, Allis	*Alosa alosa*	A-F
Shad	Shad, American	*Alosa sapidissima*	A-F
Shad	Shad, gizzard	*Dorosoma cepedianum*	A-F
Shad	Shad, hickory	*Alosa mediocris*	A-F
Shad	Shad, threadfin	*Dorosoma petenense*	A-P-F

Locations: A = Atlantic   P = Indo-Pacific   F = Freshwater
Source: F.D.A.

Market name	Common name	Scientific name	Location
Shad	Shad, twaite	*Alosa fallax*	A-F
Shark	Shark, basking	*Cetorhinus maximus*	A-P
Shark	Shark, bignose	*Carcharhinus altimus*	A
Shark	Shark, blacktip	*Carcharhinus limbatus*	A
Shark	Shark, blacktip reef	*Carcharhinus melanopterus*	A-P
Shark	Shark, blue	*Prionace glauca*	A-P
Shark	Shark, bull	*Carcharhinus leucas*	A-F-P
Shark	Shark, dusky	*Carcharhinus obscurus*	A-P
Shark	Shark, finetooth	*Carcharhinus isodon*	A
Shark	Shark, gray reef	*Carcharhinus amblyrhynchus*	P
Shark	Shark, lemon	*Negaprion brevirostris*	A-P
Shark	Shark, leopard	*Triakis semifasciata*	P
Shark	Shark, narrowtoothed	*Carcharhinus brachyurus*	P
Shark	Shark, night	*Carcharhinus signatus*	A
Shark	Shark, reef	*Carcharhinus perezi*	A
Shark	Shark, salmon	*Lamna ditropis*	P
Shark	Shark, sandbar	*Carcharhinus plumbeus*	A
Shark	Shark, sevengill	*Notorynchus cepedianus*	A-P
Shark	Shark, silky	*Carcharhinus falciformis*	A
Shark	Shark, silver tip	*Carcharhinus albimarginatus*	P
Shark	Shark, sixgill	*Hexanchus griseus*	A-P
Shark	Shark, smalltail	*Carcharhinus porosus*	A
Shark	Shark, spinner	*Carcharhinus brevipinna*	A
Shark	Shark, tiger	*Galeocerdo cuviere*	A-P
Shark	Shark, tope	*Galeorhinus galeus*	A
Shark	Shark, white	*Carcharodon carcharias*	A-P
Shark	Shark, whitetip	*Carcharhinus longimanus*	A-P
Shark	Shark, whitetip reef	*Triaenodon obesus*	A-P
Shark mako	Shark, shortfin mako	*Isurus oxyrinchus*	A-P
Shark, angel	Shark, Atlantic angel	*Squatina dumerili*	A
Shark, angel	Shark, Pacific angel	*Squatina californica*	P
Shark, mako	Shark, longfin mako	*Isurus paucus*	A-P
Shark, thresher	Shark, bigeye thresher	*Alopias superciliosus*	A-P
Shark, thresher	Shark, common thresher	*Alopias vulpinus*	A-P
Shark, thresher	Shark, pelagic thresher	*Alopias pelagicus*	P
Shark/bonnethead	Shark/bonnethead	*Sphyrna tiburo*	A-P

Market name	Common name	Scientific name	Location
Shark/hammerhead	Shark, great hammerhead	*Sphyrna mokarran*	A-P
Shark/hammerhead	Shark, scalloped hammerhead	*Sphyrna lewini*	A-P
Shark/hammerhead	Shark, smalleye hammerhead	*Sphyrna tudes*	A
Shark/hammerhead	Shark, smooth hammerhead	*Sphyrna zygaena*	A-P
Shark/porbeagle	Shark, porbeagle	*Lamna nasus*	A
Shark/smoothhound	Smoothhound, brown	*Mustelus henlei*	P
Shark/smoothhound	Smoothhound, grey	*Mustelus californicus*	P
Sheephead	Sheephead, California	*Semicossyphus pulcher*	P
Sheepshead	Sheepshead	*Archosargus probatocephalus*	A-F
Silverside	Jacksmelt	*Atherinopsis californiensis*	P
Silverside	Silverside, Atlantic	*Menidia menidia*	A
Silverside	Silverside, S. American	*Basilichthys australis*	A-F
Silverside	Topsmelt	*Atherinopsis affinis*	P
Skate	Skate	*Raja spp.*	A-P
Skate	Skate, Alaska	*Raja parmifera*	P
Skate	Skate, Aleutian	*Raja aleutica*	P
Skate	Skate, Bering	*Raja interrupta*	P
Skate	Skate, California	*Raja inornata*	P
Skate	Skate, barndoor	*Raja laevis*	A
Skate	Skate, big	*Raja binoculata*	P
Skate	Skate, clearnose	*Raja eglanteria*	A
Skate	Skate, flathead	*Raja rosispinis*	P
Skate	Skate, little	*Raja erinacea*	A
Skate	Skate, longnose	*Raja rhina*	P
Skate	Skate, rosette	*Raja garmani*	A
Skate	Skate, roughtail	*Raja trachura*	P
Skate	Skate, roundel	*Raja texana*	A
Skate	Skate, sandpaper	*Raja kincaidi*	A
Skate	Skate, smooth	*Raja senta*	A
Skate	Skate, spinytail	*Raja spinicauda*	A
Skate	Skate, spreadfin	*Raja olseni*	A
Skate	Skate, starry	*Raja stellulata*	P
Skate	Skate, thorny	*Raja radiata*	A
Skate	Skate, winter	*Raja ocellata*	A
Skilfish	Skilfish	*Erilepis zonifer*	P

Market name	Common name	Scientific name	Location
Smelt	Smelt, Arctic	*Osmerus dentex*	P-F
Smelt	Smelt, European	*Osmerus eperlanus*	A
Smelt	Smelt, common	*Retropinna retropinna*	P
Smelt	Smelt, deep sea	*Argentina semifasciata*	P
Smelt	Smelt, delta	*Hypomesus transpacificus*	P-F
Smelt	Smelt, eulachon	*Thaleichthys pacificus*	P-F
Smelt	Smelt, great silver	*Argentina silus*	A
Smelt	Smelt, lesser silver	*Argentina sphyraena*	A
Smelt	Smelt, longfin	*Spirinchus thaleichthys*	P-F
Smelt	Smelt, night	*Spirinchus starksi*	P
Smelt	Smelt, surf	*Hypomesus pretiosus*	P-F
Smelt	Smelt, whitebait	*Allosmerus elongatus*	P
Smelt/American smelt	Smelt, rainbow	*Osmerus mordax*	A-F-P
Snake eel/keoghfish	Snake eel, giant	*Ophichthus rex*	A
Snapper, Caribbean red	Snapper, Caribbean red	*Lutjanus purpureus*	A
Snapper, Pacific	Snapper, Pacific	*Lutjanus peru*	P
Snapper, Pacific dog	Snapper, Pacific dog	*Lutjanus novemfasciatus*	P
Snapper, black	Snapper, black	*Apsilus dentatus*	A
Snapper, black and white	Snapper, black and white	*Macolor niger*	P
Snapper, blackfin	Snapper, blackfin	*Lutjanus buccanella*	A
Snapper, blacktail	Snapper, blacktail	*Lutjanus fulvus*	P
Snapper, blubberlip	Snapper, blubberlip	*Lutjanus rivulatus*	P
Snapper, bluestriped	Snapper, bluestriped	*Lutjanus kasmira*	P
Snapper, cardinal	Snapper, cardinal	*Pristipomoides macrophthalmus*	A
Snapper, colorado	Snapper, colorado	*Lutjanus colorado*	P
Snapper, crimson	Snapper, crimson	*Pristipomoides filamentosus*	P
Snapper, cubera	Snapper, cubera	*Lutjanus cyanopterus*	A
Snapper, dog	Snapper, dog	*Lutjanus jocu*	A
Snapper, emperor	Snapper, emperor	*Lutjanus sebae*	P
Snapper, golden	Snapper, golden	*Lutjanus inermis*	P
Snapper, gray	Snapper, gray	*Lutjanus griseus*	A-F
Snapper, humpback	Snapper, humpback	*Lutjanus gibbus*	P
Snapper, lane	Snapper, lane	*Lutjanus synagris*	A
Snapper, mahogony	Snapper, mahogany	*Lutjanus mahogoni*	A

Market name	Common name	Scientific name	Location
Snapper, malabar	Malabar	*Lutjanus malabaricus*	P
Snapper, midnight	Snapper, midnight	*Macolor macularius*	P
Snapper, mullet	Snapper, mullet	*Lutjanus aratus*	P
Snapper, mutton	Snapper, mutton	*Lutjanus analis*	A
Snapper, onespot	Snapper, onespot	*Lutjanus monostigma*	P
Snapper, queen	Snapper, queen	*Etelis oculatus*	A
Snapper, red	Snapper, red	*Lutjanus campechanus*	A
Snapper, ruby	Snapper, ruby	*Etelis carbunculus*	P
Snapper, rufous	Snapper, rufous	*Lutjanus jordani*	P
Snapper, sailfin	Snapper, sailfin	*Symphorichthys spilurus*	P
Snapper, scarlet	Snapper, blood	*Lutjanus sanguineus*	P
Snapper, silk	Snapper, silk	*Lutjanus vivanus*	A
Snapper, spotted rose	Snapper, spotted rose	*Lutjanus guttatus*	P
Snapper, twinspot	Snapper, twinspot	*Lutjanus bohar*	P
Snapper, vermilion	Snapper, vermilion	*Rhomboplites aurorubens*	A
Snapper, yellowstriped	Snapper, yellowstriped	*Etelis coruscans*	P
Snapper, yellowtail	Snapper, yellowtail	*Ocyurus chrysurus*	A
Snook	Constintino	*Centropomus robalito*	P-F
Snook	Snook	*Centropomus nigrescens*	P-F
Snook	Snook	*Centropomus ornatus*	P-F
Snook	Snook	*Centropomus pedemacula*	P-F
Snook	Snook	*Centropomus undecimalis*	A-F
Snook	Snook	*Centropomus vindis*	P-F
Snook	Snook, fat	*Centropomus parallelus*	A-F
Snook	Snook, swordspine	*Centropomus ensiferus*	A-F
Snook	Snook, tarpon	*Centropomus pectinatus*	A-F
Sole	Sole	*Austroglossus microlepis*	A
Sole	Sole	*Austroglossus pectoralis*	A
Sole	Sole, English	*Parophrys vetulus*	P
Sole	Sole, European	*Solea vulgaris*	A
Sole	Sole, kobe	*Aseraggodes kobensis*	P
Sole	Sole, lemon	*Microstomus kitt*	A
Sole	Sole, narrowbanded	*Aseraggodes macleayanus*	P
Sole	Sole, oriental black	*Synaptura orientalis*	A
Sole	Sole, slender	*Lyopsetta exilis*	P
Sole	Sole, thickback	*Microchirus variegatus*	A
Sole dover	Sole, dover	*Microstomus pacificus*	P

Market name	Common name	Scientific name	Location
Sole/flounder	Flounder, witch/gray sole	*Glyptocephalus cynoglossus*	A
Sole/flounder	Sole, C-O	*Pleuronichthys coenosus*	P
Sole/flounder	Sole, bigmouth	*Hippoglossina stomata*	P
Sole/flounder	Sole, butter	*Isopsetta isolepis*	P
Sole/flounder	Sole, curlfin	*Pleuronichthys decurrens*	P
Sole/flounder	Sole, deepsea	*Embassichthys bathybius*	P
Sole/flounder	Sole, fantail	*Xystreurys liolepis*	P
Sole/flounder	Sole, flathead	*Hippoglossoides elassodon*	P
Sole/flounder	Sole, petrale	*Eopsetta jordani*	P
Sole/flounder	Sole, rex	*Glyptocephalus zachirus*	P
Sole/flounder	Sole, rock	*Lepidopsetta bilineata*	P
Sole/flounder	Sole, roughscale	*Clidoderma asperrimum*	P
Sole/flounder	Sole, sand	*Psettichthys melanostictus*	P
Sole/flounder	Sole, yellowfin	*Limanda aspera*	P
Spadefish	Spadefish, Atlantic	*Chaetodipterus faber*	A
Spadefish	Spadefish, Pacific	*Chaetodipterus zonatus*	P
Spearfish	Spearfish, longbill	*Tetrapturus pfluegeri*	A
Spearfish	Spearfish, shortbill	*Tetrapturus angustirostris*	P
Spinefoot	Spinefoot	*Siganus spp.*	A-P
Spot	Spot	*Leiostomus xanthurus*	A-F
Sprat/brisling	Sprat	*Sprattus spp.*	A-P
Squirrelfish	Squirrelfish	*Holocentrus ascensionis*	A
Squirrelfish	Squirrelfish	*Myripristis argyromus*	P
Squirrelfish	Squirrelfish	*Myripristis berndti*	P
Squirrelfish	Squirrelfish	*Sargocentron lacteoguttatum*	P
Squirrelfish	Squirrelfish, longspine	*Holocentrus rufus*	A
Squirrelfish	Squirrelfish, scarlet	*Sargocentron spiniferum*	P
Stargazer	Stargazer, giant	*Kathetostoma giganteum*	P
Stargazer	Stargazer, smooth	*Kathetostoma averruncus*	P
Stargazer	Stargazer, spotted	*Genyagnus monopterygius*	P
Sturgeon	Sturgeon, Atlantic	*Acipenser oxyrhynchus*	A-F
Sturgeon	Sturgeon, European	*Huso huso*	F
Sturgeon	Sturgeon, Russian	*Acipenser gueldenstaedti*	F
Sturgeon	Sturgeon, green	*Acipenser medirostris*	P-F
Sturgeon	Sturgeon, star	*Acipenser stellatus*	F

Market name	Common name	Scientific name	Location
Sturgeon	Sturgeon, white	*Acipenser transmontanus*	P-F
Sucker	Carpsucker, river	*Carpiodes carpio*	F
Sucker	Quillback	*Carpiodes cyprinus*	F
Sucker	Sucker, blue	*Cycleptus elongatus*	F
Sucker	Sucker, white	*Catostomus commersoni*	F
Sucker/redhorse	Redhorse, shorthead	*Moxostoma macrolepidotum*	F
Sunfish	Perch, Sacramento	*Archoplites interruptus*	F
Sunfish	Pumpkinseed	*Lepomis gibbosus*	F
Sunfish	Sunfish, green	*Lepomis cyanellus*	F
Sunfish	Sunfish, redbreast	*Lepomis auritus*	F
Sunfish	Sunfish, redear	*Lepomis microlophus*	F
Sunfish	Sunfish, spotted	*Lepomis punctatus*	F
Surfperch	Seaperch, rubberlip	*Rhacochilus toxotes*	P
Surfperch	Surfperch, barred	*Amphistichus argenteus*	P
Surfperch	Surfperch, black	*Embiotoca jacksoni*	P
Surfperch	Surfperch, calico	*Amphistichus koelzi*	P
Surfperch	Surfperch, redtail	*Amphistichus rhodoterus*	P
Surfperch	Surfperch, shiner	*Cymatogaster aggregata*	P-F
Surfperch	Surfperch, striped	*Embiotoca lateralis*	P
Surfperch	Surfperch, walleye	*Hypersopon argenteum*	P
Swordfish	Swordfish	*Xiphias gladius*	A-P
Tang	Doctorfish	*Acanthurus chirurgus*	A
Tang	Tang, blue	*Acanthurus coeruleus*	A
Tarpon	Tarpon, Atlantic	*Megalops atlanticus*	A-F
Tautog	Tautog	*Tautoga onitis*	A
Thornyhead	Thornyhead, longspine	*Sebastolobus altivelis*	P
Thornyhead	Thornyhead, shortspine	*Sebastolobus alascanus*	P
Tilapia	Tilapia, Mozambique	*Tilapia mossambica*	F
Tilapia	Tilapia, Nile	*Tilapia nilotica*	F
Tilapia	Tilapia, blackchin	*Tilapia melanotheron*	F
Tilapia	Tilapia, blue	*Tilapia aurea*	F
Tilapia	Tilapia, longfin	*Tilapia macrochir*	F
Tilapia	Tilapia, mango	*Tilapia galilaea*	F
Tilapia	Tilapia, redbreast	*Tilapia rendalli*	F
Tilefish	Tilefish, blueline	*Caulolatilus microps*	A
Tilefish	Tilefish, golden	*Lopholatilus chamaeleonticeps*	A
Tilefish	Tilefish, goldface	*Caulolatilus chrysops*	A

Market name	Common name	Scientific name	Location
Tilefish	Tilefish, sand	*Malacanthus plumieri*	A
Tilefish	Whitefish, ocean	*Caulolatilus princeps*	P
Toadfish	Toadfish, Gulf	*Opsanus beta*	A
Toadfish	Toadfish, oyster	*Opsanus tau*	A
Tomcod	Tomcod, Atlantic	*Microgadus tomcod*	A-F
Tomcod	Tomcod, Pacific	*Microgadus proximus*	P
Tonguesole	Tonguesole	*Cynoglossus spp.*	P
Torpedo	Torpedo, Atlantic	*Torpedo nobiliana*	A
Trevally	Trevally, bigeye	*Caranx sexfasciatus*	P
Trevally	Trevally, white	*Caranx dentex*	P
Triggerfish	Filefish, fringed	*Melichthys niger*	A-P
Triggerfish	Triggerfish	*Navodon convexirostris*	P
Triggerfish	Triggerfish	*Navodon scabra*	P
Triggerfish	Triggerfish, gray	*Balistes capriscus*	A
Triggerfish	Triggerfish, ocean	*Cantherdermis sufflamen*	A
Triggerfish	Triggerfish, queen	*Balistes vetula*	A
Tripletail	Tripletail	*Lobotes surinamensis*	A
Tripletail	Tripletail, fourband	*Datinoides quadrifasciatus*	P
Tripletail	Tripletail, west coast	*Lobotes pacificus*	P
Trout	Trout, brown	*Salmo trutta*	A-F
Trout	Trout, gila	*Salmo gilae*	F
Trout	Trout, golden	*Salmo aguabonita*	F
Trout, brook	Trout, brook	*Salvelinus fontinalis*	A-F
Trout, cutthroat	Trout, cutthroat	*Salmo clarki*	P-F
Trout, lake	Trout, lake	*Salvelinus namaycush*	F
Trout, rainbow/ steelhead	Trout, rainbow	*Salmo gairdneri**	A-F-P
Trout/Dolly Varden	Trout, Dolly Varden	*Salvelinus malma*	P-F
Trout/inconnu	Inconnu	*Stenodus leucichthys*	F
Trumpeter	Trumpeter, bastard	*Latridopsis ciliaris*	P
Trumpeter	Trumpeter, striped	*Latris lineata*	P
Tuna	Albacore	*Thunnus alalunga*	A-P
Tuna	Kawakawa	*Euthynnus affinis*	P
Tuna	Skipjack, black	*Euthynnus lineatus*	P
Tuna	Tuna, bigeye	*Thunnus obesus*	A-P
Tuna	Tuna, blackfin	*Thunnus atlanticus*	A
Tuna	Tuna, bluefin	*Thunnus thynnus*	A-P
Tuna	Tuna, bullet	*Auxis rochei*	A-P
Tuna	Tuna, longtail	*Thunnus tonggol*	P

Market name	Common name	Scientific name	Location
Tuna	Tuna, skipjack	*Euthynnus pelamis*	A-P
Tuna	Tuna, southern bluefin	*Thunnus maccoyii*	A-P
Tuna	Tuna, yellowfin	*Thunnus albacares*	A-P
Tuna	Tunny, little	*Euthynnus alletteratus*	A
Turbot	Turbot	*Scophthalmus maximus*	A
Turbot	Turbot, diamond	*Hypsopsetta guttulata*	P
Turbot	Turbot, hornyhead	*Pleuronichthys verticalis*	P
Turbot	Turbot, spotted	*Pleuronichthys ritteri*	P
Turbot	Turbot, spottedtail	*Psettodes belcheni*	A
Turbot	Turbot, spring	*Psettodes bennetti*	P
Turbot, Greenland	Halibut, Greenland	*Reinhardtius hippoglossoides*	A-P
Wahoo	Wahoo	*Acanthocybium solanderi*	A-P
Walleye	Pike, walleye	*Stizostedion vitreum*	F
Warehou	Warehou, blue	*Seriolella brama*	P
Warehou	Warehou, silver	*Seriolella punctata*	P
Warehou	Warehou, white	*Seriolella caerulee*	P
Weakfish	Weakfish	*Cynoscion spp.*	A-P
Weakfish	Weakfish, king	*Macrodon ancylodon*	A
Wenchman	Wenchman	*Pristipomoides aquilonaris*	A
Whitefish	Whitefish, humpback	*Coregonus pidschian*	F
Whitefish	Whitefish, lake	*Coregonus clupeaformis*	A-F
Whitefish	Whitefish, round	*Prosopium cylindraceum*	F
Whiting	Hake, Argentine	*Merluccius hubbsi*	A
Whiting	Hake, Cape	*Merluccius capensis*	A-P
Whiting	Hake, Chilean	*Merluccius gayi*	P
Whiting	Hake, European	*Merluccius merluccius*	A
Whiting	Hake, New Zealand	*Merluccius australis*	A
Whiting	Hake, Patagonian	*Merluccius polylepsis*	A
Whiting	Hake, silver	*Merluccius bilinearis*	A
Whiting	Whiting, European	*Merlangus merlangus*	A
Whiting New Zealand	Hoki	*Macruronus novaezealandiae*	P
Whiting blue	Poutassou	*Micromesistius poutassou*	A
Whiting blue	Whiting, southern blue	*Micromesistius australis*	A-P
Whiting/ Pacific whiting	Hake, Pacific	*Merluccius productus*	P

*Note that scientific names for some trout species have changed. See sections on Trout and Salmon.

NET SALMON: Salmon caught in gillnets or seine nets. Because the nets may bruise the flesh of the fish, net salmon gives a lower yield for smoking than troll caught fish and sells at a lower price. Most net salmon is landed with guts in while troll salmon is eviscerated before landing. Holding fish with the guts in reduces quality.

NET WEIGHTS: Net weight is very simply defined as the weight of the product without packing material or glaze.

The problem is to determine the net weight without glaze, since most seafoods drip their own moisture for days. Definitions of net weight and drained weight and disputes about them are a continual problem throughout the industry. For a full discussion of the problem, see Economic fraud in the seafood industry. For details of standard and acceptable methods for defrosting seafoods, see Defrosting methods.

N.F.I.: The National Fisheries Institute; the trade association covering importers, processors, traders, distributors and retail and restaurant chains. It is an effective body representing the industry and distributing information. Mail inquiries to: 200 M Street N.W., Washington D.C. 20036.

NILE PERCH *Scientific name: Lates niloticus:* A large (up to 300lb) freshwater bass from Africa. The flesh of larger fish is coarse, but smaller specimens are usable. Some product is offered in Europe and the U.S. from time to time.

NOBBING: Removing the head and guts from a fish without cutting the belly. This leaves the roe or milt in the fish. Nobbing is used mainly on herring.

NOMENCLATURE: See Names.

NORWAY LOBSTER: See Lobsterette.

NOVA SALMON: Nova lox. Probably an abbreviation for Nova Scotia, which was once the source of much of the smoked salmon sold on the east coast. See Smoked salmon.

NUTRITION: Seafood today is increasingly perceived as healthy and nutritious food, providing good quality proteins and minerals with only small amounts of fats. See Health and nutrition for further details.

NUTRITION LABELLING: Nutrition information on labels is not mandatory unless
- nutrients such as vitamins, minerals or proteins are added to enhance the product, or
- the product makes nutritional claims which must be backed up by information on the label.

Once a manufacturer decides to include nutritional information, he must follow certain regulations. The following is required on a nutrition label:

Serving size: A serving is a reasonable amount of food as part of a meal suited for an adult male engaged in light physical activity. Serving size is a statement of the portion size and should be a convenient measure that the consumer can easily recognize.

Servings per container: The number of portions per container.

Calories: The number of calories per serving. Calories are rounded to the nearest 2 calories up to 20 calories, to the nearest 5 calories between 20 and 50 calories and to the nearest 10 calories when over 50 calories.

Protein: The number of grams of protein per serving rounded to the nearest gram. If a serving contains less than one gram, then the statement "Contains less than one gram" or "less than one gram" may be used.

Carbohydrates: The number of grams of carbohydrates per serving rounded to the nearest gram. If a serving contains less than one gram, then the statement "Contains less than one gram" or "less than one gram" may be used.

Fat: The number of grams of fat per serving rounded to the nearest gram. If a serving contains less than one gram, then the same applies as above. Fatty acid and cholesterol content may also be declared directly following fat content information. Whenever fatty acid or cholesterol content is provided the following statement must appear either right after the information given or footnoted at the bottom of the label: "Information on fat and/or cholesterol content is provided for individuals who, on the advice of a physician, are modifying their dietary intake of fat (and/or cholesterol)."

Sodium: Sodium content has been a mandatory item on nutrition labels since April 1984. The number of milligrams of sodium per serving must appear on the label directly following the information on fat, fatty acid and/or cholesterol content. If a serving contains less than 5 milligrams per serving, it may be listed as zero content. Sodium content is rounded to the nearest 5 milligrams between 5 and 140 milligrams and to the nearest 10 milligrams when content is greater than 140 milligrams.

Potassium: Information on potassium content is not mandatory. However, when it is listed it should follow the information on sodium. Potassium is also measured in milligrams per serving.

Percentage of U.S. Recommended Daily Allowances (U.S. RDA): The amount per serving expressed as a percentage of the U.S. Recommended Daily Allowance for the following nutrients (listed in the order they must appear): protein, vitamin A, vitamin C, thiamin, riboflavin, niacin, calcium and iron. Any other vitamins or minerals added to enhance the nutritional value or which naturally occur in the product may also be included on the list. The percentages are rounded to the nearest 2 percent up to 10 percent, rounded to the nearest 5 percent from 10 percent to 50 percent and rounded to the nearest 10 percent when above the 50 percent level. Nutrients less than 2 percent may be listed as zero percent or by the statement "Contains less than two percent U.S. RDA of this (these) nutrient(s)."

A label is considered misbranded if the declared vitamin, mineral or protein content is less than 80 percent or more than 120 percent of the declared value.

For detailed information, including U.S. RDA levels, see *Seafood Nutrition* by Joyce Nettleton.

OCEAN BLOWFISH: See Monkfish. Name mainly used in New York.

OCEAN CATFISH: See Catfish.

OCEAN PERCH: See Rockfish. The Rockfish item covers ocean perch from the Atlantic as well as the Pacific rockfish under its many names.

OCEAN POUT *Scientific name: Macrozoarces americanus:*
Also called eelpout. Sea pout, muttonfish, yellow pout and viviparous blenny are other names which are not approved for interstate trade. It is more or less interchangeable with *Zoarces
viviparus*. Both are North Atlantic species.

It matters little what the name is, or how attractive the name
may sound – ocean pout is almost inedible. It is one of the more
publicized "underexploited species" of the North Atlantic. Considerable efforts have been made with Government grading to
develop a market for the fish. Presumably it was thought that if
people would eat this, they would eat anything, therefore solving
all marketing problems for foodstuffs.

Pout fillets look quite nice, but are tough and tasteless when
cooked. The fillets are boneless, long and rather thin, with a
creamy yellow color. New England packers produce ocean pout to
special order, but after the first flush of enthusiasm, no-one produces it as a regular part of their line.

Recent attempts to market the fillets centered on the discovery
that if the fillets are passed through a meat tenderizer or beaten
with a mallet they cook up without the characteristic tough,
chewy consistency. This may offer packers an opportunity to produce a pre-tenderized pack, but should leave all potential users of
the fish warned about what to look for.

OCEAN RUN: Sea run. Any product packed as caught without
grading for size.

OCTOPUS: Also called pulpo. Cephalopod with eight arms,
popular in Mediterranean cuisines. Pulpo is mostly sold head on,
beak removed, eviscerated and frozen in blocks of 10lbs. Larger
sizes are generally preferred. Grading is usually 1/2lbs, 2/4 and
4lb up. Octopus smaller than 1lb may be packed in printed cartons for retail sale.

Buyers prefer eastern Atlantic pulpo over fish from the western
Atlantic and the Gulf of Mexico. The market's order of preference
for the various origins is Spain, Portugal, Canary Islands and
Mexico. There are supplies also from Korea and other Asian
countries, usually at much lower prices. Asian octopus is small,
sometimes only two ounces.

OMEGA-3: See Health and nutrition.

OPILIO: A small snow crab from Alaska and eastern Canada. See snow crab under Crabs.

ORANGE ROUGHY *Scientific name: Hoplostethus atlanticus:* A deep-water fish from southern waters of New Zealand and Australia. It first appeared on the U.S. market about 1982 and has become a popular item. The boneless flesh is white and quite firm, with large flakes which hold together well when cooked, whatever the cooking method. It has an unobtrusive flavor which Americans seem to prefer.

The species was once known as slimehead, a name with no marketing future. New Zealanders managed to persuade the F.D.A. that their name of orange roughy was preferable. Largely because the name could not be confused with any other fish, the change was permitted and the fish rapidly became a success story.

Orange roughy run to about three pounds, giving fillets up to about 10 ounces, although most are much smaller. The fillets are usually layer-packed in 22lb (10kg) boxes, graded in two-ounce steps. Harvesters use large freezer-trawlers to catch this deep-water fish. A comparatively small quantity of the fish is processed on land. Because the species is exploited with joint-venture boats from Korea and Japan, some of the fish are frozen at sea headless and dressed, then filleted and refrozen elsewhere.

One of the many unusual aspects of the orange roughy success story is that it was first popularized through the retail trade. Supermarkets originally saw the opportunity. Foodservice sales followed after.

There appear to be large resources of orange roughy off Tasmania which are not yet fully exploited.

Because of its popularity, roughy is a target for substitutions. Oreo dory and even hoki, packed in similar New Zealand layer-packs, reportedly are used. Names like Pacific roughy or golden roughy are used to describe other species pretending to be orange roughy. Some substituters even use phoney labels purporting to be from major packers. Orange roughy, perhaps even more than many other species, should be bought only from reliable brokers and suppliers.

OYSTERS: The most expensive bivalve mollusc and still an important industry, although production has fallen from a peak of 170 million pounds in 1875 to about 40 million pounds in 1987 (figures are weights of meat). The bulk of the trade is fresh, and most of it is live oysters in the shell. The rest is shucked fresh meats. The Pacific oyster, *Crassostrea gigas*, and the eastern oyster, *Crassostrea virginica*, are similar in appearance and taste (the eastern oyster is variously called "blue point," "Cape Cod" and other names) and make up all frozen supplies. The rare and expensive Olympia oyster, *Ostreola conchaphila*, (which is the only commercial oyster species native to United States waters) and the newly introduced European flat oyster, *Ostrea edulis*, sometimes called "belon," are sold fresh.

Fresh oysters are graded as standards, about 200 to 250 per bushel, selects, about 100 to 200 per bushel, and large, under 100 per bushel. These definitions are by no means universal, though the use of the descriptive terms is widespread. If you buy live oysters, it is far better to specify weights and counts. Bushels are a volume measure and give an indeterminate weight.

Shucked oysters are defined by the F.D.A. in Title 21 of the Code of Federal Regulations. Eastern oysters and Pacific oysters are defined differently:

Pacific oysters – meat counts

Large	Not more than 64
Medium	64 to 96
Small	96 to 144
Extra small	More than 144

Eastern oysters – size definitions

Size description	Meats per gallon	Smallest meats: quart contains	Largest meats: quart contains
Extra large, counts or plants	not over 160	not over44	——
Large or extra selects	160 to 210	not over 58	not under 36
Medium or selects	210 to 300	not over 83	not under 46
Small or standards	300 to 500	not over 138	not under 68
Very small	over 500	——	not over 112

For eastern oysters, sizes are defined in terms firstly of the number of meats in one gallon, secondly by the number of meats in a quart selected from the SMALLEST meats in the gallon and another quart selected from the LARGEST meats in the gallon. This ensures that the oysters are reasonably uniform in size.

Olympia oysters, shucked, count to about 1,800 to 2,500 per gallon.

Shucked oysters present a number of problems when defining the drained weight. Meats are "blown" before packing, which means they are put in a bath of water with air bubbling through it to remove grit and sand. Addition of chemicals to the blowing bath can add to the weight of the oyster meats. A lot of work has been done on the variations of drip loss from shucked oysters. The best conclusion so far seems to be that you get what the packer put in the can.

In many ways, frozen oysters are easier to handle and use. They keep well, are easy to store and handle and allow for proper inventory control. Frozen oysters come in almost as many ways as fresh ones.

Whole frozen oysters may be used exactly like live ones. Tasting panels have been unable to tell the difference between the frozen and the live ones. But there is a strong and continuing prejudice against whole frozen. Raw, frozen on the half shell is similarly flexible in use. Whole or half-shell oysters thaw quickly. The whole ones are easy to open because the muscle is relaxed. The period in the deep-freeze serves to kill most of any remaining bacteria as well. Half-shell product may include sauces or preparations such as oysters Rockefeller, which can be cooked from the frozen state in a very short time.

Breaded oysters of all sizes are sold, usually packed in plastic trays of one dozen each. The trays give good protection to this particularly delicate product.

Frozen I.Q.F. meats are imported from Korea and Japan, but most of the breaded oysters are produced from local shellfish, with some imports being used during out of season periods. The Asian oysters are *Crassostrea gigas*, the same species as the Pacific oyster.

Different species appear on the market from time to time as oyster growers experiment with types and strains that will give faster and more even growth. Although oysters have been farmed since Roman times, great improvements in hatchery techniques as well as in on-growing have been made in the last decade. Oyster farmers could well reverse the decline in supply. One development that has attracted a lot of attention is the triploid oyster, genetically engineered so that it does not ripen and spawn. This means it can be harvested year round without at any time having the oily taste associated with ripe oysters or the thin meats that are left after spawning.

See also Shellfish Sanitation Program and Depuration.

The following is taken from the Southeastern Fisheries Association's *Seafood Product Quality Code*:

> Percent water content for oysters: The percent drain weight or percent water content (weight basis) in a package of shucked oysters should be determined by the standard procedure recommended in the Official Methods of Analysis of the Association of Official Analytical Chemists (AOAC), 1984, 14th Edition. Numerous studies have demonstrated water content in a package of shucked oysters will vary during storage due to "bleeding" or water leaching from the meats and water absorption. Water loss or uptake depends on the osmotic condition of the oyster meats. This condition can be influenced by the salinity and temperature of harvest waters, seasons, rainfall, and processing/ storage conditions. Properly shucked and packed containers of raw oysters should routinely have less than 15 percent water content. Occasionally environmental factors can cause higher water loss. In some instances a higher percent water content may denote water additions when packaged. This situation should be discussed with the supplier with reference to the prevailing state and federal regulations.
>
> Procedure (AOAC Secs. 18.014-015): Weigh tared (known weight) container with shellfish meats (entire contents of one package or container of oysters), transfer the contents to a special skimmer tray and quickly distribute meats evenly over the draining surface with a minimum of handling. Drain for 2 minutes, then return meats to the tared container and reweigh. Calculate loss of weight as percent drained liquid (or percent water content). This procedure should be conducted with product temperature

near $7 \pm 1°C$. ($45 \pm 2°F$.).

Equipment: The skimmer tray or strainer should be a flat-bottom metal pan or tray with bottom area greater than or equal to 1900 cm^2 (300 sq. inch) for each gallon of oysters to be poured on the tray. The tray should have smooth edged holes 0.6 cm (0.25 inch) diameter and 3.2 cm (1.25 inch) apart in a square pattern, or holes of equivalent area and distribution. The tray should be supported over a slightly larger tray so the liquid drains into the larger tray.

PACKING: The importance of correct packing cannot be over-emphasized. Although the primary purpose of packing material is to protect the product during storage and transportation, it is also a vital part of the display for marketing purposes and for foodservice. The size, shape and type of pack are important aspects for every buyer. Some buyers require units of certain sizes to aid inventory control; others prefer certain shapes or packing styles, to aid their distribution and selling efforts. Many buyers look for familiar labels as well as familiar packs and are content with something they recognize.

Introduction of non-standard packs immediately creates suspicion in the mind of the buyer. For example, Argentine shrimp is sometimes packed in square boxes, instead of the more familiar rectangular shrimp boxes. Receipt of these square boxes is likely to cause the buyer to thaw and check the product carefully, just because it is unfamiliar. The same product packed in normal shrimp boxes is more likely to pass without inspection.

The same is true for familiar labels: Canadian scallop packs, for example, are seldom queried because the buyers recognize the labels and have confidence in them.

Many product packs are standardized. Scallops from Canada and U.S.A. are invariably 10/5lb blocks; shell-on shrimp is normally 10/5lb or 10/2kg blocks; cellos are always 10/5lb or 5/10lb. Throughout this book, the standard packs for each product, if they are standardized, are mentioned. If you are offered packs that vary from the normal, it is your choice whether or not to use them. If you follow the advice of checking everything you receive, then the pack is less important, provided your own customers are not concerned by variations. However, it is always easier to sell the same pack and brand, time after time, than to introduce variety.

The value of packaging for marketing is not always realized by the seafood industry. In Japan, retail packs must be transparent or have a window so that the customer can see the product. In the U.S.A., attractive packaging sells many products, in and out of freezer cases.

PACKING STYLES: Product may be packed in blocks, in layer or shatter packs, be cello wrapped or I.Q.F. Each of these packing styles is covered separately below.

Block frozen: Product is placed in a form or carton, topped up with water and frozen in a plate freezer (all references to freezing can be followed up in the item Freezing processes). This technique is probably the one most often used for seafood. It gives good product protection and because cartons are solidly filled it makes transportation and storage easier, with less chance of damaging cartons or contents. The product is protected because a relatively small surface area is exposed and this is easy to cover with glaze.

Block-frozen product is the least convenient to use, because it is not possible to thaw less than a block, which is usually five pounds, so the end user must be able to handle this amount each time. Do not confuse block-frozen with fish blocks, which are the raw material for portions of all kinds. Block frozen product includes most shell-on shrimp, most peeled shrimp, most scallops, all king crab and snow crab meat and also cheap fish such as herring when frozen for bait or animal food.

Cello wraps: Fillets wrapped together in cellophane or polyethylene film. Each wrap is usually labelled with the type of fish, the packer and the brand. Six polywraps per 5lb box is standard. Cellos may also be unlabelled (blanks) to permit tray packing and labelling by the retail seller. In this case they are usually packed in 10lb inner boxes instead of fives with 12 cellos per 10lb inner box. Master cartons are a standard 50lbs (10/5 or 5/10lbs). Very occasionally cellos will be packed for retail sale in 2½lb inner boxes, with four cello wraps per innerbox. Outer cartons will usually conform to retail standard, that is one dozen packs, giving a master carton of 12/2½lbs, 30lbs total weight.

Weights of the individual cellos are irregular, approximately 14 ounces. The pack is cheap partly because these inner packs do not have to be weighed and also because the contents are ungraded. Fillets and pieces of widely differing sizes may be used within a wrap. If a size grade is quoted, it will usually be in terms of count per wrap. So, 2/4 count means that there are two, three or four pieces in each wrap, and these pieces may be of quite unequal size. There is no offer of nor requirement for uniformity of size in cello wrapped product.

Cellos are widely used for retail sale and may be displayed as they are packed, or they may instead be traypacked, with one, two or three cellos per tray. Cellos are also very popular with institutional caterers who are not particularly concerned with exact portion control. For example, they are ideal for a fast food fish-and-chip operation, where variations in the size of the portions is of little importance and can be compensated with more or fewer pieces on the plate.

Cellos are the cheapest pack available because the processor does not have to undertake the expensive grading and weighing processes needed for, say, 1lb retail boxes and can utilize small and irregular pieces that would not be acceptable in other packs. In recent years a better cello pack has appeared, using bags instead of wraps. The bags are printed in color. Fish is put into the bags, the tops rolled over and three bags placed on the bottom layer of the carton. A card divider is placed on top, then three more bags of fillets. This is quicker to pack than the traditional cellos and has found increasing markets among both foodservice and retail buyers.

The practice of packing blank cellos for retailer labelling has led to abuses. Although labels are packed in the top of each box with the cellos for the final seller to put on, there is nothing to prevent the seller substituting his own labels and calling cheap pollock expensive haddock, or labelling cheap hake as expensive ocean catfish. As with all substitutions, the best defenses are to know how the fish should look and taste and to deal with reputable suppliers.

To produce cellos, the processor wraps approximately fourteen ounces of fish, places six of these wraps in a five pound box, checks the weight, then freezes the box using a plate freezer which compresses the fish slightly, making the cellos fit together snugly and squaring the box (see Freezing processes). Cello fives with a bulge on top were probably frozen in a blast freezer, which does not compress the box. This is an inferior method for this type of pack, but should be perfectly good if it was done properly. Stacking the cartons can become difficult, however, since the bulging boxes do not fit snugly into the normal standard outer carton.

Some product other than fillets may be cello wrapped. Scallops and lobster meat are examples. This is generally done for retail sale. The packs are likely to be close to one pound each, packed 5 per inner box.

I.Q.F. – Individually Quick Frozen: Product frozen piece by piece, each piece glazed, then bagged and boxed. I.Q.F. product is particularly desirable for retail sale since it can be easily tray-packed or otherwise repackaged. It is also good for certain processing applications and for institutional use since a small amount can be taken from the box. Most I.Q.F. seafood can be cooked without prior defrosting.

The disadvantages of the I.Q.F. product are:

• Difficulty in stacking cartons, because they are not solidly filled. This creates problems in transportation and storage. Cartons damage much more easily than containers of block frozen product.

• Shorter storage life, partly because of the poorer protection from damaged boxes, but mainly because the I.Q.F. form exposes the whole surface of the product to the air and dehydration. Very little of the total surface area of the block frozen product is exposed. It is very important that I.Q.F. product be packed in thick inner bags or wraps and in solid cartons.

• Good glaze is essential but it is easy to overglaze and give short weight. Therefore it is particularly important with I.Q.F. product to determine that you are getting good weights. See Economic fraud in the seafood business.

The disadvantages are, for many users, outweighed by the advantages of minimum waste and convenience in use. Good I.Q.F. packs do not distort the product but retain the natural shape. This is also an advantage where the product is resold frozen.

All product has to be frozen very quickly and the newer technologies of nitrogen and carbon dioxide tunnels do a much better job than the traditional method of laying product on trays in a blast freezer. Product that has been frozen in a storage freezer is not acceptable.

Among products frequently sold in I.Q.F. form are:
- fillets; ideal if the user cannot forecast demand too closely, but less good for battering or breading since the glaze can prevent proper adherence of the covering. Also ideal for traypacking for retail sale since the fillet retains its natural shape.
- small dressed and whole fish such as whiting, herring and smelts.
- peeled shrimp for retail and institutional use.
- shell-on shrimp, especially for retail sale (see Shrimp for problems with this type of pack).
- crab products in shell. These are often brine frozen. Snow crab clusters, king crab legs and claws and similar product is always I.Q.F.
- large dressed or whole fish such as salmon, which are usually blast frozen, then glazed and individually bagged. Since this sort of fish is used one by one, I.Q.F. pack is a necessary convenience.
- scallops for retail sale. Scallops can absorb a great deal of glaze without it being obvious and this is a product to check with particular care. Block frozen scallops tend to give better net weights.
- miscellaneous product such as frogs legs, conch and soft-shell crabs.

Interleaved: Fillets packed in layers with a continuous sheet of polyethylene film between the layers. There is no significant difference between this and layer pack or shatterpack product (see below).

Layer packs: Product, usually fillets, put into a carton in layers with a sheet of polythene between each layer of product. This enables the fish to be separated easily while still frozen, so avoiding the waste of time and product involved in thawing blocks when less than the full block is required. Layer packs provide better product protection than I.Q.F. since less of the product is exposed to the air and the risk of dehydration is reduced. Layer packs are also easier to stack and handle in storage and transportation than I.Q.F. packs.

Layer packs are commonly 10lbs or 15lbs, or close metric equivalents. They are long flat boxes with not more than four layers of fillets. They are usually packed three or four to a master carton. Some layer packs are 14lbs, which is one English stone.

A good layer pack has the fillets placed so that their edges are barely touching. If the fish overlap at the edges or are packed too closely together, they become difficult to separate, so negating the whole idea of the layer pack. Poor quality packing of this nature is a frequent problem with supplies from certain countries.

A properly made layer pack is expensive to produce, so tends to contain carefully graded, good quality fish. The pack is used by institutions and caterers concerned with portion control and consistent grading: generally, layer packs will contain the best fish available to the packer and be the best handled and processed of the catch. (This is changing as I.Q.F. becomes more widespread).

Layer packs are plate frozen in the box, so the fish is slightly compressed and the individual fillets are pushed into rather odd shapes, which they lose when thawed or cooked. For this reason, layer pack product is not much used for retail trade, since the fillets, if traypacked in frozen state, look unattractive. Retailers selling "previously frozen" fish, however, will do well to consider using layer pack rather than I.Q.F. product.

Shatterpack: To separate fillets in a less than perfect layer pack, you may have to hurl the whole box at the concrete floor to break it apart. This explains the name. Some customers insist on shatterpacks, some on layerpacks. The two are the same for all practical purposes. There is also no significant difference between interleaved and layer pack products.

PADDLEFISH *Scientific name: Polyodon spathula:* Also called spoonbill catfish, though this is not an approved name. Paddlefish is a freshwater fish sometimes sold hot smoked. Its roe is used as a caviar substitute. Found throughout the central part of the U.S.A., it grows as large as 90lbs. It is not normally offered frozen.

PAINTED SWEETLIPS *Scientific name: Diagramma pictum:* A previous scientific name was *Plectorhynchus pictum.* This fish is also known as morwong and thicklip bream. It is an important food fish throughout the Indo-Pacific from the Red Sea and eastern Africa to northern and western Australia, the Philippines, the Sea of Japan and even into Polynesia. It grows to about 15lbs. Small quantities appear in New York's Fulton Fish Market from time to time. The fish has a growing local following. It is not highly regarded by Australians, who refer to it as a "Mother-in-law fish" implying that it is fit only to be given to that much-abused relation.

PALE KINGS: Also called tullies. King salmon close to spawning. Flesh color is very pale pink to grey and skin is heavily watermarked. It is cheap and fairly nasty.

PALOMETA: See Pompano.

PAN-READY: Pan fish. Any small fish prepared for the pan by removing head, guts and scales and trimming off the tail and fins. Croaker, blue runner, small flounder, butterfish, scup and other small fish are often prepared in this way, especially for retail sale. They should be I.Q.F. since block freezing results in deformation which detracts from their visual appeal.

Headless, dressed fish may be trimmed after freezing into pan-ready form, using a bandsaw to remove any yellowing or other signs of deterioration as well as the fins and belly flaps. Some pan-ready flounder prepared in this way can be surprisingly bad.

PARALYTIC SHELLFISH POISONING: P.S.P. See Seafood safety and Red tide.

PARASITES: Tapeworms (Cestodes), flukes (Trematodes) and roundworms (Nematodes).

• Tapeworm infection causes pernicious anemia, a deficiency of vitamin B_{12}. The tapeworm depletes this source of vitamin as well as other nutrients from the host's gut.

• Flukes are most common throughout Asia where eating raw fish, using human feces as fertilizer and drinking fecally contaminated water encourage the continuous cycle of the parasite. Importing live fish or shellfish which may contain flukes is prohibited.

• Roundworms appear occasionally at retail level. As revolting as they may seem, they are harmless.

These are worms or other unwanted creatures that may be found in or on the flesh of seafood. Southern scallops suffer from worms and swordfish may have enormous worms embedded in the sides. Cod and similar groundfish fillets are normally candled, that is, inspected with a light behind each piece before packing. Candling is a requirement of good packing-house procedure.

Most parasites are rendered invisible by cooking, so the main objection is aesthetic. Fish stocks which have been little exploited are likely to have parasites. As the fish are caught and the resource is reduced, the food supply of the fish improves, they become stronger and healthier and are better able to resist parasites. Labrador cod and Peru whiting were heavily infested when first exploited, but are now good. A previously clean resource can become infested rapidly if a seal population moves into the area. Seals carry codworms and are a major cause of infestation of fish. Do not assume that parasites will always be present on fish from a particular origin. This is one problem that time heals or at any rate that changes over time.

Parasites are a potential problem for the seafood industry because of the increasing consumption of raw fish in the forms of sushi and carpaccio. Although there have been very few cases notified to the Centers for Disease Control, the risk of picking up a parasitic worm from many species of raw fish is very real. Parasites are not restricted to inshore fish, as many believe. Even tunas often have parasites. The rapid spread of sushi restaurants has outstripped the supply of experienced sushi chefs trained to look for and remove parasites.

The solution is actually very easy: use only fish that has been frozen for at least a week. Frozen fish is widely used in Japan for sushi, partly to avoid parasite problems. Parasites will be killed in properly frozen fish held at 0°F. for one week. Americans tend to subscribe to the myth that unfrozen fish is "fresher" than frozen fish, making it difficult to sell them on the idea of using frozen product. However, anyone selling sushi should seriously consider the idea of using frozen fish. Give the idea extra consideration when renewing your liability insurance. For more information on the health aspects of parasites, see Seafood safety.

PASTEURIZING: Heating product sufficiently to kill most bacteria, but not enough to cook (or re-cook) the meat. Pasteurizing is used on blue crab meat, which can then be refrigerated for lengthy periods and on cooked langostinos which are then frozen. The texture of langos is definitely softened by pasteurizing. Cooked product is especially vulnerable to bacterial contamination, but pasteurizing is a technique that requires skill and care in its use, so is not widely applicable for many seafood origins.

PEELED FROM COUNTS: Applies to peeled shrimp. The labelled count is the size of the shell-on shrimp tails which were used to make the peeled product. The actual count (finished count) will generally be about one or two sizes smaller, depending on the thickness of the shell and the size and depth of the vein. See Shrimp.

PERCH: For freshwater perch, see Lake perch. For ocean perch (Atlantic and Pacific), see Rockfish.

PERIWINKLE *Scientific name: Littorina littorea:* A small sea snail, sold fresh (alive) in parts of the northeast. There is no market for frozen winkles in the U.S.A. The name is sometimes given to conch in certain localities.

PERMIT: See Pompano.

PETRALE SOLE: A west coast flatfish. See Flatfish.

PICKEREL: See Pike.

PICKING SECTIONS: Dungeness crabs, cut in half. See Crabs.

PICOWAVED: See Irradiation.

PIKE AND PICKEREL: Because of the confusion of many names, it is convenient to cover these different fish in one item. **Pike** *Scientific name: Stizostedion vitreum:* The fish called walleye or walleye pike in the U.S.A. is also known (but not with F.D.A. approval) as pike-perch, yellow pickerel and doré. It grows to about six pounds and commercial quantities come mainly from the lakes of northern Canada. The sauger (*Stizostedion canadense*) is very similar but slightly smaller. This is also known as sand pike, yellow walleye and again as doré.

There are other names as well, but these are the most frequently encountered. The names cover a number of different fish, all of which taste very similar and are commercially available from Canada. Most U.S. supplies are taken by sport fishermen.

Walleye gives a sweet, finely flaked fillet similar to sole in taste and usage. The flesh is lean and stores well when frozen.

Frozen Canadian pike is available dressed; headless and dressed; as fillets with skin on packed in blocks; I.Q.F. and in retail boxes; as steaks and also as minced fish blocks.

Similar fish, often called yellow pike, is imported as I.Q.F. skinless and boneless fillets from Holland, Turkey and Rumania. All these fish carry high prices and are particularly prized in the mid-section of the country.

A number of similar fish called variously pike, pickerel and other names are all available similarly, mostly from Canadian lakes.

Northern pike *Scientific name: Esox lucius:* This species is normally 5-10lbs.

Muskellunge *Scientific name: Esox masquinongy:* This is a much larger fish, sometimes reaching 30lbs. Its eating qualities are perhaps a little inferior to the walleye.

Pickerel *Scientific name: Esox americanus:* The pickerel is the smallest member of the pike family, seldom exceeding 12 inches in length. It is a popular gamefish.

PILCHARD: Small sardine-like fishes about six inches long. If available frozen they are used for bait and animal food. Pilchards are an important resource for the canning industry in many countries.

PILLOW PACK: A frozen pillow-shaped block, used for containing wet items such as chopped clams.

PINBONES: A row of small bones running horizontally along the mid-line of the sides of most fish from the nape for about one third the length of the fish. In most species, unless the fish is large, the pinbones soften sufficiently in cooking to become almost or completely undetectable. Pinbones can be removed by making a V-shaped cut at the nape end of the fillet, but since this removes meat from the thickest part, the yield is reduced and the cost of V-cut (boneless) fillets is therefore higher. In some species, like snapper, the pinbones and the belly flap are removed together with a single diagonal cut. See also Fillets.

PINK SALMON: Also called humpback. The smallest and most abundant Pacific salmon. See Salmon.

PLAICE: See Flatfish. European plaice is a superior flounder distinguished by red spots on the skin. It is occasionally offered either as plaice or as flounder in headless dressed or fillet forms. American plaice is more commonly called dab.

POGY: A name for menhaden. Do not confuse with porgy, which is scup.

POLLOCK: Also spelled pollack. There are many other names given to these fish, none of them approved for interstate trade, including Boston bluefish, (which is deliberately misleading), saithe, coalfish or coley (which are the British names) and walleye pollock (for the Pacific species).
Atlantic pollock *Scientific name: Pollachius virens:* Cod-like fish with rather darker flesh and more pronounced flavor than cod or haddock. It is always less expensive than cod and is sometimes substituted for it, especially in cello blanks. When cooked, the flesh is still not as white as that of cod or haddock. It is excellent for fish and chips or for baked and steamed preparations with heavy sauces.

Atlantic pollock comes from the U.S.A. and Canada and from Northern Europe (where there is an additional and very similar species, *Pollachius pollachius*). It is generally caught at about four pounds, though may grow as large as 35 pounds. Fillets are invariably packed skinless, but may be pinbone in or boneless. Cellos are frequently used. Layer pack pollock is usually graded in ounces, 4/8, 8/12, 12/16 and 16oz up.

Headless, dressed fish are sometimes available frozen for specialized markets.

Pacific pollock *Scientific name: Theragra chalcogramma:*
This is a similar fish but has whiter and softer flesh, much more
like Pacific cod. It is now widely used as an alternative to cod and
haddock. It is abundant throughout the north Pacific, where it is
by far the most important bottomfish species harvested. Much of
it is made into blocks and it has become the most important block
material on the U.S. market. Fillets are readily available from
domestic packers as well as from imports. They are normally
skinless and boneless, packed in 25lb polylined cartons with each
fillet individually wrapped. Grading is 1/2, 2/4, 4/8, 8/16 and 16/
32 ounces, with the middle sizes the most common.

Pollock is heavily fished for surimi production and is the most
important raw material for that industry. Pollock roe is an important item, sold to Taiwan and Japan.

Although the fish has proved its quality and value, some packers still like to offer it under misleading names. Snow cod and
snow scrod are among the less palatable. Pollock is a fine and
inexpensive fish in its own right. Paying more for it under a different name makes no sense.

POLYPHOSPHATE: See Dips.

POMFRET *Scientific names: Brama brama* (Atlantic) and
Brama japonica (Pacific): A sea bream, shaped like a large butterfish. Frozen fillets with skin on are sometimes available from
India and Thailand and may be used as an inexpensive alternative to pompano. The Pacific species is abundant off California. It
can be caught by high-seas gillnetting, but as there are few boats
equipped for this the catch is small. The species is potentially
important and produces good quality meat, similar to pompano.

POMPANO *Scientific name: Trachinotus carolinus:* Also
called Carolina pompano, Florida pompano and cobbler. This is a
thin silvery fish with a deep body. Pompano is a member of the
very large jack family. It has oily flesh and grows to about 2lbs
and eighteen inches. Pompano are excellent broiled, cooked in
pouches and baked. It is highly esteemed as a food fish. In Florida, where much of it is caught, it is an important commercial and
sport fish. Most of it is sold fresh. There is a similar Pacific
species.

Frozen pompano is available whole, packed 1/25lb and as raw or breaded fillets. Larger fish are poorer eating than the smaller ones. Although permit is a different fish, larger pompano are frequently called permit, which grow to much larger sizes.

The high price of pompano has attracted imports from various places, none with long-term success. There are well flavored pompanos from Ecuador and large permit from India. One problem is that worldwide there are so many different species that a description such as "Indian permit" could refer to many different fish and not identify precisely what you are offered. It is essential to look at samples and compare them with what you know to be regular domestic pompano. This is not a question of improper substitutions, but simply that the range of fish described by these names is so great that you have to see it yourself to determine if any particular one is acceptable.

The so-called African pompano (*Alectis ciliaris*) is another jack very similar to the pompano. It grows to over 30 pounds and is caught on both sides of the tropical and subtropical Atlantic. It is usable with and as regular pompano.

Permit *Scientific name: Trachinotus falcatus:* This fish is remarkably similar to the pompano. The only external difference is the number of rays on the second dorsal fin: the permit has one spine and 17 to 21 soft rays; the pompano has one shorter spine and 22-27 soft rays. (Rays are the rib-like rods in the fin.) To the layman, the only noticeable difference is that the pompano has a long dorsal fin which reaches almost to the back of the fish (unless, as happens frequently, this has broken off). Permit and pompano are found in the same waters.

While pompano seldom grow larger than five pounds, permit may reach 50lbs. Pompano, however, cost much more. Pompano gets a little drier and coarser as it gets larger, but is always considered better eating than permit. Commercially, the smaller fish of either type are offered as pompano and the larger fish are called permit.

Palometa *Scientific name: Trachinotus goodei:* This fish may be called pompano legally, as well as palometa. It is sometimes called longfin pompano. It is distinguished from the pompano by four dark gray bars vertically on each side and a very long dorsal spine which extends behind the tail when flattened against the fish. It is slightly thinner than the pompano, so yields a little less fillet meat. In practice, this fish may also be called permit.

PORGY *Scientific name: Stenotomus chrysops:* Also called scup. It is a sea bream. Do not confuse the name porgy with pogy, which is menhaden. Scup is a small bony fish, usually sold fresh in the U.S.A. Substantial quantities are frozen for export. It is caught off the Atlantic coast (it ranges from the Gulf of Maine to the Gulf of Mexico) and grows to about 1½lbs.

The fish is abundant off the east coast. The flesh is light and delicate but because of the many small bones it is quite difficult to eat. The scales must be removed soon after the fish is caught, or the skin becomes difficult to remove.

Sometimes called red porgy, *Pagrus pagrus* is a similar, smaller fish which is also thought to be abundant off the middle and south Atlantic coasts.

Small quantities of frozen scup are sold, chiefly in New York. Frozen product is usually intended for export but sold domestically from time to time. It is usually packed in 10kg or 20kg boxes. Quality of product packed for export is usually excellent because of the quality standards required by Japan, the main market. Avoid product frozen in large domestic boxes. This was probably intended for fresh sale and was frozen because it remained unsold for too long. If so, it is very poor product.

There are a number of similar fish with different market characteristics.

PORTIONS: Regularly shaped pieces of fish flesh, cut or formed from a fish block. Portions are frequently breaded or battered. Portions of all types are the largest single constituent of the seafood industry, using in excess of a million pounds a day of fish blocks.

Portions are nearly always sold as exact weights. Almost any size you need is available, from fish sticks under one ounce to portions of six ounces. Portions may be of any fish which is made into blocks – cod, pollock, whiting, haddock, flounder, Greenland turbot or any other white-fleshed fish. Many are also sold under the generic description "fish portions" which allows the processor to work to a price specification and use whatever is cheapest from time to time.

Portions are available in many shapes, as well as sizes. The standard rectangular shape, which is obviously easy to cut from a block, is joined by wedges and fillet shaped pieces of all descriptions.

Portions may be covered with breading or with a batter. Breaded types are generally raw but battered portions are pre-cooked to set the batter. There are numerous types, thicknesses and colors of breadings and batterings. Many processors use special coverings to make their product distinctive.

Some processors pack under U.S. inspection to enable them to put the Grade A shield on their product (see U.S. Grade Standards) This means that their product conforms to the specifications in Title 50 of the Code of Federal Regulations. Product without the Grade A marking is not necessarily inferior. Some packers have their own standards which in many cases are at least as high as the Federal requirements. Protection of a brand name identity and reputation is of the utmost importance in the portion business.

There are some scallop portions cut from blocks of scallops or scallop pieces. Portions made of minced crabmeat and minced shrimp are also available.

For both institutional and retail use, irregular portions are often acceptable. Many irregulars fail the rigorous tests required by the individual processor, but may nonetheless be perfectly wholesome and usable. For example, small gaps in breading or battering may render portions useless for deep-fat frying, but entirely usable for domestic consumption. Such items can be bought very cheaply, usually in bulk packs of six or ten pounds and traypacked for retail sale. Other irregulars may be slightly misshapen, undersized or oversized, unevenly coated, or have other minor defects that preclude the processor from packing them under his brand name, but leave them perfectly good and wholesome if appropriately used. Irregulars are always sold on detailed descriptions and against samples.

PORTION PACK: Product graded so that all pieces in a package are of specified weight or within a specified range of weights. For example, steaks may be graded 4/6oz, or exact weight 4oz, 5oz and 6oz. Either of these is a portion pack. A random pack has a range of sizes mixed together in one package.

POTASSIUM PYROPHOSPHATE: See Dips.

POUT: See Ocean pout.

POUTASSOU: See Blue whiting.

P.P.M.: Parts per million. Used as a measurement of mercury and other contaminants in foods.

PRAWN: Shrimp. The word is used to describe quite different types of shrimp. Usage varies around the world. The following is from *An Illustrated Guide to Shrimp of the World* (Osprey Books, 1987):

> In the United Kingdom, prawns tend to be larger than shrimp. Originally, *Crangon crangon*, the common shrimp, was called "shrimp" and *Palaemon serratus*, the common prawn, was called "prawn." However, both names are applied to many other species. "Dublin Bay prawn" is even used to describe *Nephrops norvegicus*, which is a langoustine or Norway lobster. The only consistent pattern in British usage is that "prawn" is not used for the very small species. The Oxford dictionary defines prawn as "larger than shrimp."
>
> In the United States, prawn is sometimes used on restaurant menus in some areas to mean large shrimp, and in other places to mean small shrimp. Norwegian producers have been promoting northern shrimp, *Pandalus borealis*, as prawns. Webster's Dictionary describes prawn as "a small edible crustacean of the shrimp family." In Bengal and Bangladesh, the word prawn is often used to label the large freshwater shrimp from the region's huge estuaries. Australians call their extensive shrimp resources "prawns." In South Africa, larger animals are called prawns and smaller ones shrimp. In Australia and New Zealand, crangonids are called shrimps and palaemonid and penaeids are called prawns, irrespective of size.
>
> The only point on which everyone can surely agree is that the use of the word "prawn" in the English language is confusing and unclear. It should be avoided. Anyone involved in using English in international trading of

shrimp or prawns will do better to ignore the term "prawn" and stick to "shrimp."

For canned shrimp, the F.D.A. states in Title 21 of the Federal Code:

> The name of the food is "Shrimp" or "shrimps." The word "prawns" may appear on the label in parentheses immediately after the name "shrimp" or "shrimps" if the shrimp are of large or extra large size as designated...

Clearly, the F.D.A. regards prawns as larger shrimp. The confusions are such that use of the word prawn should be avoided wherever possible.

PRECOOKED: A portion or other product which is cooked or partially cooked, so requires only heating or minimal cooking for serving. See Portions.

P.S.P.: Paralytic shellfish poisoning. See Seafood safety and Red tide.

P.U.D.: Shrimp that is peeled but not deveined; peeled-only shrimp.

PUFFER *Scientific name: Sphoeroides spp.:* These small fish are usually marketed as sea squab. Other names are globefish and blowfish. The best known name is the Japanese, fugu. Puffers are poisonous: their internal organs and viscera can be deadly. Provided the fish is properly prepared, it is supposed to be non-toxic. Nevertheless, Japanese gourmets die from puffer poisoning every year, despite stringent licensing and training of fugu chefs. The F.D.A. refuses to allow importation of Japanese puffer.

The Atlantic northern puffer is said to be fairly non-toxic. Cleaned, skinned butterfly fillets are sometimes sold in fishmarkets.

PULPO: See Octopus.

PURIFICATION OF SHELLFISH: See Depuration.

QUAHOG: Hard-shell east coast clam. See Clams.

QUEEN CRAB: See Snow crab under Crabs.

QUEEN SCALLOP: Types of bay scallops from Australia and Great Britain. See Scallops.

QUINAULT: An Indian word for salmon. See Salmon.

QUINNAT: New Zealand name for king salmon, which was transplanted from the U.S.A. in the nineteenth century. A few of these fish still survive and there is currently an expanding program to increase the resource and develop it for commercial purposes. Salmon is also being farmed in New Zealand. Salmon are not found naturally in the southern hemisphere.

RAJAFISH: See Skate.

RANCIDITY: Oxidation. The oxidation of the natural oil in the fish, making the fish unpalatable. Rancidity is obviously more of a problem with oily fish than with lean fish. It is easily detectable by smelling the fish – even when frozen hard, the flesh will still emit a rancid odor. Also, the oxidized oil on the surface of the fish turns yellow, especially around the edges of the belly flaps where the fish was cut as well as in the body cavity. This yellowing is instantly recognizable.

On some fish, of which salmon is an important example, drops of oil ooze through the skin making "rust spots" in or on the glaze. This is a symptom of improper storage – if temperatures in the freezer fluctuate, the cells of the flesh expand and contract and oil is squeezed to the surface where it goes rancid in contact with the oxygen in the air.

Freezing slows oxidation, but does not prevent it and fluctuations in storage temperatures, as mentioned, can make matters worse. Note that these fluctuations are at temperatures below freezing. The fish appears to be hard frozen at all times. Nevertheless, slight changes in temperature affect it and considerably reduce the storage life of the product.

RANDOM PACK: Either:
- Ungraded product, all sizes in the same pack without regard to size grading; or
- Graded product in boxes containing varied weights. This makes life easy for the packer, but makes the distributor's inventory control and billing problems unnecessarily complicated.

RATPACKING: Putting the good, well prepared product on top, the inferior product underneath.

RAYS: See Skate.

RECALL: If unfit product is found in distribution, for example where a case of food poisoning is traced to a particular food, the Food and Drug Administration (F.D.A.) can request the recall of every remaining piece from that batch. The product is traced from the importer or packer through the distribution chain to each end user and must be located, separated from other batches and held for the F.D.A.'s inspection or disposal. Although the F.D.A. does not have power to order a recall, their requests are treated very seriously. If a recall request is refused, the F.D.A. can seek court action to enforce the procedure.

Recalls are rare, but very expensive. Class One recalls apply to product which may cause death or serious health problems. A case of botulism poisoning traced to a food, or accidental mislabelling of a powerful drug, are examples of possible Class One recalls. Class Two recalls apply if there is a possible health problem; Class Three recalls apply to almost any other infringement of the Pure Food and Drug laws, including false or incorrect labelling.

The recalls that hit the headlines are the Class One type. Often, publicity is sought for these if product has already reached some consumers: the publicity can help to secure the return of the product.

Whatever the recall type, make sure that sales invoices identify product by lot numbers and that you maintain internal records showing which lots were shipped to which customers. With this information you can trace back with the least amount of effort. Also check that your product liability insurance covers the identifiable costs of a recall.

RECONDITIONING: See Irradiation.

REDFISH *Scientific name: Sciaenops ocellatus:* Also called red drum. Incorrectly called channel bass and red bass. A large lean fish, growing sometimes as large as 70lbs, caught mainly inshore in the Gulf of Mexico and also on the Atlantic coast of Florida. Mostly sold fresh, some redfish is filleted and sold frozen in 10lb boxes, usually I.Q.F.

Because of declining catches, most states have either banned commercial fishing for redfish or reserved the fish for sportfishermen. Such action came at the time when "blackened redfish" was becoming the country's most fashionable seafood preparation. Importers have searched for similar fish around the world, mostly without success. Aquaculture of redfish is beginning, in response to the high price and unmet demand for the fish.

Redfish is also a name used in Europe for ocean perch. See Rockfish.

RED ROCK LOBSTER *Scientific name: Linuparus trigonus:* A rock lobster with a deep red color which is imported from Japan. Both tails and meat are graded in 2oz steps from 2/4oz up to 10/12oz. Sizes in the middle of this range are preferred.

Generally, red rock products are more expensive than other warm water lobster tails. They have a small but devoted market following, especially with some Chinese restaurants. Although the meat is normally produced from cracked or discolored tails, the quality of red rock product from Japan is high, with only an occasional incidence of black spot (melanosis). Watch out for reglazed and repacked product.

RED SALMON: Sockeye. See Salmon.

RED SNAPPER: See Snapper.

RED TIDE: A group of planktons which cause paralytic shellfish poisoning (P.S.P.). At certain times, a particular algae eaten by clams, mussels and oysters multiplies very rapidly and is visible as a reddish carpet below the surface of the sea. This is "red tide".

The plankton is not harmful to the shellfish, but leaves a toxin in them that causes a severe poisoning reaction in humans who eat the shellfish. There is no antidote to this poison and the only preventive measure possible is to avoid the contaminated shellfish, which cleanse themselves very quickly once the algal "bloom" passes.

State authorities on both Atlantic and Pacific Coasts monitor very carefully for signs of P.S.P. and close shellfishing areas as soon as it is suspected. Because of this program, P.S.P. is not a problem for the industry. You must, of course, ensure that all your shellfish come only from shippers approved under the Shellfish Sanitation Program. See also Seafood safety and Shellfish Sanitation.

REDUCTION: Use of fish or fish wastes for fish meal or oil.

REJECTION AND REJECTION INSURANCE: All imported foodstuffs are subject to inspection by the Food and Drug Administration. Imported product may not be sold in the U.S.A. without F.D.A. approval.

The F.D.A. samples imports on a random basis qualified by its experience. Obviously it is more sensible to sample product with a history of being unfit. In extreme cases, where the experience has been very bad, the F.D.A. will "blocklist" a particularly type of product, a specific origin, or even the product of an individual overseas packer. If a shipment comes under a blocklisted category the import is automatically detained until the importer proves that it conforms to required sanitary and other standards, by means of analyses performed by a recognized U.S. laboratory.

Product that the F.D.A. does not wish to sample enters the U.S. on a "green ticket" which is the color of the notice telling the importer that he "may proceed" with selling the goods.

For an importer, the risk of rejection is substantial, since he is usually liable to pay for goods when they are shipped from the producing country. Rejected product normally must be re-exported and is saleable at only a fraction of its original cost. Even if rejection is for a reason that can be corrected – that is the product can be brought "into compliance" with the laws – the cost of the necessary reconditioning work is always high. This might be cooking in the case of raw shrimp rejected for salmonella contamination, or repacking product found to be short weight or relabelling product which fails to list ingredients correctly. With such exceptions, rejected product has to be removed from the country promptly and usually only can be sold to overseas customers at reduced prices.

To reduce losses from rejections, importers began insuring against this risk. Underwriters soon learned not to insure product unless they first inspected the packer's plant to be reasonably sure that sanitary conditions there would mean the production of wholesome product. Since insurance without plant inspection is impossible, the process has resulted in improved quality of imported supplies.

Even in the best run plant, there is always a chance of some contamination, but the risk is much higher if the plant is unsanitary. Insurance premiums reflect the experience of the underwriters with particular plants. Insurance is restricted to rejection only for reasons connected with unwholesomeness of the product. If the product is packed short weight, this was obviously a deliberate decision by the packer and not an accidental, insurable risk.

The F.D.A. inspection process has much to commend it, but importers complain because of its random effect. This would be cured if all import shipments were routinely examined, as is done in Canada. However, the present system gives good protection to the consumer and costs far less than total inspection.

Microbiological standards have been established for certain products, such as fish sticks, fish cakes and crab cakes. Standards for foods in general are not established: all imported foodstuffs must conform to the Food, Drug and Cosmetic Act which requires that they be prepared, packed and held under sanitary conditions; that the food itself be safe, clean and wholesome, and that its labelling be truthful and informative. Title 21 of the Code of Federal Regulations, Part 110 defines good manufacturing practices and these form the basis for the F.D.A.'s examination of product.

The F.D.A. will train personnel and assist foreign plants in designing and operating their facilities to upgrade product for sale to the U.S.A.

For further information, see items Defect action levels and Inspection.

RELEASE: Instruction to a warehouse to permit named customer or carrier to collect product. Title passes upon pick-up. See Delivery terms.

RETAIL FILLET PACKS: Apart from cellos, the most popular retail consumer pack for fillets is the familiar rectangular box, overwrapped in printed paper, containing 1lb of product. These are packed 12 per case and are available for most popular fillets, with packers' labels, distributors' labels and for own label use.

Contents of 1lb packs may be fillets cut from blocks, or fillets specially packed into the carton, or interleaved fillets. Specifications can be adapted to individual requirements. Because the overwrap paper is expensive to produce and print, 1lb packs normally require large production runs to be economical. If sales are sufficient to justify their use, they are a much more attractive and saleable pack than a cello wrap in a tray.

REX SOLE: A Pacific coast flatfish. See Flatfish.

RIGOR MORTIS: Stiffening of a body after death. Fillets cut before or during rigor may tear apart. For a full discussion, see Gaping.

RIPE FISH: Fish, containing roe or milt, about to spawn. Because much of the fish's reserves are put into the production of roe, the flesh of ripe fish is soft and poor and oil content is low.

RIVER HERRING: See Alewife.

ROCK COD: Name sometimes given to Rockfishes.

ROCKFISH: Also called redfish, ocean perch, perch, Pacific snapper, rock cod and many other names. See below for which names are legal. These names cover a variety of different fish most of which have red skin. Ocean perch is often sold as a substitute for lake perch. North Atlantic and Pacific product differ and should be considered as separate items. Striped bass is called rockfish in some areas.

North Atlantic ocean perch *Scientific name: Sebastes marinus:* A slow-growing deepwater fish reaching eight pounds, but usually much smaller. It is called redfish in Britain, perch or ocean perch in the U.S.A. and Canada. Although this is the main species, there are two others which co-exist with it and are so similar that the differences require a trained scientist to distinguish them: *Sebastes mentella* is the deepwater redfish; *Sebastes fasciatus* is the Labrador redfish. These species are always filleted before freezing and are available in the following forms:

- 10/5 cellos, skin on. Grading is usually count per wrap, from 2/4, the largest, down to 8/10, the smallest normally found. Smaller sizes, that is larger counts, are preferred.
- 10lb and 15lb layer packs, skin on, usually graded in ounces, though some packers retain the older style of counts per pound. This is confusing so make sure you know what you are getting.
- I.Q.F. skin on fillets, in 4/10lb or 1/25lb boxes. Grades may be very precise, such as 1½ to 2oz and fish so graded is used for breading.
- Perch blocks, usually skin on. The blocks are thawed and the fillets used individually.

Some skinless perch is offered, but since the main feature of perch is its attractive skin, the market for skinless product, which may be packed in any of the above forms, is small and erratic.

North Atlantic ocean perch comes from the U.S., Canada, Germany, Norway and Iceland. Fresh Icelandic perch is available by air freight. This is sold in the north-east as red snapper. Since the color of perch skin fades with time, it is probable that slow handling, rather than the basic nature of the fish, accounts for the skin color problem traditionally associated with some perch.

A great deal of perch is breaded and sold as "breaded perch" which confuses buyers into thinking they are getting the much more expensive lake perch.

Pacific rockfish: A large group of fish found the length of the west coast. The naming and identification of this group has become extremely complex. The next table shows the species and the names permitted by the F.D.A. for interstate commerce. In general, they can all be called rockfish. The only one that may be called "Pacific ocean perch" is *Sebastes alutus*.

Rockfish: Common Name and Market Name

Market name	Common name	Scientific name	Location
Perch, ocean	Deepwater, redfish	*Sebastes mentella*	A
Perch, ocean	Ocean perch, Pacific	*Sebastes alutus*	P
Perch, ocean	Redfish, Labrador	*Sebastes fasciatus*	A
Perch, ocean	Redfish, Norway	*Sebastes viviparus*	A
Perch, ocean	Redfish/ocean perch	*Sebastes marinus*	A
Rockfish	Bocaccio	*Sebastes paucispinis*	P
Rockfish	Chilipepper	*Sebastes goodei*	P
Rockfish	Cowcod	*Sebastes levis*	P
Rockfish	Rockfish	*Helicolenus papillosus*	P
Rockfish	Rockfish, Mexican	*Sebastes macdonaldi*	P
Rockfish	Rockfish, Puget Sound	*Sebastes emphaeus*	P
Rockfish	Rockfish, aurora	*Sebastes aurora*	P
Rockfish	Rockfish, bank	*Sebastes rufus*	P
Rockfish	Rockfish, black	*Sebastes melanops*	P
Rockfish	Rockfish, black & yellow	*Sebastes chrysomelas*	P
Rockfish	Rockfish, blackgill	*Sebastes melanostomus*	P
Rockfish	Rockfish, blue	*Sebastes mystinus*	P
Rockfish	Rockfish, bronzespotted	*Sebastes gilli*	P
Rockfish	Rockfish, brown	*Sebastes auriculatus*	P
Rockfish	Rockfish, calico	*Sebastes dalli*	P
Rockfish	Rockfish, canary	*Sebastes pinniger*	P
Rockfish	Rockfish, chameleon	*Sebastes phillipsi*	P
Rockfish	Rockfish, china	*Sebastes nebulosus*	P
Rockfish	Rockfish, copper	*Sebastes caurinus*	P
Rockfish	Rockfish, darkblotched	*Sebastes crameri*	P
Rockfish	Rockfish, dusky	*Sebastes ciliatus*	P
Rockfish	Rockfish, dwarf-red	*Sebastes rufinanus*	P
Rockfish	Rockfish, flag	*Sebastes rubrivinctus*	P
Rockfish	Rockfish, freckled	*Sebastes lentiginosus*	P
Rockfish	Rockfish, gopher	*Sebastes carnatus*	P
Rockfish	Rockfish, grass	*Sebastes rastrelliger*	P
Rockfish	Rockfish, greenblotched	*Sebastes rosenblatti*	P
Rockfish	Rockfish, greenspotted	*Sebastes chlorostictus*	P
Rockfish	Rockfish, greenstriped	*Sebastes elongatus*	P
Rockfish	Rockfish, halfbanded	*Sebastes semicinctus*	P
Rockfish	Rockfish, honeycomb	*Sebastes umbrosus*	P

Market name	Common name	Scientific name	Location
Rockfish	Rockfish, kelp	*Sebastes atrovirens*	P
Rockfish	Rockfish, northern	*Sebastes polyspinis*	P
Rockfish	Rockfish, olive	*Sebastes serranoides*	P
Rockfish	Rockfish, pink	*Sebastes eos*	P
Rockfish	Rockfish, pinkrose	*Sebastes simulator*	P
Rockfish	Rockfish, pygmy	*Sebastes wilsoni*	P
Rockfish	Rockfish, quillback	*Sebastes maliger*	P
Rockfish	Rockfish, red	*Scorpaena cardinalis*	P
Rockfish	Rockfish, redbanded	*Sebastes babcocki*	P
Rockfish	Rockfish, redstripe	*Sebastes proriger*	P
Rockfish	Rockfish, rosethorn	*Sebastes helvomaculatus*	P
Rockfish	Rockfish, rosy	*Sebastes rosaceus*	P
Rockfish	Rockfish, rougheye	*Sebastes aleutianus*	P
Rockfish	Rockfish, semaphore	*Sebastes melanosema*	P
Rockfish	Rockfish, sharpchin	*Sebastes zacentrus*	P
Rockfish	Rockfish, shortbelly	*Sebastes jordani*	P
Rockfish	Rockfish, shortraker	*Sebastes borealis*	P
Rockfish	Rockfish, silvergray	*Sebastes brevispinis*	P
Rockfish	Rockfish, speckled	*Sebastes ovalis*	P
Rockfish	Rockfish, splitnose	*Sebastes diploproa*	P
Rockfish	Rockfish, squarespot	*Sebastes hopkinsi*	P
Rockfish	Rockfish, starry	*Sebastes constellatus*	P
Rockfish	Rockfish, stripetail	*Sebastes saxicola*	P
Rockfish	Rockfish, swordspine	*Sebastes ensifer*	P
Rockfish	Rockfish, tiger	*Sebastes nigrocinctus*	P
Rockfish	Rockfish, vermillion	*Sebastes miniatus*	P
Rockfish	Rockfish, widow	*Sebastes entomelas*	P
Rockfish	Rockfish, yelloweye	*Sebastes ruberrimus*	P
Rockfish	Rockfish, yellowmouth	*Sebastes reedi*	P
Rockfish	Rockfish, yellowtail	*Sebastes flavidus*	P
Rockfish	Treefish	*Sebastes serriceps*	P
Rosefish	Rosefish, blackbelly	*Helicolenus dactylopterus*	A
Scorpionfish	Scorpionfish, orange	*Scorpaena scrofa*	A
Thornyhead	Thornyhead, longspine	*Sebastolobus altivelis*	P
Thornyhead	Thornyhead, shortspine	*Sebastolobus alascanus*	P

Locations: A = Atlantic   P = Indo-Pacific   F = Freshwater
Source: F.D.A.

However, California has its own rules and permits twelve species to be labelled and sold as "Pacific red snapper." These include the rose rockfish, the splitnose rockfish and the chilipepper rockfish. Pacific red snapper is also permitted as a name in Oregon and Washington. Because the name is not approved for interstate trade, however, it should not be used on fish transported between these states, although it is legal locally in each of them.

Of course, the rockfishes are quite unlike genuine red snapper.

To compound the confusion, marketers also use other names for rockfish. Rock cod is quite common in both Canada and the U.S.A. Channel rockfish is used also. Generally, the redskinned species are sold as Pacific red snapper or perch and the brown skinned species are skinned and sold as rock cod.

Fillets of the redskinned fish are highly marketable throughout the country. Usual pack is I.Q.F. skin on fillets in 25lb or 10lb boxes. Fillets should be individually wrapped. Grading is usually in two ounce steps, 2/4, 4/6 and 6/8oz. Domestic, Canadian and Japanese origins are essentially similar in quality and price and sell at around the same level as I.Q.F. Canadian Atlantic ocean perch.

Rockfish quality varies. Skin should be taut and shiny. Loose skin is a sign of product that was stale before it was frozen. Line-caught fish can be very good, provided the fish is brought to the boat alive so it can be bled. Most rockfish, though, are dead when landed.

Once rockfish are filleted it is almost impossible to distinguish between species without laboratory tests such as iso-electric focussing.

ROCK LOBSTER: See Lobster.

ROCK SALMON: Name formerly used in the UK for dogfish.

ROCK SHRIMP *Scientific name: Sicyonia brevirostris:* A shrimp with a particularly thick, hard shell, caught in the Gulf of Mexico from the Yucatan and around the Florida Atlantic coast northwards through the Carolinas. Most U.S. supplies come from the Gulf coast of Florida and it is often called "Florida rock shrimp" even if imported from Mexico. A closely related species, *Sicyonia ingentis*, is fished in small quantities off California and

Baja California. It is known locally as "ridgeback prawn."

Rock shrimp tastes rather like lobster, with firm white flesh when cooked. The shell is so thick that a raw tail will yield only about 50 percent meat. Sizes range from 21/25 to 70/80 count per pound. Grading is exactly the same as for regular shrimp.

Available packs include raw whole tails, split and deveined tails, split peeled and deveined tails and tail-on configurations like regular shrimp. Packs are 4lb and 5lb blocks, or 1lb and 2lb I.Q.F. packs for retail use. Breaded rock shrimp packed in 2½lb boxes is also available.

This market has remained small, despite the clear appeal of the product and its cheap price, because of the difficulty of large scale peeling of the tails. Peeling machinery developed in the last few years is helping to put more product on the market. Rock shrimp are an excellent retail item, since the price and flavor are most attractive and the problem of peeling them is less serious for retail customers, who are more willing to use split tails. Breeders like to use them when peeled product is available because they are comparatively inexpensive and well flavored.

Rock shrimp should have clean white or transparent flesh, with no discoloration. Shell color varies from pink to grayish-brown, often with some green tint on the back of the shell. All these colors are normal and are not a sign of deterioration. However, rock shrimp deteriorate rapidly so must be handled promptly.

ROE: Fish eggs, the female gonads. Most fish species grow their eggs in a sac in the lower part of the abdomen. When ripe, that is when the eggs are about to be laid, the roe can amount to one third of the weight of the fish. Some fish roe is very valuable. Sturgeon roe is the most valuable. See Caviar. Others follow in alphabetical order.

Cod roe is not much seen in the U.S. but is a regular part of northern European cuisine. It is often smoked and can be frozen successfully in this form.

Herring roe from both Atlantic and Pacific coasts is salted and frozen for the Japanese market. Atlantic herring roe and milt are both sold frozen in various European countries. Japanese buyers often prefer the female fish frozen whole so that the preparation of the roe product can be done closer to the market. Machines have been devised to distinguish between male and female herring for this trade.

A variation of the sale of herring roe to Japan is the "kelp herring" from Alaska, which is a small, highly specialized and very valuable fishery, with a short season lasting only hours. The roe is collected with the kelp seaweed to which it is fastened just after it is spawned by the fish. The Japanese market pays a very high price for this item.

Mullet roe from the Gulf and South Atlantic areas is sold mainly to Taiwan and other areas with Chinese culture. See Mullet. Mullet roe is also used in the eastern Mediterranean.

Pollock roe from the Pacific pollock is prized in Japan, salted.

Salmon roe is the basis of Japanese sujiko and in some years is a vital part of the west coast salmon fishery. When the eggs are salted and frozen for sale in Japan, they may be worth more than the fish that contained them. This market is highly volatile and has recently been adversely affected by warnings of health risks from high-salt foods.

Salmon eggs are used in the U.S.A. as bait by anglers. This is an expensive product, using eggs that are dyed and packed in small jars. It cannot be processed in frozen form without bursting the eggs. Some "salmon caviar" is also sold (fresh, salted) in the U.S.A.

Scallop roe is half-moon shaped, red or brown, and sometimes seen attached to the scallop muscle. It is not eaten in the U.S.A. and many buyers will reject scallops with roe attached as unfit. In Europe the scallop roe is a delicacy, and larger shellfish are handshucked to ensure that the roe remains attached and intact.

Sea urchin roe is the only edible part of the sea urchin and is a very valuable product in fresh form. Frozen sea urchin roe is inferior in quality and price to fresh but is occasionally available.

Shad roe is one of the few roes eaten in the U.S.A. and one that can be frozen if care is taken. Shad are available from both coasts. Roes are normally sold in natural pairs, that is, intact as removed from the fish. It is important that the sac is not torn or broken in any way. Because of the very high oil content, frozen shad roe has a very short shelf life.

Whitefish roe is sold as an inexpensive and mild tasting alternative to caviar.

ROUGHY: See Orange roughy.

ROUND FISH: Whole fish, complete with viscera.

SABLEFISH *Scientific name: Anoplopoma fimbria:* The only officially approved name for this species in interstate trade is sablefish, but it is widely known along the west coast as black cod. In California it is sometimes called butterfish, although it is totally unlike the real butterfish. (The name butterfish appears to be related to the shiny, buttery appearance of the fresh fillets).

Sablefish average about eight pounds and range between two pounds and twelve pounds. They are caught the entire length of the Pacific coast, from Alaska to California. Sable has dark grey to black skin with a very distinctive furry texture. The flesh is fairly oily, but when cooked is pearly white with large flakes and a flavor close to that of salmon. Most sablefish sold in the U.S.A. is smoked, though fillets are eaten in many restaurants on the west coast and are becoming more common in retail outlets. Smoked sable is offered as sides (called "sable plate" on the east coast) and chunks.

The market is heavily influenced by Japan, which buys headless dressed fish, preferring those over 5lb (when available), and generally refusing anything under 2½lbs. For Japan the fish is usually packed in 15kg trays, semidressed (that is napes on) and graded in pounds 2/3, 3/4, 4/5, 5/7 and 7-up. Japan buys most of the world catch (the U.S.A. is the largest producer). Smokers in the U.S. have similar preferences for size. Sable may be I.Q.F., individually wrapped, or frozen in small glazed blocks, laid head to tail in the style used for the Japanese market.

Fillets are generally pinbone-in, skin-on. The fish is caught on lines, in pots and by trawling. Although the line-caught fish is traditionally preferred, the frozen-at-sea trawled fish is also very good. Sable has a lot of oil and spoils quickly, so must be handled with speed and care.

SAINT PETER'S FISH: See St. Peter's fish.

SAITHE: See Pollock.

SALAD MEAT: Crab body meat chunks frozen in blocks. See King crab and Snow crab under Crabs.

SALMON: The name refers to seven different species of anadromous fish (all start their lives in fresh water and travel into the oceans to grow). One species is from the Atlantic, the others from the Pacific. True salmon are only found naturally in the northern hemisphere. Salmon farming is now big business. Atlantic salmon are farmed in the Pacific Ocean and several species are now regularly sold from the southern hemisphere. This is an important and rapidly changing piece of the seafood business.

The life cycle of the salmon, much televised and dramatized in glossy magazines, is important to the fish buyer because salmon are mostly caught on their way to or up their home river when they are intending to spawn. The fish stop feeding when they leave the sea and enter fresh water. Consequently the energy the fish use to swim up the river is all taken from their stored fat. A salmon caught in the ocean will be fat, silver skinned and moist to eat. The same salmon taken hundreds of miles up river, just before spawning, will have pale, soft watery flesh, black or red skin and will be almost inedible. In between are many grades of salmon which the buyer has to learn to recognize and differentiate.

There are landlocked populations of several salmon species in large American and Canadian lakes. These fish are not available in commercial quantities.

Salmon are distinguished in the market by species and by different designations given as they get further from the sea. There are also some differences among fish caught in different areas. There is a great deal of myth and prejudice – or tradition if you prefer – in the salmon trade, but all of it is based on the unique life cycle and habits of the salmon and the adaptations man has made to exploit these fish.

Farmed salmon is increasingly important. Norway started the industry and developed the basic techniques. Some two dozen countries now profess to be farming salmon. Perhaps half of these have product to sell. There is no doubt that farmed salmon will be increasingly available – and possibly less expensive – as the 1990s progress. Atlantic salmon is the major farmed species, but coho, kings and chums are also grown.

Pacific salmon, of which there are five main species, come from California and the whole length of the western North American coastline around Alaska to the U.S.S.R., Japan, Korea and northern China. (The different species have different ranges, as will be indicated in the section on each). Man has destroyed fewer of the habitats of the Pacific salmon than of the Atlantic species and has also successfully restored and restocked many rivers with fish – a process which has barely begun with the Atlantic fish.

Atlantic salmon, *Scientific name: Salmo salar,* is one single species. It starts its life in rivers all around the North Atlantic from the middle of the U.S.A. up around Canada, Greenland, Iceland, the United Kingdom, Norway and down the European coastline to Spain and Portugal. There probably was a time when salmon lived in every river of the North Atlantic but pollution and man-made obstructions to the passage of the fish to their spawning grounds have greatly reduced the number of rivers in which salmon now live.

The fish is sometimes called eastern salmon in the U.S.A. and various origin names may also qualify it, such as Newfoundland salmon, Icelandic salmon or Norwegian salmon. All of them are the same species of fish. Wild Atlantic salmon when caught weigh from 3lbs upwards. Fish of 20-30lbs are not uncommon. In Norway the fish is farmed to 60lbs. For most commercial uses, fish of 6-12lbs are preferred.

The flesh of the Atlantic salmon is deep pink to red, the skin color is silver and distinguished by small black crosses. The taste is delicate and the fish is favored by many smokers for the quality of product it allows.

Steelhead *Scientific name: Oncorhynchus mykiss/Salmo gairdneri:* Also called steelie, salmon trout and sea trout. The A.F.S. changed the scientific name to *O. mykiss* at the beginning of 1989. This is the same species as freshwater rainbow trout, but an anadromous variety. It is called steelhead trout in the U.S.A. and steelhead salmon in Canada. In terms of marketability, however, it is an Atlantic salmon living in the Pacific. Along parts of the Pacific coast, especially in Canada, rainbow trout have developed a life cycle similar to that of salmon, living in the ocean and returning to rivers to spawn. Steelhead is almost indistinguishable from Atlantic salmon in size, appearance and taste.

In western Europe, you may be offered sea trout, which is an anadromous rainbow just like steelhead. In the U.S.A. sea trout refers to a totally different selection of white-fleshed fish, described under Sea trout.

239

Only small quantities of steelhead are frozen, but it is one of the best salmons, worth trying when available.

Sockeye *Scientific name: Oncorhynchus nerka:* Also called red salmon, blueback and quinault. A fine silver fish with deep red meat ranging from 3lbs to 8lbs, usually graded headless and dressed at 3/5lbs and 5/8lbs. It is caught from Washington north to Alaska. Much of the catch is canned as red or blueback salmon, or frozen in special packs for the Japanese market.

Sockeye is a little small for economical steaking. It has a limited market in frozen headless and dressed form, but if delicately cooked it is very fine eating and the deep color makes it an attractive fish on retail display. Northwest smokers use a lot of sockeye for hot-smoking. European smokers prefer kings and Atlantic salmon for their traditional smoked salmon methods.

King salmon *Scientific name: Oncorhynchus tshawytscha:* Also called chinook, spring, tyee and blackmouth. The last two names are not officially recognized. Kings are the largest of the Pacific salmon, averaging 20lbs and ranging commercially from 4lbs up to 30lbs. The usual grading for kings, headless and dressed, is 4/7lbs, 7/11lbs, 11/18lbs and 18lbs up. Kings are landed from California to Canada, Alaska to Asia.

Kings run at different times in different areas. Some places have spring runs and others fall or early winter runs. The Columbia river has a large and important king salmon fishery.

Kings are good eating and excellent smoking fish. In Europe, many smokers prize them as highly as their local Atlantic salmon. Many kings are sold fresh, but the high price makes them unsuitable for steaking and fresh fish generally goes to smokers and institutional customers.

King salmon caught in the ocean or while preparing to enter their river have red flesh and silver skin. As they stop feeding and enter fresher water the skin starts to darken and black and red vertical bands and patches begin to appear. At the same time, the flesh loses color and softens as the fat in it is consumed by the efforts of the fish to swim upstream. By the time the fish reaches its spawning ground, the flesh is greyish white and the skin mottled black, grey and red. At this point it is very poor eating. In some areas these fish are known as tullies, which have a limited low-priced market for smoking and processing.

Smokers particularly are fussy customers and will have knowledge of fish from different river systems. They tend to prefer some origins to others. These preferences may be due to the intrinsic flesh quality of fish entering certain rivers, or to the way the fish is handled in different places – some salmon catching areas are very far from processing plants. It is therefore necessary to know the river from which the fish originated. The main determinant of flesh quality, however, is the distance from the sea when the fish was caught: the further up the river, the poorer the flesh is likely to be and the less attractive the skin.

The best and most expensive kings are the troll-caught fish from the ocean. These always have bright silver skins and red flesh. Because troll fish is gutted immediately after it is caught it is generally superior to even the best net-caught fish. Net red kings should be a little cheaper than trolls. Some packers may distinguish between gillnet and seined fish, but this is of minor importance. Because net fish may be caught anywhere from the estuary upwards, the quality varies and sampling is more important. Netted fish often suffocate in the nets and are more likely to be bruised. Both of these aspects lead to lower-quality fish. Kings caught fairly far up river are known as pale kings which have badly marked skins and pale pink flesh. These are slightly superior to the tullies mentioned above.

Pale kings must not be confused with white kings which are a white fleshed sub-species with silver skin and good salmon flavor. Because the market expects salmon to be red, white kings have a limited market near to the areas where they are caught and known.

Kings, like most salmon, are generally packed in boxes of 100lbs. Each fish should be polybagged separately, though some packers do this only for export. It is essential that the fish has a proper glaze to protect it. Salmon should be reglazed every three months or so as the ice covering evaporates. Otherwise, rancidity occurs quickly. The largest kings may be packed in 200lb boxes, or in random weight packs of approximately 200lbs. King salmon fillets or sides are available, usually well wrapped and packed in 50lb boxes. Because this increases the risk of dehydration, most users prefer to buy the fish in headless dressed form.

Coho *Scientific name: Oncorhynchus kisutch:* Also called silver, medium red (canned), blueback (an incorrect name used on some canned product) and jack salmon (young mature males). Coho or silver salmon average 8 to 10 pounds when caught and are found throughout the range of Pacific salmon. The two names are equally used but it is preferable to say "coho" to avoid the possibility of confusion with silverbrights, which are not cohos but chums (see below).

Coho meat is a little less robust than that of the king salmon, and a little less red. Like kings, the skins start to darken and redden when the fish enter the rivers. Redskin silvers are an inferior grade of coho, but the flesh color remains reasonable. The larger fish of this type are a popular buy for steaking, where the skin appearance is less important. Some producers pack "blush" fish separately from red skins. This is supposedly a little better, being fish that is less red and less heavily watermarked.

Headless dressed cohos are normally graded 2/4lbs, 4/6lbs, 6/9lbs and 9/12lbs. Fish over 9lbs are not common. Most cohos are packed in 100lb boxes, with the fish individually polybagged. 2/4lb fish may be packed in 50lb boxes which are preferred by some retail outlets.

Cohos make good smoked salmon and are especially liked by European smokers. As with kings, the fish that is troll caught in the ocean is superior to the net caught fish that is landed later. Although smokers rarely use fish under 6lbs, cohos of all sizes are taken on lines.

Pink salmon *Scientific name: Oncorhynchus gorbuscha:* Also called humpback and humpie. Pinks are the most abundant salmon. They are caught between Oregon and Alaska and average five to six pounds when landed. Most pinks are canned, though plenty are frozen and are especially popular for retail use.

As the name suggests, the flesh is pink rather than red. It is less moist than king or coho salmon meat. The skin is silvery grey – less bright and not as attractive as the skins of the sockeye and king. Catches of pinks tend to be very heavy in alternate years; the fish is usually a good, inexpensive buy during the big seasons.

Pinks are normally graded 2/5lb or 3/5lb and 5lb up. Smaller fish predominate. Packing is 50lb or 100lb boxes and the fish, like all salmon, should be well glazed and polywrapped. Pinks are sometimes used to make salmon roasts.

Oxidation of pinks is particularly noticeable along the belly cuts as a yellow stain. Trimmed fish may be offered and should be carefully inspected for further rancidity.

Nearly all pinks are net-caught in estuaries. A small number of fish are troll-caught but since the fish is seldom used for smoking there is little advantage to troll pinks. Watermarked fish is unusual.

Chum salmon *Scientific name: Oncorhynchus keta:* The official names for the fish are chum salmon and keta salmon. In the market, you may hear many others, including dog salmon, silverbright, semibright, falls, calico and darks. Most of these names refer to quality grades rather than to the species in general.

Chums average 10 to 12 pounds when caught and are found in the Pacific from Washington to Alaska and down to Japan, where they are particularly prized. This species is always net caught.

Chums are graded the same way as cohos, that is 2/4lb, 4/6lb, 6/9lb and 9lb up or 9/12lb. Packing is 100lb cartons, individually bagged fish.

Chums are the most complex salmon to buy because of the wide range of names and quality designations. As with all seafood, a full description is essential.

The best grade of chum is called silverbright or silverbrite chum. This has shiny silver skin, red flesh color and according to purists comes only from the Johnstone Strait in British Columbia, between northern Vancouver Island and the mainland. However, most packers use the term silverbright to describe any chum with silver skin all over and good quality meat. It is important not to confuse this name with silver salmon, which is coho.

As chums move into fresh water, the skin starts to turn red and black and the flesh becomes paler. The skin watermarkings begin at the top of the fish. Semibright chums are those fish where the watermarking does not extend below the lateral line that runs from just behind the eye to the center of the tail. Fish may be described as "bright chums" and this will normally be semibright fish, since if the fish are full silverbrights the packer can be expected to say so to sell for the higher price.

Once the watermarking spreads below the lateral line, nomenclature gets confused. The fish may be called a fall chum or just a chum. When the skin is almost black and the flesh color is pale grey rather than pink, the fish is called by its lowest quality designation, that is a dark chum. These fish are cheap and have a limited use for steaking and in some parts of the midwest for smoking.

The price differential between dark chums and silverbrights may be as much as 300 percent, so it is important to know what you want as well as what you are actually getting.

There are local names such as "river chum" used from time to time and these are a source of confusion. Whatever the fish is called, it is important to know the flesh color and the degree of watermarking in order to make a sensible buying decision.

Cherry salmon *Scientific name: Oncorhynchus masou:* Also called masou and Japanese salmon. This species is found only on the Asian side of the North Pacific and is unknown in the U.S.A.

Other salmon: There are no other salmon species. Some salmon have been transplanted to other parts of the world with limited success. Schemes to undertake large scale relocating of salmon are often suggested, but so far none have been brought to fruition. Fish called salmon in other parts of the world are not salmon. For example, Australians have a fish called beach salmon, also known as silver salmon or salmon trout, which is in no way related to a salmon. Now that several salmon species are being farmed as far away from their original habitats as New Zealand and Chile, it must be expected that some of these fish will escape and find congenial environments in which to establish new wild stocks. To date, though, this does not seem to have happened.

Hatchery salmon: Fish which has spawned. This has very soft meat and is suitable only for animal feed or the production of spreads or stuffings. The name derives from the conservation practice of taking fish about to spawn and placing the eggs in a hatchery so that the baby fish are protected through the earliest and most vulnerable stages of their life cycle. It is this technique which has given the Pacific salmon its continued existence as an important fishery resource and is now also applied to Atlantic salmon.

Number 1 and Number 2 salmon: Descriptions such as "No.1 net silvers" are common and while number one fish is clearly supposed to be better than number two fish, each packer has his own definitions. There are no universal standards.

In general, fish sold as No.1 quality should be fresh, clean and carefully handled, with no indications of cuts, belly burn, rancidity or other defects. Anything else should be sold as No.2 fish. Some fish may be damaged by seal bites, for example, making the fish difficult to use. This is no reflection on the ability of the packer, just a fact of nature.

Packing salmon: Headless dressed salmon is almost always individually polybagged and packed in 100lb cartons, double strapped each way. This is sometimes called "export pack" because at one time some domestically marketed fish was not polybagged. Almost all fish is now packed with the wrapping.

Smaller salmon, especially 2/4lb and 3/5lb fish may be packed in 50lb containers which are more convenient for retail use. Large fish such as 18-up kings and cheap fish such as dark chums may be packed in random weight boxes. Weights recorded on random weight cartons usually include glaze. The recorded weights are the gross weight of the fish, not the net weight. It is normal practice to allow three percent of the gross weight for the glaze and to invoice therefore for three percent less. Exact weight boxes should contain the marked net weight of fish.

Cartons should always be marked with the count of fish in the box as well as the usual information on type, size and quality.

Troll and net caught salmon: As mentioned earlier, a troll has nothing to do with Nordic folklore, but is a fish caught on a hook and line. Troll-caught salmon are superior since the fish are handled individually when caught and are landed with minimal bruising. Bruised flesh has dark areas which are particularly noticeable if the fish is smoked. These patches are unappealing and detract from the value of the final product.

Net fish are caught by gillnets or seines, or by any of the other methods used to catch salmon in the Pacific, such as dip-nets, fish-wheels and traps. Gillnets are hung vertically in the water to entangle the fish. Seines are similar but are closed around the fish to prevent its escape. Both techniques are liable to cause some bruising. A few buyers have preferences for one technique over the other. Net caught fish are usually landed whole with the guts in, since the rate of catching is too high to permit the fishermen to eviscerate them on the boat. Consequently, the fish may begin to deteriorate a little before they can be processed. Net fish are more likely to suffer from belly burn than troll fish.

Silvers and kings are the main species caught on lines. A few pinks are also landed this way, but the majority of pinks, and almost all sockeyes and chums, are net caught.

Salmon seasons: In theory and often in fact, you could put a net across a river and catch almost every salmon that swims into that river, which would completely destroy the salmon population of the river; salmon return to spawn in the river in which they were born. If none are born there, none return. It might be difficult to net the whole of the Columbia, but it can be done and has been done on many smaller rivers.

Wild salmon stocks are maintained by allowing a certain number of fish each year to swim up their rivers to spawn. This is called "escapement" and is achieved generally by designating closed seasons when fish may not be caught. Seasons are designated for particular species in particular rivers and vary widely according to the local requirements and the habits of the fish.

In general, salmon are caught throughout the year but the great bulk of production is in the summer and fall.

The period of strongest demand for salmon is the two weeks leading up to the Fourth of July, when only a limited number of areas are available for fishing.

Salmon farming: Aquaculture is changing the seasonal nature of the salmon business. Although wild Pacific stocks are still the major part of the business, more and more farmed salmon is being sold. Much of this can be harvested at times when wild salmon is in short supply. Norwegian salmon is most heavily marketed in the winter months. Salmon from the southern hemisphere, which is beginning to appear on the market, can quite easily be harvested and sold when the wild supplies are at their lowest winter point.

Aquaculture is also changing the frozen market, because European smokers, who were its mainstay, are now able to buy fresh Atlantic salmon virtually year round from the farms. Although wild, frozen salmon is still important to this market, it seems that the cream of the market is going to the farmers.

Salmon bellies: Pickled salmon. Usually made from king salmon, they are the center sections of the fish which are hard salted in barrels. This used to be exported to Scandinavia but is a dying, perhaps dead, process.

Salmon eggs: Sujiko. In the U.S.A. salmon eggs are cured, often colored and packed into small jars to be used as bait by anglers. The industry came to realize that salmon eggs are a high priced delicacy in Japan. Japanese buyers were taking the eggs and discarding the fish. The export of salmon eggs is now an important part of the industry's income.

Sujiko is a special preparation of salmon eggs but the name is often used in the U.S.A. to describe the unprocessed roe as well as the finished product. See also Roe.

Salmon roasts: Also called barbecue roasts. Start with a headless dressed fish. Cut the collar off with a straight cut. Cut off the tail. Split the body in two vertically with half the backbone in each part. This makes two roasts. Polybagged with cooking instructions, this has become a useful retail item in parts of the west, but has never become popular throughout the country.

Pinks, small chums, or any salmon with reasonable color can be used. Because the bellies can easily be trimmed while cutting roasts, salmon showing signs of rancidity can be used. Roasts should not be regarded as a salvage product and retailers may prefer to cut their own from cheap fish when this is available.

SALMONELLA: A micro-organism causing food poisoning in humans, salmonella is very common and is found widely on meat, poultry and seafoods. Fortunately it is easily destroyed by heat, being killed at 145°F. in 60 seconds, at 155°F. in six seconds and at 165°F. in one second. Normal cooking will therefore destroy the bugs.

The risks from salmonella are firstly from insufficient cooking, and secondly from contamination of surfaces in kitchens which may transmit the organism to foods that are eaten raw. For example, if a product with salmonella on it is prepared on a surface that is shortly afterwards used to cut up salads, the salmonella may infect the consumer via the salad, although originally starting on a foodstuff of a quite different type.

Salmonella poisoning rarely if ever kills, but can be nasty. The F.D.A. checks imports for salmonella contamination. There is no similar screening applied to domestic product.

Frog legs are particularly prone to salmonella and F.D.A. checks most import batches, sometimes rejecting very high proportions of shipments from south Asia. Canada has even more stringent standards and it is possible for product approved for sale in the U.S.A. to be shipped to Canada and rejected there. (In this event, the product is not allowed to return to the U.S.A.).

Shrimp found to contain salmonella can be cleaned by cooking to a sufficient temperature. The F.D.A. permits this to be done under its supervision and control.

SALT COD: Also called bacalao. See Curing.

SALTING AND BRINING: Using salt to draw moisture from flesh, so making it unattractive to the growth of spoilage bacteria, thereby preserving it.

SALTONSTALL-KENNEDY: A Federal law awarding grants to promote the development and use of the fisheries of the United States. Research has been supported under the Act to resolve problems associated with harvesting, processing and marketing fish and shellfish, to improve the quality and safety of processed fishery products and to develop information for and about the industry. Grants are made after an annual application and review process. Funding derives from fees levied on foreign fishermen for permits to fish within the U.S. 200-mile zone.

SARDINE: This name is given to a number of small herrings and herring-like fish. In Maine, small or young herrings are canned as Maine sardines. In Europe, mostly, sardines are a different species which looks exactly like a small herring. Brisling is also a different fish. All are virtually indistinguishable in normal trading situations.

Frozen sardines are imported in small quantities from France, Spain and Portugal. Usually these are whole, sometimes dressed, packed in 1kg (2.2lb), 5kg (11lb) and 10kg (22lb) boxes. Some buyers will specify length (5/7 inches, 7/9 inches) and generally prefer smaller sizes to larger.

The Pacific or California sardine (*Sardinops sagax*) used to be a major fishery, but the resource was replaced decades ago by the anchovy. Although it occasionally shows signs of returning, it is still a protected species which may be taken only as a by-catch of mackerel fishing.

The Spanish sardine from Florida covers two species: *Sardinella aurita* and *Sardinella anchovia*. These fish are also caught on the European side of the Atlantic, where they support a major fishery. In Florida, although the resource is thought to be large, there is little market and therefore not much fishing for sardines.

SASHIMI: Raw fish and shellfish sliced thinly and eaten. See Sushi.

SATSUMA-AGE: See Surimi.

SAUGER: See Pike.

SCALLOPS: The scallop is a bivalve mollusc, that is a mollusc with two shells. The part eaten is the muscle that holds the two shells together. In Europe and Japan the roe is also eaten, but in the U.S.A. the presence of the half-moon shaped red or brown roe will cause customers to reject scallops. The roe is lost in mechanical shucking, so is only found on imported hand-shucked scallops. Most sellers are aware of the market requirement in the U.S.A. for roe-free scallops.

Scallops are a major seafood commodity in the U.S.A. The market standard is set by the large sea scallops from the northeast. Smaller bay scallops, also from the northeast, are an important high quality product, though sold in much smaller quantities. Calico scallops, mainly from the Carolinas and Florida, are smaller, cheaper and less well regarded than bays but account for substantial volume in some years. There are a number of other scallops from domestic and overseas waters. All of them more or less fit into one of these three categories: seas, bays and calicos.

Sea Scallop *Scientific name: Placopecten magellanicus:* The largest proportion of the scallops sold in the U.S.A. are caught on or near the Georges Bank fishing grounds in the northeast Atlantic close to New England and the Canadian Maritimes. Scallops from this area are landed in Canada, Massachusetts and Virginia. Historically, these scallops have been mainly between 20 and 40 count per pound. They started to get much smaller in the early 1980s, resulting in conservation measures restricting the use of smaller shellfish. In practice, 40 count per pound is about the smallest seen on the U.S. market, resulting from a practical interpretation of a rule that says 30 count is the smallest allowed. Despite resource problems, the fishery for this species is still the largest scallop fishery in the world, although the Japanese scallop is now produced in larger quantities thanks to aquaculture.

The sea scallop is creamy colored, sometimes with pinkish or brownish marks. It is shaped like a small patty. Sometimes, incomplete cleaning leaves a small piece of white gristle attached to the side of the meat. This is a different part of the muscle, is entirely edible and is a positive indicator that you have a real scallop, not one made from surimi.

Frozen scallops packed in Canada normally sell at a premium over similar product packed in the U.S.A. because Canadian packers are considered to give better weights. This distinction is probably invalid, but regard must be paid to market prejudices. Similarly, New Bedford scallops often sell for slightly more than Virginia scallops. Grading in Virginia tends to be less precise, but no packers do a particularly good job grading scallops.

The European common scallop, *Pecten maximus*, is very similar. Brisk demand in Europe makes it unlikely that this species will be offered in the U.S.A. If it is, however, it is readily usable as a sea scallop. Just make sure that the roe is removed before processing, since many European markets prefer scallops with the roe still attached.

Sea scallops are the major market supply and in many ways are the standard against which all other scallops are compared. Mostly they are packed in 10/5lb blocks. Some are packed in 10/5/1lb cellos for retail use. Large scallops may be I.Q.F. in 5lb bags. Scallop pieces are sometimes frozen in 15lb blocks for further processing.

Bay scallops *Scientific name: Argopecten irradians:* Probably the best flavored of all scallops is the inshore bay scallop caught around Cape Cod, Rhode Island and Long Island (Peconic Bay especially). There is also some small production from Virginia. The bay scallop is creamy colored and shaped like the sea scallop. Production varies greatly from year to year and most of them are sold fresh in gallon containers, except in years of surplus production. They are usually about 70/90 count, ranging from 50/60 to about 100 per pound. Many substitutes are sold as Cape Cod bays, including thawed imported scallops of various types. Product offered as frozen Cape Cod bays is very likely to be something else.

Bay scallops have been hard hit in recent years by "brown tide" algae, which grows abundantly in the water and being too large for the scallops to absorb, causes the scallops to starve for lack of other food (the brown tide displaces the usual algae in the sea).

Calico scallops *Scientific name: Argopecten gibbus:* Every few years a huge quantity of small scallops from the Carolinas and Florida appear as cheap alternatives to bays. Calicos tend to be rather smaller and browner than bays. They are also longer and thinner than bay scallops. The flavor and texture are rather moderate, not nearly as good as bays. Calicos are sold fresh in gallons and frozen in numerous different packs. Calicos are sometimes offered as Cape scallops, presumably referring to Cape Canaveral rather than Cape Cod.

Weathervane scallops *Scientific name: Patinopecten caurinus:* Alaskan scallop beds are extensive, but fishing is restricted to small areas because the scallop dredges damage the more important king crab resources. The Alaskan scallop is similar to the eastern sea scallop, with good flavor. They are available packed 10/5lb blocks or 6/5lb I.Q.F. polybags. Sizes, like those of seas, range from 10/20 to 30/40 count per pound.

Queen scallops *Scientific name: Chlamys opercularis:* The United Kingdom ships queen scallops which are similar to bays and usually count between 60/80 and 90/110 per pound. They may be block frozen or I.Q.F. packed 6/5lb, 8/5lb or 10/5lb. Other packs also appear. These scallops come mainly from one area in the Irish Sea and may be packed in Scotland, England, Ireland or the Isle of Man (Manx scallops). Many buyers have preferences for one of these origins over others, but brand differentiation is more important than the regional since some packers are very good and others poor. The queen scallop has good flavor and texture, unless too much phosphate dip is used. The better packs are often substituted for bay scallops.

Icelandic scallops *Scientific name: Chlamys islandica:* This is a northern scallop found not only off Iceland but also in the Arctic Ocean and northern waters of the Pacific as well as the Atlantic. Exported to the U.S.A. from Norway and the Faroe Islands as well as from Iceland, these are generally 40/60 and 60/80 count, block frozen or I.Q.F. in 5lb and 2kg units, or bulk packed I.Q.F. in polylined boxes. The Icelandic scallop is good eating but may be pink or brown in color due to the roe "bleeding" into the muscle. The scallops are not shucked until after landing, so there is time for this to happen, while domestic and Canadian scallops are normally shucked on the fishing boat. Icelandic scallops are white when cooked, but some buyers will reject them if colored meats are noticeable. Norwegian scallops from the Barents Sea, even though shucked and frozen on board the fishing vessel, also tend to be brown. Bleaching removes the tint. Repackers sometimes do this. The flavor and texture of this scallop is good. Unless you need them for retail display, do not be deterred by the color.

Japanese scallops *Scientific name: Patinopecten yessoensis* or *Pecten yessoensis:* This is now the most important commercial scallop species in the world, because it is being farmed in large quantities. The scallop meats tend to be large, often 10/20 count, but sell at a discount compared to east coast seas because the drip loss is generally greater. This scallop is rather large in diameter and flat for its size, but otherwise the appearance is good. It toughens quickly if overcooked. Packs are generally I.Q.F. and may be 2kg, 2½lb, or 5lb units. Expect more of these if supplies of large scallops from other sources fall.

Peruvian scallops *Scientific name: Chlamys purpuratus:* This is a calico scallop, subject like most of its kind to boom-and-bust cycles. Importers first noticed the species during the unusual weather patterns following the El Niño episode in the early 1980s. The fishery produced huge quantities of scallops for a couple of years, then died. The industry is being revived with aquaculture techniques, based on those used in Japan.

Processing of Peruvian scallops is haphazard. It is important to check shipments carefully for freshness, weight, size grading and color. Provided it is properly handled, the product is fine.

The same species is found in northern Chile and some small quantities of product are already available from that source.

Panama scallops *Scientific name: Argopecten circularis:* This is another calico-type scallop found through central America as well as off the Pacific coast of Mexico and California. Panama supplies large quantities of scallops, although this species also seems to have a boom-and-bust cycle. The product can be terrible: grey and stale, poor grading and poor net weight. It can also be acceptable. Check it carefully.

Australian scallops: These are similar to Icelandic in size and appearance. They are also reasonably good to eat. Some packs have been consistently short weight and careful checking is essential. There are some unusual packs such as 2½kg and 5½lb, but there has been a marked lack of relationship between labelled and actual weights.

Brazil scallops: The late 1970s saw the development of a major scallop resource in Brazil. This is warm water material, and although cold water scallops are generally superior, the Brazil scallop, if properly handled, is reasonably good. Sizes range from 30 count down to 90 or 100. Block frozen and I.Q.F. are shipped in a variety of different packs.

Scallops tend to be a secondary business for Brazilian packers, taking a back seat to shrimp. Weights and counts range from very good to awful, use of dips is erratic and freshness cannot be guaranteed. When Brazil scallops are substantially cheaper than Canadian they are probably worth the hassle. At small discounts, the effort is hardly worthwhile. Several Brazil brands have established reasonable and consistent quality. Find them and stay with those labels.

The general advice on scallops is to use block frozen rather than I.Q.F. but with Brazilian it is better to stay with I.Q.F. packs. Often the blocks are packed in shrimp plants that are fully occupied with freezing shrimp so that the scallops may be frozen in the storage freezer instead of the plate freezer (see Freezing processes). In this case the centers of the blocks can turn bad before they finally freeze, while the outer parts of the blocks appear to be satisfactory. Checking freshness of block-frozen scallops should be done by breaking the block or boring a hole into the center with an icepick to ascertain if there is any unpleasant odor coming from inside the pack.

Other origins: Scallops are sometimes offered from Thailand or the Philippines. These scallops are basically terrible: poor texture and flavor, greyish color and often poorly packed without regard for freshness. It is unfortunate for the seafood industry that such product can be sold as scallops.

New Zealand has a sea scallop (*Pecten novaezealandiae*) and a queen (*Chlamys delicatula*). The queen scallop may be offered for export. It is similar to the European species and is usually processed with the roe attached.

There are numerous species of scallop in all the seas of the world. Any that are offered for sale in the U.S.A. will necessarily be marketed as seas, bays or calicos. All need careful inspection to ensure that they meet the quality standards that are traditional in this market.

The following section discusses these quality features of scallops.

- Quality in scallops relates to meats with creamy white color, of consistent size within a pack, of regular shape, and of course, of good flavor. The domestic or Canadian scallop from the Georges Bank in the Atlantic is the "normal" product against which other scallops are measured. Brownish, pinkish or mottled scallops are usually a sign that roe pigment has leaked into the muscle. This is totally harmless and the scallop will cook up quite white, but it is unattractive in frozen form and may be a reason for rejection by some customers. Regularity of shape and thickness is also important, since scallops require very little cooking and it is important that all of a batch should cook in the same time.

  Weight of packs of frozen scallops is a difficult and contentious topic. Scallop muscle consists of tiny fibers parallel to each other. This construction enables the shucked meats to draw up moisture by capillary action and also to release both this moisture and inherent moisture at a later time. It is possible to thaw scallops slowly over a long period so that they effectively evaporate. This feature gives rise to endless and repeated disputes about the actual weight of scallops in a frozen pack.

  Title 50 of the Code of Federal Regulations includes recommendations for thawing scallops to arrive at a fair estimation of the true weight. This technique may not be perfect but it is reasonable. In the absence of anything proven better it should be used to settle disputes. For a detailed description of thawing techniques, see Defrosting methods.

  - Because of their capillary construction, scallops respond well to the use of dips, which help them to absorb water before freezing and to retain it afterward. Dips can also whiten scallops a little. The use of dips should always be listed on the label's ingredients panel, but this rule is not always obeyed. It is probably safe to assume that almost all scallops are dipped.

Using too high a concentration of dips can toughen scallops and also make them foam like detergent if they are thawed in water.

• Size grading of scallops is not standardized, but the generally-used size ranges are counts per pound as follows:

Under 10 (rare)	50/70
10/20 or 10/25	70/90
15/25 (mainly from Virginia)	90/110 or 80/100 Pieces
20/30	
30/40	

Grading is often done by eye and tends to be approximate. Most packers allow 10 to 15 percent pieces with regular scallops and tend not to pack pieces separately if possible.

Packing for scallops is also varied. The standard is probably 10/5lb blocks, which is the pack used for almost all domestic and Canadian scallops. Imported scallops come in various packing forms including 1lb and 5lb bags of I.Q.F. scallops and blocks of 2kg, 2½kg and 5lb.

• Blocks or I.Q.F.? Because of the need to glaze scallops for protection and the tendency of scallops to absorb water, block frozen scallops are often a better buy than I.Q.F. simply because there is less water around them in the form of glaze. You generally get more edible weight from a 5lb block than from 5lb of I.Q.F. scallops. I.Q.F. meats have to be well thawed before frying or the glaze will sublimate in the cooking oil and blow off the breading, spoiling both the food and the oil. If your application permits the use of block frozen scallops, these are generally better value, except where packers have expertise with I.Q.F. but not with block freezing (see Brazil, above).

Sea and bay scallops are distinguished biologically as different species, but market designation is mainly related to size: larger scallops are called sea scallops and smaller ones are called bay scallops or calicos. The standard domestic scallop between 20 and 40 count per pound is always called a "sea" and small scallops such as the Scottish 70/90 count are called "bays" while the medium sizes are not always designated. In any case, it is preferable to use counts rather than descriptive words to ensure understanding.

Broken scallops tend to be packed with the whole ones, but if packed separately may be I.Q.F. which is a good cheap item for certain uses, or in 5lb or 15lb blocks. The large blocks are for processors who can stamp out a desired shape for breading, so getting cheaper raw material than by using regular whole scallops. Pieces are also useful for chowders, for stuffings and similar applications.

Substitutions for scallops may be less prevalent than is generally believed. Some imported scallops may be repacked into domestic or Canadian boxes. Cartons marked "packed in U.S.A." rather than "product of U.S.A." may be an indication of repacked product.

Most of the substitutions in scallops relate to Cape Cod bays. Both calicos and U.K. queens may be thawed and passed off as the superior domestic bay, though no-one accustomed to the real thing would be deceived for long by the calicos.

It is widely believed that cod cheeks and pieces of skate wings are used as substitutes for scallops. It is perhaps possible to do this at a restaurant level if there is extremely cheap labor available, but the chances of receiving such items in a commercially frozen form are non-existent. Further, the texture of such fishy substitutes is totally different from the texture of a scallop. This is a long-lived, repeated myth about seafoods that will not go away but contains no element of truth.

SCAMPI: See Lobsterette.

SCIENTIFIC NAMES: Latin names for species are a universally understood naming convention. All scientists, whatever their native tongue, use the same scientific name to describe the same creature or organism. The system was first codified and agreed upon in 1901.

Each species is (generally) referred to by two Latin words. The first word is capitalized and represents the genus. The two words together name the species. For example, the scientific name *Gadus morhua* shows that the fish is a member of the genus

Gadus and that the name of the species is *Gadus morhua*. If there are subsequent references to other members of the same genus, the first word is often abbreviated to its initial letter. *G. macrocephalus* then indicates another member of the same genus Gadus. In this book, we normally spell out the name in full to avoid any possible confusion.

You will occasionally see three-word names. The third word, if in Latin, indicates a subspecies. Atlantic herring is *Clupea harengus harengus* while the virtually identical Pacific herring is *Clupea harengus palassi*. For all commercial purposes, the first two words are sufficient. Sometimes, the third word is not italicized but is the name of the scientist who first defined the species. This is valuable for other scientists, making it easier to check the original sources to review the work. Again, for commercial purposes it is not significant.

Using scientific names clarifies which fish or shellfish is being discussed. A seabass could be one of several hundred different species. Only the scientific name will give the precise animal. The system, like every system, is not perfect. Sometimes names are changed as more information develops about a family, genus or species, or mistakes are made in classifying species. But in general, the convention works well.

SCHILLERLOCKEN: Smoked dogfish belly-flaps.

SCOMBROID POISONING: See Histamines.

SCROD: Also spelled schrod. Not a fish, but a size used on the Boston fish pier to classify cod, haddock or similar fish that are between small and market in size. That is, scrod is 1½lb to 2½lb. Massachusetts has definitions for scrod, as a size, applying to cod, haddock, pollock and cusk. The use of the word for sizes of other fish is illegal.

A menu dish calling for scrod can use cod, haddock, pollock, ling, hake or some other similar fish equally well. Consumers believe in the Boston scrod as a separate species, but anyone working in or with the seafood industry should know better. Nevertheless, many people, inside and outside the industry, will tell you they prefer scrod to cod. Others prefer scrod to haddock.

The F.D.A. and the National Marine Fisheries Service regard the use of the term "scrod" on its own as mislabelling. Action has been taken against the use of the word for ocean pout and wolf-fish. Remember, scrod is a size description, not a fish.

SCUNGILI: See Conch.

SCUP: See Porgy.

SEA BASS: See Bass.

SEA DEVIL: A non-approved name for monkfish. The name is also used for the manta ray. See Monkfish.

SEA EGGS: See Sea urchin.

SEAFOOD SAFETY: To put this topic in perspective, the U.S. General Accounting Office, in a 1988 report, said that there is no need for a mandatory Federal inspection program for sea-food, because seafood was implicated in very few incidents of food-borne diseases. The G.A.O. reported that under 5 percent of food-related illnesses reported to the Centers for Disease Control were caused by seafood. The largest part of these were from eating raw shellfish illegally harvested from polluted waters.

Nevertheless, consumers are concerned. Ocean dumping, polluted beaches and PCBs make headlines. The fact that the chances of harm from eating fish are minimal is less publicized.
Bugs: Raw or lightly cooked molluscs eaten whole are the likeliest seafoods to cause a problem. Oysters, clams and mussels are the main shellfish in this category. There is a comprehensive, federally supervised system for ensuring that these shellfish are taken only from clean water and are properly handled after harvest. The problem is that it is very difficult to ensure that no one breaks these rules. (See the items on Inspection, Shellfish Sanitation and Depuration for more details).

These shellfish can contain bacteria and viruses that cause nasty diseases including gastroenteritis, hepatitis or even cholera. The one certain solution to this problem is to cook all molluscs thoroughly. Also, make sure that you buy only from reputable dealers, or from fishermen you can trust to be honest about where they caught the product.

Parasites: Parasites are another safety hazard. All fish MAY have parasites. It is more common in fish from fresh water than in fish from the ocean. Most of these parasites are not harmful to humans. The incidence of parasites varies with the season, the water the fish is in, the food it is eating and many other factors such as the size of the local seal population (seals are responsible for passing on the worms in cod).

Illnesses caused by ingesting parasites are very rare in the U.S.A. The main problem with parasites is that consumers are terrified of them.

Fish fillets should always be candled by the processor. This entails passing them over a lighted glass table so that any parasites can be seen and cut out.

There are three types of parasitic worms occasionally found in fish: tapeworms (cestodes) flukes (trematodes) and roundworms (nematodes). All of them can be killed by cooking the fish to a (quite low) internal temperature of 140°F. None of them will survive proper freezing. To kill the parasite, freeze the fish to −20°F. and hold it there for 72 hours.

The moral of this: do not eat raw fish. Encourage your customers not to eat raw fish. If you supply fish for sushi, or serve sushi, follow a common Japanese practice and use top quality frozen fish. It is probably fresher and may be cheaper. If using frozen fish saves a customer from contracting anisikiasis, it will have saved you a lot of grief.

Contaminants: Heavy metals (mercury, arsenic, lead, cadmium and others) may be introduced into the sea from industrial wastes, although far larger quantities result from the natural flow of rivers and rainwater and from other natural processes. Mercury in swordfish has been a well-known problem for many years. Swordfish, and other large, long-lived species that eat other fish, may accumulate mercury and other metals in their flesh. The older and larger the fish, the more likely it is to be contaminated. Freshwater fish such as muskellunge and yellow perch are also vulnerable to mercury accumulation.

Most, if not all, mercury problems can be avoided by using smaller fish. With swordfish, those over approximately 100lbs are more likely to be contaminated. To keep the problem in proportion, bear in mind that there is no record in this country of anyone ever being harmed by absorbing mercury from fish.

PCBs (polychlorinated biphenyls) are synthetic compounds used industrially since 1929. They break down very slowly and are absorbed through the skin, the lungs, or from foods. PCBs accumulate in fatty fish, mainly those that feed inshore or in fresh water where the compounds have reached. PCBs are highly toxic, although little is known about the effects of low-level contamination.

The F.D.A. enforces a tolerance level for PCBs in fish and shellfish of 2.0 parts per million. States close areas known to be affected and issue warnings against eating certain species too often. Since the chemical accumulates mostly in fatty tissues and the organs, exposure can be reduced by avoiding fish livers and cutting out the darker strips of meat.

There are numerous chemicals which might be found in fish, as in other foods. Those thought to be harmful are listed by the F.D.A., which monitors fish and fishing grounds. Action levels for these substances are listed below.

F.D.A Action levels for poisonous or deleterious substances in seafood

Aldrin	(fish & shellfish)	0.3 ppm
Dieldrin	(fish & shellfish)	0.3 ppm
Benzene Hexachloride	(frogs legs)	0.5 ppm
Chlordane	(fish)	0.3 ppm
DDT,DDE,TDE	(fish)	5.0 ppm
Endrin	(fish & shellfish)	0.3 ppm
Heptachlor	(fish & shellfish)	0.3 ppm
Kepone	(crabmeat)	0.4 ppm
Kepone	(fish & shellfish)	0.3 ppm
Mercury (measured as methyl mercury)	(fish & shellfish & crustaceans)	1.0 ppm
Mirex	(fish)	0.1 ppm
PCB	(fish)	2.0 ppm
Toxaphene	(fish)	5.0 ppm
Paralytic Shellfish Toxin	(clams)	80mg/100g meat
Paralytic Shellfish Toxin	(mussels)	80mg/100g meat
Paralytic Shellfish Toxin	(oysters)	80mg/100g meat

Note: ppm means parts per million, mg means micrograms

Marine toxins occur naturally in certain fish and shellfish. The best known is probably red tide, which causes paralytic shellfish poisoning (PSP) in humans. It is caused by a bloom of dinoflagellate algae, which are eaten by filter-feeding molluscs such as mussels, oysters and clams. The algae produces a toxin in the shellfish which does not harm the shellfish but is very poisonous to anyone eating the whole mollusc.

The problem occurs from the Canadian Maritimes to southern New England, on most of the Pacific coast from California to Alaska, and in parts of the Gulf of Mexico, mainly the west coast of Florida. In each area a different plankton is to blame. The effects are the same everywhere.

Coastal waters in vulnerable areas are monitored very carefully by state authorities responsible for shellfish sanitation (see Shellfish sanitation). There is no reason for anyone to suffer from PSP provided they do not eat shellfish from restricted waters. People gathering shellfish on the beach are at the most risk, since those outside the industry may be unaware of the existence of restricted areas and the reasons for having such rules.

Some toxins may be present in the muscle of a few fish or shellfish species. Ciguatoxin is fairly common. It has been found in over 400 different species in subtropical and tropical waters. Grouper, snapper and other reef fish may be affected. Barracuda in the Caribbean is a risk, although barracuda from the Pacific coast is safe to eat.

The only way to prevent ciguatera is to avoid possibly toxic species.

Scombroid poisoning (also called histamine poisoning) is mainly found in scombroid fish – tunas and mackerels – but may also occur in some other pelagic species such as mahi-mahi. It results from poor handling after the fish is caught. If the fish is not properly chilled and iced, histamines are produced in the flesh. These trigger strong allergic reactions in some people. The best way to avoid scombroid poisoning is to inspect your fish for signs of spoilage. Also, know your fish and how it was handled. See also Histamines.

Most marine toxins are not destroyed by cooking.

Seafood safety also covers hazards that might be introduced during processing: for example, botulism is a risk in low-acid canned foods and some vacuum packed foods. But these risks are common to all food industries.

Overall, seafood is extremely safe. Most of the (few) reported cases involve a very few species; many of these cases involve shellfish harvested illegally from restricted waters. Almost 50 percent of all seafood-related illnesses are reported from Hawaii, Guam, Puerto Rico and the Virgin Islands, all of which are far away from the major populations centers of the U.S.A. As the industry becomes increasingly aware of the potential problems, seafood will no doubt become safer still.

SEA RUN: Ocean run. Product packed as caught, without grading for size.

SEA SNAIL: See Conch and Periwinkle.

SEA TROUT: In the U.S.A., this generally means certain species of drum from the Atlantic coast. The F.D.A.'s Fishlist (see Names) suggests that they may all be called weakfish and sea bass. However, normal usage restricts the name weakfish to the grey seatrout and sea bass is seldom if ever applied to any of these species commercially. Other names are striped trout and Mexican trout. In this section, we continue to use the names that are customary in commerce.

The name can also cover anadromous brown trout and rainbow trout. For information on these fish see Salmon and Trout. **Spotted seatrout** *Scientific name: Cynoscion nebulosus:* Also called speckled seatrout. Most production comes from the Gulf states, although the fish ranges from Texas to Virginia. The species is also imported from Mexico. It is an important recreational fish and grows to about seven pounds. Frozen fish is sold either headless and dressed in 25lb boxes, or as skin-on fillets, usually I.Q.F. in 5lb packages. Graded fillets from Mexico are a premium product.

The flesh is lean, delicately flavored and has a small flake. The fish does not keep well, needing fast, careful handling. Imported product from Argentina and Uruguay is cheaper and generally inferior. This is usually layer packed in 10lb or 15lb boxes. Boneless fillets are offered but may contain pin-bones, which are small and cook out easily.

Grey seatrout *Scientific name: Cynoscion regalis:* Also called weakfish, squeteague, yellow fin trout and tide runner. This is a similar fish with a more northerly range. Most commercial catches originate between New York and North Carolina. It, too, is important for recreational fishermen. It is similar to the spotted seatrout in eating characteristics and available commercially in similar forms.

Silver seatrout *Scientific name: Cynoscion nothus:* Also called white seatrout. It is very similar to sand seatrout (*Cynoscion arenarius*) and the two fish are frequently mixed together. These fish are small, usually under 1½lbs, sold pan-ready. Large quantities of very small fish are caught and used for fish meal.

SEA URCHIN: An expensive shellfish, found in most seas, the sea urchin (or sea egg) is spherical and covered with sharp spines. The only edible part is the large gonad which is normally sold fresh. Frozen sea urchin roes are considered inferior to fresh but can be produced.

SECTIONS: See Crabs.

SEMIBRIGHT: See Salmon.

SEPIA: See Cuttlefish.

SEVICHE: Fish "cooked" in acid, namely lemon juice, lime juice or vinegar, instead of heat. Fish must marinate in the acid for at least four hours in the refrigerator.

SHAD *Scientific name: Alosa sapidissima:* Also called American shad. An anadromous Atlantic species that was successfully introduced into the Pacific last century. The roe is a delicacy and can be frozen. Boned fish is also used, mainly fresh but sometimes frozen. The hickory shad (*Alosa mediocris*) is a smaller but similar fish, mainly caught and eaten by game fishermen.

Shad roe should be in unbroken sacs, frozen in pairs. If the fish is ready to spawn the eggs may be large and soft and will break when frozen. Frozen shad roe can be used much as fresh. It should not be kept in storage for more than a month or two as it turns rancid fast.

263

SHARK: Increasing quantities and more species of shark are being eaten in the U.S.A. Mako is a substitute for and alternative to swordfish. Thresher shark is an alternative to mako. Dogfish is an important food fish in some European countries, though has not yet caught the imagination of American marketers.

Shark is generally not expensive and many species are good eating. The meat varies from light to very dark, but most cooks up attractively light. All sharks have cartilage, not bones, so the absence of pinbones and other small bones can be guaranteed. Sharks must be handled very carefully. They lack a urinary tract, excreting wastes through the skin. Wastes remaining in the body after capture turn to ammonia very quickly: the fish must be cleaned and well iced as soon as it is caught and killed or it will smell bad. Sharks should always be bled, which helps to remove the urea that turns to ammonia in the bloodstream. Bleeding also whitens the meat. Longline-caught fish may be inferior to those taken on rods, since the longline fish often die on the hook before being landed, so cannot be bled.

Residual ammonia smell in shark meat can sometimes be removed by soaking it in a weak acid/brine solution for several hours.

Because of the big differences in eating quality between different species and the difficulty of identifying the species once the shark is dressed, it is important to buy shark from a knowledgeable supplier who really knows the species that he is shipping.

The following table shows the fifty-one sharks in the Fishlist with their approved common names and market names. Of these, perhaps half are used or usable as food.

Sharks: Market Names and Common Names

Market name	Common name	Scientific name	Location
Dogfish	Catshark	*Centrophorus squamosus*	P
Dogfish	Dogfish	*Mustelus antarcticus*	P
Dogfish	Dogfish, black	*Centroscymnus fabricii*	A
Dogfish	Dogfish, large spotted	*Scyliorhinus stellaris*	A
Dogfish	Dogfish, lesser spotted	*Scyliorhinus canicula*	A
Dogfish	Dogfish, northern	*Squalus blainvillei*	A-P
Dogfish	Dogfish, smooth	*Mustelus canis*	A
Dogfish	Dogfish, spiny/spring	*Squalus acanthias*	A-P
Dogfish	Shark, dogfish	*Mustelus lenticulatus*	P
Shark	Shark, basking	*Cetorhinus maximus*	A-P
Shark	Shark, bignose	*Carcharhinus altimus*	A
Shark	Shark, blacktip	*Carcharhinus limbatus*	A
Shark	Shark, blacktip reef	*Carcharhinus melanopterus*	A-P
Shark	Shark, blue	*Prionace glauca*	A-P
Shark	Shark, bull	*Carcharhinus leucas*	A-F-P
Shark	Shark, dusky	*Carcharhinus obscurus*	A-P
Shark	Shark, finetooth	*Carcharhinus isodon*	A
Shark	Shark, gray reef	*Carcharhinus amblyrhynchus*	P
Shark	Shark, lemon	*Negaprion brevirostris*	A-P
Shark	Shark, leopard	*Triakis semifasciata*	P
Shark	Shark, narrowtoothed	*Carcharhinus brachyurus*	P
Shark	Shark, night	*Carcharhinus signatus*	A
Shark	Shark, reef	*Carcharhinus perezi*	A
Shark	Shark, salmon	*Lamna ditropis*	P
Shark	Shark, sandbar	*Carcharhinus plumbeus*	A
Shark	Shark, sevengill	*Notorynchus cepedianus*	A-P
Shark	Shark, silky	*Carcharhinus falciformis*	A
Shark	Shark, silver tip	*Carcharhinus albimarginatus*	P

Locations: A = Atlantic   P = Indo-Pacific   F = Freshwater
Source: F.D.A.

265

Market name	Common name	Scientific name	Location
Shark	Shark, sixgill	*Hexanchus griseus*	A-P
Shark	Shark, smalltail	*Carcharhinus porosus*	A
Shark	Shark, spinner	*Carcharhinus brevipinna*	A
Shark	Shark, tiger	*Galeocerdo cuviere*	A-P
Shark	Shark, tope	*Galeorhinus galeus*	A
Shark	Shark, white	*Carcharodon carcharias*	A-P
Shark	Shark, whitetip	*Carcharhinus longimanus*	A-P
Shark	Shark, whitetip reef	*Triaenodon obesus*	A-P
Shark mako	Shark, shortfin mako	*Isurus oxyrinchus*	A-P
Shark, angel	Shark, Atlantic angel	*Squatina dumerili*	A
Shark, angel	Shark, Pacific angel	*Squatina californica*	P
Shark, mako	Shark, longfin mako	*Isurus paucus*	A-P
Shark, thresher	Shark, bigeye thresher	*Alopias superciliosus*	A-P
Shark, thresher	Shark, common thresher	*Alopias vulpinus*	A-P
Shark, thresher	Shark, pelagic thresher	*Alopias pelagicus*	P
Shark/bonnethead	Shark/bonnethead	*Sphyrna tiburo*	A-P
Shark/hammerhead	Shark, great hammerhead	*Sphyrna mokarran*	A-P
Shark/hammerhead	Shark, scalloped hammerhead	*Sphyrna lewini*	A-P
Shark/hammerhead	Shark, smalleye hammerhead	*Sphyrna tudes*	A
Shark/hammerhead	Shark, smooth hammerhead	*Sphyrna zygaena*	A-P
Shark/porbeagle	Shark, porbeagle	*Lamna nasus*	A
Shark/smoothhound	Smoothhound, brown	*Mustelus henlei*	P
Shark/smoothhound	Smoothhound, grey	*Mustelus californicus*	P

Locations: A = Atlantic   P = Indo-Pacific   F = Freshwater
Source: F.D.A.

In general, avoid sharks with red meat and particularly thick skin. Most white-fleshed sharks are good. Sharks are shipped dressed or as slabs (fillets) or chunks. Handling and preparation rules that apply to swordfish also apply to shark. Consumer acceptance of shark meat seems to be growing. The product is complex and demands some learning and care, but can be very profitable.

Those sharks generally considered to be good for the table include the following:

Name	Location
Shortfin mako	Atlantic - Pacific
Longfin mako	Atlantic - Pacific
Lemon	Atlantic
Blacktip	Atlantic
Sandbar	Atlantic
Smooth dogfish	Atlantic - Pacific
Spiny dogfish	Atlantic - Pacific
Bonnethead	Atlantic
Sharpnose	Atlantic
Angel	Pacific
Common thresher	Pacific
Soupfin	Pacific
Whitetip	Pacific
Salmon	Pacific
Blue	Atlantic - Pacific
Silky	Atlantic
Spinner	Atlantic

Among those not recommended are:

Name	Location
Atlantic thresher	Atlantic
Pelagic thresher	-
Nurse	Atlantic - Pacific
Bull	Atlantic
Dusky	Atlantic - Pacific
Tiger	Atlantic - Pacific
Hammerheads	Atlantic - Pacific

SHATTERPACK: Another name for layer pack. Fillets in a good layer pack can be separated easily, perhaps after banging the block against a hard surface. See Packing.

SHEEPSHEAD *Scientific name: Archosargus probatocephalus:* An Atlantic and gulf fish popular in the New York area as well as Florida. It is mostly sold fresh, dressed. It has good, firm flesh and is abundant and inexpensive. Frozen product is unusual but the resource is capable of greater exploitation if a market develops.

The name sheephead (without an "s" in the middle) is also given to a California wrasse.

SHELLFISH SANITATION PROGRAM: The F.D.A. monitors all interstate shipments of fresh and frozen clams, mussels and oysters to ensure that no product containing harmful organisms reaches the consumer. State authorities administer the Program by inspecting and licensing shellfish shippers and packers and by implementing State cleanliness standards, based on the F.D.A. guidelines for growing areas. The State agencies are also responsible for inspecting shellfish to ensure it is clean. Some foreign governments and growing areas are included in the Program.

The Program is, in general, effective. All containers of the molluscs covered by the system have to be labelled with the licence number of the originating plant. To check these licence numbers and ensure that they are valid, write for a free copy of the Interstate Certified Shellfish Shippers List to:

> Chief, Fishery Technology Branch,
> F.D.A. 200 "C" Street SW,
> Washington, D.C. 20204

This shows the name of every approved U.S. and foreign shipper and packer of the three shellfish species, so is a useful catalog of suppliers as well as a check on the validity of shellfish licenses. The Program is being reviewed and updated to deal with the never-ending problem of environmental contamination. See also Depuration.

SHRIMP: The most important seafood commodity in the U.S.A. and in the world. The market is supplied from almost everywhere. It is a highly competitive sector of the seafood business. Because of its size, complexity and value it is vital to understand what you are buying.

Prices for shrimp depend on a world market in which Japanese demand is an even more important factor than U.S. demand. Japan consumes more shrimp than the U.S. and produces virtually none of its own, while the U.S.A. is a major producer as well as consumer. Price trends reflect world demand and supply. It is possible to have poor demand in the U.S.A. together with very high prices at times when Japanese demand is strong.

Green headless shrimp: The standard form of shrimp on the U.S. market is raw, frozen shell-on tails. This is also the major internationally traded commodity. It is known variously as green headless, headless or shell-on shrimp. It consists of the six tail segments of the shrimp, complete with shell, tail fin and vein. Larger sizes of domestic shrimp are landed in this form by the fishermen. The processor only has to grade and pack them for freezing.

Almost all green headless shrimp is packed in 5lb and 2kg blocks, 6, 8, or 10 to the master carton. The standard pack is 10/5lb or 10/2kg. Small quantities of headless shrimp are packed in 2lb blocks for retail sale. Increasing quantities of headless shrimp are packed I.Q.F. which gives the advantage that you only have to thaw the exact amount you need; it is not necessary to defrost a whole block. However, the I.Q.F. shrimp must be well glazed to protect it and packaging needs to be of good quality and secure. Even so, it has a much shorter shelf life than block frozen product.

Whole: Some shrimp is frozen whole, known also as heads-on shrimp. Whole shrimp is little used in the U.S.A. and can be disregarded in normal trade. It is important in some specialty markets and is a premium commodity in Japan and other Asian countries. Because whole shrimp develops melanosis (blackening) very quickly it must be frozen immediately after catching and must be handled with care. Whole shrimp are brittle. Legs and antennas break off easily, spoiling the attractiveness and reducing the value of the shrimp.

PRODUCT FORMS OF FROZEN SHRIMP: The following U.S. standards of product forms is taken from the Code of Federal Regulations: Title 50, 265.102.

Product forms: Types: (1) Fresh (2)Frozen individually (IQF) glazed or unglazed. (3)Frozen solid pack, glazed or unglazed.

Styles: (1) Raw (uncoagulated protein). (2) "Parboiled" – heated for a period of time such that the surface of the product reaches a temperature adequate to coagulate the protein. (3) "Cooked" – heated for a period of time such that the thermal center of the shrimp reaches a temperature adequate to coagulate the protein.

Market forms: (1) Heads on (head, shell, tail fins on). (2) Headless (only head removed; shell, tail fins on). (3) Peeled, round, tail off (all shell and tail fins removed with segments unslit and vein not removed). (4) Peeled, round, tail on (all shell except last shell segment and tail fins removed, with segment unslit and vein not removed). (5) Peeled and deveined, round, tail off (all shell and tail fins removed with segments shallowly slit to last segment and vein removed to last segment). (6) Peeled and deveined, round, tail on (all shell removed except last shell segment, and tail fins, with segments shallowly slit to last segment and vein removed to last segment). (7) Peeled and deveined, fantail or butterfly tail off (all shell and tail fin removed with segments deeply slit to last segment and vein removed to last segment). (8) Peeled and deveined, fantail or butterfly, tail on (all shell removed except last shell segment and tail fins, with segments deeply slit to last segment and vein removed to last segment). (9) Peeled and deveined, western (all shell removed except last shell segment and tail fins, with segments split completely to last segment and vein removed to last segment). (10) Shell on pieces (head removed, shell and tail fins when existing not removed). (11) Peeled and deveined, round pieces (all shell removed with segments shallowly slit except last segment when existing: vein removed except last segment when existing). (12)Peeled and deveined butterfly pieces (all shell removed with segments deeply slit except last segment when existing: vein removed except last segment when existing). (13) Peeled undeveined pieces (all shell removed). (14) Other forms of shrimp as specified and so designated on the label.

The Japanese market sometimes uses a special pack for large, whole shrimp. The shrimp are laid side by side in the carton. Water is added so the container is one-third full. The pack is then frozen and the upper parts of the shrimp above the ice line are glazed. This is called a semi-block and protects the fragile appendages while allowing buyers to see the individual shrimp.

Split tails: This form is used mainly for rock shrimp. The back of the shell is split to make it easy to prepare, cook and remove the meat. Split tails may also be deveined. For full details, see Rock shrimp.

Peeled shrimp: Peeled shrimp is green headless without the shell and is known also as peeled only, peeled undeveined or p.u.d. The vein (the intestine) which runs the full length of the tail remains in the meat. Shrimp may be hand peeled or machine peeled. Hand peeled may command a higher price. Machinery removes the whole of the telson, which is the pointed end between the fans of the tail. Careful hand peeling removes the shell from the telson, leaving it attached to the last segment of the tail meat. This looks a little more attractive.

Peeled shrimp is mainly packed in blocks, in the same sizes and combination as green headless product. Peeled shrimp other than blocks is I.Q.F. in a variety of packs. Small shrimp is often packed in 1lb bags for retail sale. Medium sizes may be packed in 1½lb bags for similar use. Most larger I.Q.F. shrimp is packed in 3lb bags. With all of these, master carton sizes vary, but packs for retail are generally in multiples of a dozen.

Peeled and deveined shrimp: Because most people dislike the appearance of the vein, the U.S. market generally prefers its peeled shrimp to be deveined also. This is achieved either by cutting the shrimp tail along the back and washing out the vein, or by vacuuming it out of the tail without cutting into the flesh. This is an expensive operation involving the handling of each tail individually, so most shrimp is mechanically deveined through a cut into the flesh. This form is known as peeled and deveined or p&d shrimp.

The appearance of the vein differs between species. Some shrimp have black, very pronounced, veins. Others have light colored veins which are not noticeable. The vein's appearance also depends partly on what the shrimp eats.

271

Peeled and deveined shrimp is packed exactly as peeled shrimp: blocks and I.Q.F. See the previous heading for details.

Cleaned shrimp: Peeled shrimp that have been washed to remove some of the veins. The process is usually applied to small, inexpensive shrimp. There is not much difference between peeled-only and cleaned product in practice. To avoid problems, treat cleaned shrimp as p.u.d. and not as p&d.

Peeled, deveined and split: Larger peeled shrimp may be deveined with a deep cut along the back, then laid flat with the two halves side by side but still joined. This is sometimes described as butterfly.

Western style: The same as peeled, deveined and split except that only the first four of the six segments are split.

Peeled, tail-on: This is peeled except for the last segment. The shell remains on the last segment and the tail fan is attached. In larger sizes, this form is favored for breading. It is a premium product produced by hand.

Pieces: Also called broken shrimp (see the following paragraph). In the U.S.A. a piece is a shrimp that has fewer than five segments of the original six segments of the abdomen (the tail). Pieces are both shell-on and peeled. Very small peeled shrimp are often pieces because they are almost impossible to peel without damaging them. Note that they may not always be described as pieces by the packer.

There is an international definition of peeled shrimp pieces from the Codex Alimentarius, the international food products code assembled under the auspices of two United Nations agencies. This definition depends on the size of the shrimp before it was broken. If the count is smaller than 70 per pound, four segments or fewer constitute broken shrimp. For larger shrimp (those larger than 70 count per pound) pieces have five segments or fewer. This definition means that large peeled shrimp can lack one segment to qualify as whole shrimp. Small peeled shrimp can lack two segments and still be called whole.

Broken shrimp: Usually the term is applied to shrimp that is not whole, although U.S. Grade Standards specify broken shrimp as tails with a break in the flesh greater than one third of the thickness of the shrimp at the point of the break. Broken peeled and peeled and deveined shrimp is readily available, especially in very small sizes and is a cheap material for uses where the appearance is not important. Broken shell-on shrimp is less common, but has a ready market for institutional use.

Prawn balls are not seen much anymore. The term refers to p&d shrimp pieces, usually from China, sometimes from Hong Kong between U/15 (under 15) and 41/50. Generally, prawn balls have only one or two segments missing. They were a good, economical product.

Class A shrimp: A term for Brazil shell-on pinks packed to include damaged tails, broken tails and pieces. These are roughly graded as small, medium and large. Mostly, these are now sold as second-grade brands. Sizes vary and you should check the actual counts from each batch offered. Packing is 10/2kg or 6/2kg.

Breaded shrimp comes in a wide variety of forms. It is a very important foodservice item. Both peeled and peeled and deveined shrimp are used for breading. So are pieces, which may be ground up and extruded or reformed in shrimp-like shapes, giving a uniform and inexpensive product.

Peeled tail-on shrimp are used to make a premium product. The breading may cover the whole tail but a better product is breading which does not extend to the sixth (tail) segment. This gives the consumer the option of picking up the item by the unbreaded piece of shell. This product is called "clean tail."

Breaded product with shrimp equaling less than half of the final weight must be called imitation breaded shrimp. Regular breaded shrimp has at least 50 percent shrimp and "lightly breaded" has at least 65 percent shrimp.

Whole cooked shrimp are not used very much in the U.S. Northern shrimp (*Pandalus borealis*) is the major product, frozen at sea in 11lb (5 kilo) boxes.

Cooked and peeled shrimp are an important item. The northern shrimp dominates the premium end of the business. Although it is not actually deveined, the veins are largely washed away during processing. Retail packs are often produced in the U.S. from imported peeled raw shrimp. Cooked, peeled and deveined shrimp are used in the same way as cooked and peeled. I.Q.F. cooked and peeled giant tigers, often with tail-fan left on, are a newly popular product. Specify finished counts, not made from sizes and watch the quality carefully.

Which product to use?: Determining which form of shrimp to use is complex and depends on available skills, menu requirements and cost control. Some of the considerations are outlined in the following paragraphs.

• The shell and vein of a domestic green headless shrimp represents about 15 percent of the weight. Most regular imported shrimp will give about the same yield, but there are some types of shrimp with much thicker shells that give lower yields. The labor cost of peeling and deveining may be substantial, or may be effectively free if kitchen help is on site and otherwise unutilized. Green headless shrimp is nearly always cheaper than peeled and deveined shrimp of the same type and size, so the cost of each as an alternative has to be checked carefully from time to time.

• Block frozen headless shrimp holds its quality much better than I.Q.F. p&d and rather better than block frozen p&d. It also has more versatility in use. Many restaurants prefer to restrict the number of different types of shrimp they keep to reduce inventory costs and control problems, so shell-on shrimp meets more menu requirements than other forms.

• Waste potential is another complex factor. I.Q.F. shrimp can be used frozen, so there is no loss due to thawing, while the loss on block frozen peeled shrimp can be substantial, especially if thawing procedures are unsatisfactory. An inexpert peeler in the kitchen can also waste a lot of shrimp.

Whether you use breaded shrimp clearly depends on costs compared to convenience, given the fact that the consistent and superior breading that can be assured in a factory is much more reliable than that of an individual unmechanized kitchen.

Any and all of these considerations may be less important than choice of a particular origin or type of shrimp, desire for a specific flavor, or the natural preference for retaining satisfactory methods and product in preference to change and experimentation.

Shrimp packs are remarkably standardized. Nearly all blocks are 5lb or 2kg (the 2kg blocks being especially popular with middlemen who resell them as 5lb blocks, so making a dishonest profit of 12 percent). Nearly all I.Q.F. shrimp are packed in 1lb, 1½lb and 3lb bags.

SHRIMP QUALITY: There are two aspects to shrimp quality; the intrinsic nature of the shrimp and the handling, processing and packing standards that have been applied to it.

Intrinsic quality: Shrimp from different origins have different characteristics and it is important to get to know how each type should look, taste and smell. Good freshwater shrimp will not have the same firm texture as good Central American shrimp; northern shrimp tastes a little sweeter and has softer texture than white shrimp. Such aspects can only be judged from experience.

Shrimp origins play a major part in quality expectations. Australian banana prawns are more highly regarded in the U.S.A. than Indian white shrimp. Both are the same species, *Penaeus indicus*. Chinese white shrimp sells for a substantial discount against domestic white shrimp. Yet they are so similar that repacking of the Chinese shrimp as domestic product goes unnoticed. The smart user looks at the product and decides its quality objectively. There are many differences between species which are important. There are also differences in how most shrimp is packed by one origin compared with the product from another. But every packer is an individual human operation. Generalizations may tell you which origins need the most scrutiny and no one should stop you from looking.

Product quality: Leaving aside the inherent characteristics of whatever shrimp you are examining, there are a number of common features that you should check, whatever the origin. These are similar to quality considerations of other seafood product.

Frozen blocks should be in sound packages, polywrapped inside inner cartons. Glaze should completely seal the block's upper side as the box is opened. Larger shrimp is generally "finger packed" meaning that the visible layer of the block has shrimp laid out neatly side by side. "Jumble" packs are less attractive and demonstrate less care by the packer.

I.Q.F. packs should be in strong, undamaged bags, with no signs of ice crystals or frost inside the bag. Individual shrimp should be evenly glazed all over and should be separate, with no clumping. Clumping indicates that the product has warmed since it was first frozen. This adversely affects the quality and storage life of the shrimp.

General features: All shrimp products should have fresh odor and flavor. Experience in judging taste and texture is necessary, but off odors are readily apparent.

There should be no signs of dehydration (see Freezer burn) represented by woolly or white patches around edges, or softness of unglazed parts. There should also be no black spots or patches (see Melanosis). If any spots are present, they should not extend to the meat. Shrimp not described as broken or as pieces should of course be whole. See the definitions earlier in this section.

Packs should not contain pieces of shell, shrimp legs, feelers, seaweed or other foreign matter.

It is also, of course, vitally important that the shrimp in the pack should be the shrimp described on the label and in the invoice. Apart from checking weights, to ensure that 5lb blocks are not really 2kg blocks (see above), you should check that the shrimp is really what it is claimed to be in terms of count, color, type and origin.

There are well-documented instances of Chinese white shell-on shrimp being thawed and repacked as domestic whites. The advantages to the repacker are that he is making a substantial profit because of the difference in price between Chinese and domestic shrimp. There is a subsidiary advantage that the Chinese packs are frequently overweight, so yielding even more shrimp to repack. However, if Chinese shrimp is good enough to pass as domestic – and it is – then why does it sell at a discount? The smart buyer will use the Chinese product at the lower price, leaving the more expensive alternative for the designer label purchaser.

There are honest repacks of shrimp, which state "packed in U.S.A." on the label and use different shrimp from time to time. These packs are usually I.Q.F. p&d and often consist of reprocessed block frozen shrimp that has been thawed, checked, regraded and refrozen for packing into 1½lb and 3lb bags. The advantages of this product include reasonable consistency of quality and complete consistency in the label that you use, which helps to build customer confidence. These repacks sell as such and are a useful source of supply especially for distributors with little demand for shrimp who carry it mainly as a customer service and lack the time to learn enough about the product to buy it properly.

The little word "shrimp" covers such a huge variety of product that it is clearly impossible to lay down any absolutes about quality. In one important respect, good quality means product that is suitable for its specific use and successful in pleasing the customers. With this in mind, it is often possible to cut costs by using alternative product that is just as good for a specific use, but may be perhaps less flexible in the variety of its uses, or may be cheaper simply because it is less well known. For example, freshwater shrimp is a cheaper alternative for certain recipes, but cannot be used for others; Brazil shrimp when first offered in the U.S.A. was cheaper than domestic shrimp because few users had experience with it and were cautious about trying it. Now that it is well known, it is a premium shrimp selling at a consistently higher price than domestic product.

COLORS AND TYPES OF SHRIMP: The Food and Agriculture Organization of the United Nations (F.A.O.) has identified over 340 species of shrimp that are or could be commercially important. In *An Illustrated Guide to Shrimp of the World* we selected 70 of these as the most important currently. The following section describes the major categories of shrimp and the major species within those categories, as guidance for the seafood user. For much more detail and information on shrimp, refer to *An Illustrated Guide to Shrimp of the World*.

In this section, the English names given to the numerous shrimp species are those used by F.A.O. Where other names are used in the U.S.A., these are noted also.

Northern (cold water) shrimp: These are known variously as Alaskan shrimp, Oregon shrimp, or by other origin names including Arctic, Greenland, Norway, Canada and Maine. They vary in size from about 26/30 downwards, but the majority are very small. Almost all are sold cooked and peeled since these species are difficult to peel when raw. Usual counts of cooked and peeled are 200/400 per lb, though little attempt is made at grading and it is often sold as "sea run" meaning ungraded.

Usual pack is 5lb block or I.Q.F., 6 per master. Some 5lb cold pack cans are used as well. Retail packs of 1lb and 8oz are available.

Some Canadian and Greenland shrimp is frozen whole, sometimes raw and sometimes cooked. This is sold mainly in Europe and Japan but small quantities are available in the U.S.A. and sell to zoos and aquaria for special diets. Because of its pink color when raw, it is not much liked for angling bait.

There are a few restaurant operators who have realized the advantages of using these whole shrimp for salad bars and similar applications. Whole, raw or cooked, they are generally graded 35/45 and 45/55 per lb, which look a reasonable size on the plate and take a long time to eat if diners are given the task of beheading and peeling the shrimp themselves. The bonuses are the low cost and the excellent taste of the product – this is one of the best of all shrimp to eat in any form – and the delicate pink color which is also most attractive.

The major species is *Pandalus borealis*, which is found in all sub-arctic waters and as far south as Oregon on the Pacific coast and Cape Cod on the Atlantic. This is perhaps the most important cold water species in the world and is certainly the most important in the U.S.A. This species is called Northern shrimp. There are several other pandalid shrimp species that may be sold separately or may be mixed in with the northern shrimp. All of these species have similar taste and texture.

Coonstripe is *Pandalus hypsinotus*, a larger cold water shrimp found on both sides of the North Pacific. It supports a major fishery in Korea and is well-known in British Columbia. It is sometimes called humpback shrimp in the U.S.A.

Ocean shrimp is *Pandalus jordani*. It is found only from Alaska to southern California. It used to be an important California resource, but catches now are small.

Spot shrimp, *Pandalus platyceros*, is the largest Pacific pandalid species, reaching ten inches in overall length and yielding 7/10 shell-on tails per pound. It is found on both sides of the Pacific as far south as Japan in the west and southern California in the east. It is an important species in British Columbia, where it is sometimes shipped live in tanks. Part of the catch is frozen in semi-blocks for Japanese buyers.

Sidestripe, *Pandalopsis dispar,* lives in the eastern Pacific from Alaska to Oregon. It is quite large (8 inches long) and highly esteemed for its eating qualities. Catches are small.

California shrimp, also called gray or bay shrimp is *Crangon franciscorum* and is another northeastern Pacific species. It was a major fishery in California but the pandalid species have displaced it. It is very small, growing to about 3 inches, less than half the size of the northern shrimp.

White shrimp: Most of the time, white shrimp sells at a small premium above the prices for pink and brown shrimp. White domestic and Mexican shrimp are the standard for headless product. Prices of most other headless shrimp relate to these.

Some white shrimp are whiter than others. Gulf of Mexico domestic and Mexican whites are a reasonable shade of white; some Central and South American whites are whiter whereas some east coast domestic shrimp is tan rather than white, although sold as white. White shrimp is preferred because it is thought to have less of an iodine flavor than pink or brown shrimp. Japanese buyers select brown shrimp because they like the slight iodine flavor.

Domestic and Gulf white shrimp is *Penaeus setiferus*. It is caught from the Carolinas southwards through the Gulf of Mexico, where most is landed. This is one of the world's most important commercial shrimp species. Mexican and U.S. fishermen both depend on it heavily.

The southern white shrimp, *Penaeus schmitti*, is so similar that it can only be distinguished from the Gulf white by the shape of the genitals. It is found from the Caribbean around the coast of northern South America to southern Brazil. Brazil is the major producer, but white shrimp from the Caribbean coast of Central America is also most likely to be this species.

West coast white shrimp from Mexico is mainly *Penaeus stylirostris*. U.S.A. importers may call these Mexican whites or west coast whites. The F.A.O. name is blue shrimp, which is also the common name in Mexico. El Salvador, Guatemala and Honduras produce significant quantities of this species, which is one of the mainstays of shrimp aquaculture, so may be imported from a wider range of countries as farming develops.

The Central American white shrimp, called Western white by F.A.O, is *Penaeus occidentalis*. This is caught from southern Mexico to Peru and is especially important in Panama, El Salvador, Columbia and Ecuador.

The whiteleg shrimp is *Penaeus vannamei*, and is the third most important of the west coast wild species. It is important in southern Mexico, Guatemala and El Salvador and is the major aquaculture species in Ecuador. Its full natural range is from Baja California to Peru. Because of the enormous growth of shrimp farming in Ecuador and Central America, much of it based on this species, this is now one of the commonest whites available on the U.S. market.

Chinese white shrimp has become a major factor, also because of the development of shrimp aquaculture. The Chinese species is *Penaeus chinensis* (an incorrect but still widely used scientific name is *Penaeus orientalis*). It is an excellent shrimp in shell-on form, though careless processing and overuse of dips and additives have spoiled its reputation somewhat for the peeled shrimp trade.

Indian white shrimp, *Penaeus indicus*, is an important species from much of the Indian Ocean and southwestern Pacific region. In addition to being the most important shrimp caught by Indian fishermen, it is also the largest catch of east African countries. Large quantities come from Bangladesh, Malaysia, Thailand and the Philippines. Vietnam and other parts of Indochina have large resources. It is also important in northern Australia, where it is one of several species called banana prawn. It is a good quality, well flavored shrimp.

Australian banana shrimp, including the Indian white, are perhaps off-white, but so are many other whites. *Penaeus merguiensis* is an important catch in northern and western parts of Australia. It is found from Australia throughout southeast and south Asia to the Arabian Gulf. It is the main farmed species in Thailand. Large quantities are landed in the Philippines, Malaysia and Indonesia. The meat is firm and well flavored.

Pakistan white shrimp includes *Penaeus penicillatus* known under the F.A.O. name of redtail prawn. The species is found from the Red Sea to Taiwan and throughout south and southeast Asia. However, Pakistan is the only significant producer of the species, which is very similar to the Indian white.

There are, of course, many other species of white shrimp. Those mentioned above are the major commercially exploited ones.

Brown shrimp: These often have a brownish shell when raw. When cooked they are slightly darker than whites and more similar to pinks. The flavor is generally stronger than either whites or pinks, possibly due to the higher iodine content. Peeled browns look unattractive and are not easy to sell. Some west coast browns from Mexico are quite pale and a little more acceptable.

Although brown shrimp, especially larger sizes, sells for a little less than white, it is still a major supplier of market volume. The effect of the prejudices should not be overestimated: most buyers who dislike browns will allow their dislike to be overcome for a differential of 10 or 15 cents a pound.

It is not always easy to tell browns and whites apart. Gulf fishermen look for a groove in the last segment of the tail shell of the Gulf brown shrimp to distinguish the two. They cannot be identified by color alone.

The major brown species used commercially are:

Gulf brown shrimp is *Penaeus aztecus*. It is caught from North Carolina southwards throughout the Gulf. Texas is the major producing state. Mexico produces more pinks and whites than browns. The meat is firm and the taste quite mild. As mentioned above, the colors of Gulf whites and browns (as of most shrimp) vary a lot. They cannot be distinguished just by the color of either the shell or the meat.

The west coast Mexican brown shrimp is *Penaeus californiensis*. This is called yellowleg shrimp by F.A.O. It ranges from southern California to northern Peru. It is of great commercial importance in Mexico, where in some years it accounts for three quarters of the country's Pacific shrimp catch. A large percentage of the Mexican catch is sold to Japan. Guatemala, Costa Rica, Panama and Ecuador also produce large quantities. It is an excellent quality shrimp.

Indian brown shrimp, *Metapenaeus affinis*, called Jinga shrimp by F.A.O., is also an important species in world trade. Pakistan, the west and southeast coasts of India, Malaya and Hong Kong are important sources. The species is very similar to the greasyback shrimp, *Metapenaeus ensis* and the endeavour shrimp, *Metapenaeus endeavouri*. The endeavour is limited to northern Australia, but the greasyback is found in India, southeast Asia including the Malay archipelago and Australia. Greasyback and Indian browns are often caught together and are not distinguished in practice.

The kuruma shrimp, *Penaeus japonicus*, is very important in Japan. It is found over a huge range, from Japan to Australia, westwards around eastern and southern Africa and northwards into the Mediterranean. The species is sometimes called the flower shrimp. The shell is striped, but it is treated basically as a brown and not as a tiger. The western king prawn, which covers a similar range and is important in Australia, is very similar.

Pink shrimp: These have pink shells when raw. When cooked they are slightly deeper in color than whites. The highest priced pinks come from the Guyanas. Slightly paler and slightly less expensive pinks come from the adjacent coast of Brazil. Both of these often sell for more than domestic whites. Domestic and other pinks are less highly regarded.

Pinks are frequently the preferred color for I.Q.F. p&d product, especially with buyers who favor whites for the shell-on form. Pinks are less desirable in block peeled forms.

Domestic pink shrimp, called northern pink shrimp by F.A.O., is *Penaeus duorarum*. It is fished on the Atlantic coast of Florida and throughout the Gulf. It is a major commercial resource for both the U.S.A. and Mexico. The Campeche Banks in the southern Gulf of Mexico account for a lot of the catch. Mexican processors used to pack superlative p&d shrimp made from this species but processing facilities have declined and there is now little or no production. The Tortugas area of the Florida Keys produces pink shrimp throughout the year.

The redspotted shrimp, *Penaeus brasiliensis*, is very similar: the differences between the two are mainly in the shapes of the genitals. However, the redspotted shrimp has a greater range, from Florida, through the Gulf and as far south as southern Brazil. It is very important in the Guianas and northeastern Brazil.

The southern pink shrimp, *Penaeus notialis* is also very similar to domestic pink shrimp. Until 1939, it was considered to be the same species as *Penaeus duorarum*. This ranges from the Caribbean to southern Brazil. Although it is usually called Brazil pink in the U.S.A., it is the most important commercial shrimp in the Caribbean and Venezuela as well as northern Brazil. Across the Atlantic, it is fished in West Africa from Mauretania to the Congo.

The caramote, *Penaeus kerathurus*, is another pink from the eastern Atlantic. It is caught from Spain, the entire Mediterranean and southwards along the coast of Africa to Angola. It is a highly prized species in the southern Mediterranean. It is not often sold in the U.S.A. because it is so highly valued in Europe and most supplies remain there.

European consumers value shrimp with deep pink color. There are a number of other species of very fine shrimp which are used mainly in Europe.

The deep-water rose shrimp, *Parapenaeus longirostris*, is usually sold whole, raw or cooked, in Europe and North Africa.

The striped soldier shrimp or barber pole shrimp, *Plesionika edwardsii*, is a similar pink from the same region. This species is found in the Gulf of Mexico also, where it is not exploited although there are indications of commercial quantities.

Asian pink shrimp species are mainly small and used for peeling.

Red rice shrimp, *Metapenaeopsis barbata* (the F.A.O. name is whiskered velvet shrimp), ranging from southern China to Taiwan, has a hard shell which reduces the peeled yield and so is normally sold shell-on. This is an important species in Japan, where it is caught in the Inland Sea.

Tiger shrimp is so-called because it has colored stripes around the shell and associated stripes on the meat when peeled. The shell is generally thick. In the last few years, one species of tiger has become a major product of aquaculture and a major shrimp in world markets. This is the giant tiger, black tiger or leader prawn, *Penaeus monodon*. It is the largest commercially available shrimp, growing to 13 inches in length. It grows fast and is easy to farm. Its natural range is the whole Indo-Pacific region from eastern Africa to eastern Australia. It was always commercially important in India, Bangladesh and Malaysia. Now, with aquaculture output increasing all the time, it is being farmed in Hawaii, South and North America and many other places far from its natural habitat.

Giant tigers are comparatively inexpensive and have developed new markets for shrimp and shrimp products. The best way to buy them is cooked, peeled and deveined, I.Q.F. They shrink when slightly overcooked. It is better to let the processor handle them and for you to buy them in ready-to-use form. The best packers (there are even very good ones in Taiwan) produce good, consistent, well flavored product. Less adept processors use too many additives, which results in poorer flavor and texture. Using shrimp that is past its peak freshness also shows up in the product.

Giant tigers turn bright red when cooked and retain their color for several days if refrigerated. The texture is a little softer than domestic shrimp, but is acceptable. The flavor is good. Check that sizes quoted are finished count. Made-from sizes can vary enormously.

Other tiger shrimp are used as less-expensive alternatives to other colors of shell-on product. Brown tigers (*Penaeus esculentus*) and green tigers (*Penaeus semisulcatus*) are exported from Australia and their light markings make them a reasonable alternative to browns. Green tigers are caught throughout the Indo-Pacific region and are important from Taiwan, Pakistan and other countries. The species has migrated from the Red Sea through the Suez Canal into the eastern Mediterranean. From most origins other than Australia it has more intense markings. In Taiwan and Thailand the species is being used for aquaculture. The meat is firm and mild.

Red shrimp: **The royal red,** *Pleoticus robustus*, is a domestic red shrimp which is caught off Florida, the Atlantic side of the Caribbean and the northern coast of South America. It is a deep-water species with rather soft but sweet flesh. It needs swift and careful handling and light cooking. The resource is thought to be underexploited and the shrimp is good, well worth some effort.

The Argentine red or pink shrimp, *Pleoticus muelleri* is a similar species cyclically available from Argentina. The resource seems to vary greatly in size so supplies are not reliable. It is a well-flavored species with soft flesh, also requiring gentle and brief cooking. It has better flavor than many species which cost more. Packing, grading and processing are not consistent. Buy these shrimp with great care.

The giant red shrimp, known in the U.S.A. as Spanish red, is *Aristaeomorpha foliacea*. It is found mainly in the Mediterranean and off northwest Africa. However, there are small concentrations of the same species off the Atlantic coast of the U.S.A. and Venezuela and what is probably the same species off New Zealand, Australia, Japan and parts of east Africa. Most commercial supplies come from Spanish sources. The meat is soft and tastes more like lobster than shrimp. This is a high-priced premium shrimp for specific gourmet markets. Packing is 10/5lb blocks and sizes range from under-7 to about 26/30, though shrimp smaller than 15 count is difficult to sell in the U.S.A.

Weights tend to be marginal to poor and counts tend to the smaller end of the labelled scale. Since the shrimp is particularly expensive, special care should be taken to check them.

There are a number of other commercial species of red shrimp. Most of these are sold mainly in Europe.

The blue and red shrimp, *Aristeus antennatus*, is caught with the Spanish red and often sold with it.

Freshwater shrimp: The F.A.O. name is "giant river prawn." The species is *Macrobrachium rosenbergii*. Thick brown-gray shrimp found in fresh and brackish water in southern Asia, the Malay archipelago and northern Australia. Freshwaters are cheap, generally the cheapest shell-on shrimp available in quantity. A favored aquaculture product, it is now found in many other places. There are, however, differences between the traditional freshwater shrimp and the farmed product.

Bangladesh, India and Burma are the main suppliers of wild freshwaters, fishing the enormous deltas of the Ganges, Brahmaputra and Irrawaddy rivers. Indonesia, Thailand and other Asian countries ship small quantities. Indo-China has some resources which are little fished. Hong Kong and Singapore are significant shippers of freshwater shrimp, most of which is reconsigned merchandise originating in Burma. This is not done with intent to deceive, but for legitimate reasons related to the isolation and trading practices of Burma.

Burmese shrimp is always packed in 2kg blocks and heavily glazed for protection. Gross weight of a block may exceed 7lb. If you are offered Burmese or reconsigned Burmese shrimp in 5lb units you can be certain that you are being offered marked up product. The economic and political situation in Burma is currently changing. The freshwater shrimp situation there may well change also.

Freshwater shrimp runs very large – as big as under 3 to the pound. The largest sizes are preferred in the U.S. The tails are shorter and thicker than most other shrimp and the flavor is less than outstanding. They should not be boiled, since this cooking method produces an unpleasant smell. They are perfectly good broiled or baked and are used generally for baked stuffed shrimp, or "scampi" dishes. Make sure your customers understand this restriction on the use of freshwaters or you will have unwarranted complaints of decomposed product.

Larger sizes of freshwater shrimp sell at substantial discounts under the price for the same size of domestic whites. Freshwater shipments are erratic and fluctuate seasonally. Rejections by the F.D.A. can also be high. A combination of factors has in the past pushed the price of freshwaters above that of whites. The intrinsic qualities of the products makes this an unlikely situation, but no price relationships in seafood can ever be assumed to be permanent.

Because freshwater shrimp comes from very hot, damp climates in some of the world's poorest regions which lack amenities such as adequate refrigeration, roads and water, it is inevitable that quality varies. At its best it is rather soft, but a mushy texture is an early sign of decomposition, so you need to familiarize yourself with the characteristics of the shrimp. Because of the inherent variability of the product, you cannot assume that shrimp within a batch will be consistent and should restrict purchases to importers capable of replacing defective product.

The species is a prime aquaculture shrimp. It was traditionally grown in the Malay islands in ponds but has now moved into the mainstream of modern aquaculture. It is easy to grow partly because it does not need a marine environment. Giant river prawns produced by competent shrimp farmers have the same intrinsic characteristics as commodity-traded freshwater shrimp – they should not be boiled and the appearance is a little different from regular white or brown shrimp. But aquaculture product can be shipped fresh or even alive, opening up new markets for what was a second-class product.

Seabob *Scientific name: Xiphopenaeus kroyeri:* A small brown shrimp with a thick shell found from Florida to Brazil. Imports are usually peeled shrimp from Brazil which can be used by processors, although the shrinkage rate is high. I.Q.F. peeled seabobs in 1lb bags are an adequate retail item. Seabobs used to be mainly canned, but the decline of the domestic shrimp canning industry left more of the resource for the frozen market. The species may be offered from Central American sources as a fidel.

Peeled shrimp: There are numerous species that go into the packs of smaller peeled shrimp. Various names are used, such as TDs, "tele" shrimp and salad shrimp. Peeled TD shrimp from India and Central America tends to be brownish in color and often broken because of the difficulty of peeling. When cooked, this shrimp shrinks more than most. Tiny "tele" shrimp from India is sold as p.u.d. broken, counting about 500 per pound. This very cheap product is used by processors who grind and extrude it or for institutional use in stuffings and flavorings.

Salad shrimp covers peeled, p&d or cooked peeled shrimp smaller than 100 count. This is not a precise term since it might cover Alaskan cooked shrimp or Hong Kong I.Q.F. p.u.d. shrimp – a price differential of several hundred percent. It is essential to get a clearer definition of the term if it is used.

Peeled shrimp, especially from Asian origins where there are many species, often consists of a mixture of species in the same box. Some origins distinguish between pinks, browns and sand shrimp, although the distinctions are not always readily apparent to the eye. For information on the species that might be used, see *An Illustrated Guide to Shrimp of the World*.

SHRIMP COUNTS: Shrimp are invariably graded in numbers per pound and there is substantial standardization:

Counts per pound
Under 3
Under 4
Under 6 or 4/6
Under 8 or 6/8
Under 10 or 8/10
Under 12 or 8/12
Under 15 or 11/15 or 13/15
16/20
21/25
26/30
31/35 or31/40
36/40
41/50
51/60
61/70
71/80 or 71/90
91/110
110/130 or 100/200
130/200 sometimes 130/150 and 150/200
200/300
300/500
500 up

Most sales of shell-on shrimp are U/15 through 61/70. Shell-on smaller than 71/90 is very unusual. Most peeled shrimp larger than 100 count is deveined. Smaller peeled shrimp may or may not be deveined.

Peeled shrimp may be graded as finished count, where you get the number it says on the label, or as "peeled-from" count, where the label shows the size of shell-on tail from which the shrimp was peeled. The actual count in this case is usually one or two sizes smaller. There is usually no indication given as to which you may be getting, but assume "peeled from" counts unless you are told to the contrary, as these are more usual. It is better to receive shrimp larger than you expected than to pay too much for shrimp smaller than you wanted.

Word descriptions are sometimes used instead of numerical counts. Some states have rules on what names may be used for certain sizes also. It is confusing to use word descriptions. These should be avoided, or at least be supported with numerical counts. The U.S. Grade specification (which says "Descriptive size names are not recommended") used to define the names for those who insisted on using them. The definitions were dropped in 1982 to discourage use. The potential for confusion is considerable. For example, "extra large" was bigger than "large" but "extra small" was smaller than "small". The value of words to describe sizes is mainly in the retail area. Consumers buying shrimp occasionally will not necessarily realize that 10/15 is a count and is bigger than a 31/35, but it is clear that "colossal" is bigger than "large."

Counts of broken shrimp and pieces are not defined in any standard way. Some packers may offer a 16/20 broken to indicate that the box contains shrimp that would have been 16/20 count if whole. Others will quote a wider range such as 20/40 count, indicating that number of pieces per pound. It is most common to grade broken shrimp as large, medium or small, but there are no standards for these. It is necessary to inspect product and to gain experience with a particular packer to be confident of what you are buying.

Uniformity ratios for shrimp: Counts should be correct (see below) and the shrimp should also be reasonably uniform in size. U.S. Grade Standards define uniformity, but for most purposes it can be checked by eye and only needs to be measured if you have to prove or disprove a complaint. The rules on uniformity are as follows:

Uniformity ratios (UR) provide a measure for the size composition within a designated count for a package of shrimp. The lower the ratio then the more uniform the count. For example a UR = 1.0 means all shrimp in the package are the same size. Realizing a 1.0 UR is impractical, higher ratios (i.e. 1.5, 1.75, etc) allow some tolerance for natural variation.

UR Procedures: Visually select and weigh not more than 10 percent by count (10 percent of the total number of individual shrimp in one package) of the largest shrimp. Do the same for 10 percent by count of the smallest shrimp. The shrimp selected should be whole, unbroken and undamaged. Calculate the UR.

$$UR = \frac{\text{Weight for 10\% (by count) of largest}}{\text{Weight for 10\% (by count) of smallest}}$$

Theoretical example of probable mix for different uniformity ratios for a 5 pound package of 16 to 20 count shrimp. The example is arranged to show the possible variation in the size or count for the smallest shrimp assuming the large shrimp are at maximum grade (16 count) or minimum grade (20 count).

10% Largest		Different	10% Smallest	
Count	Weight	UR s	Count	Weight
16	8oz	1.25	20	6.40oz
16	8oz	1.50	23	5.33oz
16	8oz	1.75	28	4.56oz
20	8oz	1.25	25	6.40oz
20	8oz	1.5	25	5.33oz
20	8oz	1.75	35	4.56oz

Counts should be consistent, so that the shrimp in a given pack are similarly sized. For U.S. Grade Standards the count of shell-on shrimp is determined by dividing the number of shrimp in the package by the net weight of the package in pounds. Therefore a 5lb pack of 16/20 count shrimp must contain 80 to 100 shrimp. Many processors and large users have additional requirements relating the size of the largest and smallest shrimp in a pack in order to keep the shrimp as consistently sized as possible.

SHRIMP AQUACULTURE: Production of farmed shrimp is changing the world shrimp business, partly because more shrimp is available and partly because so far it is not economical to grow shrimp larger than medium sizes. Buyers are becoming accustomed to using medium sizes rather than large ones and are also adapting to the major farmed species in quantities never before used in the trade, including the tiger shrimp. The giant tiger shrimp is thought to account for one third of the total output of the world's shrimp farms.

Shrimp farming requires hatcheries to produce juvenile shrimp and growout facilities to raise them to marketable size. Infrastructure such as processing facilities, transportation and ice is also essential and sometimes forgotten by eager investors in new shrimp farms.

Hatchery technique is developing rapidly and is effective for a number of species. Where hatcheries are not available, growers must rely on wild juveniles, which can only be captured for a short period each season.

Growout operations come in three densities. **Intensive** farming uses heavy densities of shrimp designed to produce the greatest weight for the size of the growing area. The technology is the most demanding but in some ways the most controllable. The shrimp must be fed and carefully pampered. The trend is likely to be towards increasing densities and higher yields. The risks from disease or mechanical problems are, of course, greater in intensive operations. **Extensive** shrimp farming uses very light densities of shrimp and the simplest techniques. Shrimp farming began this way, with farmers impounding seawater containing juvenile shrimp. The growing shrimp feed naturally on what is in the water. In between, **semi-intensive** farming uses a mixture of the two other techniques.

Giant tigers (*Penaeus monodon*) are the main product of shrimp aquaculture and the species is predominant throughout southeast Asia and Taiwan. China is the world's largest producer of aquaculture shrimp, concentrating on Chinese white shrimp (*Penaeus chinensis*) which is very similar to Gulf domestic white. In South America, where Ecuador is currently by far the largest shrimp farming country, the western white shrimp, *Penaeus vannamei*, is the main species. This species is well known on the U.S. market with an established reputation.

Many other species are farmed in smaller but still significant quantities, including the freshwater shrimp. In Indonesia, which has enormous potential, the Indian white shrimp *Penaeus indicus* is the main farmed species. Work with most of the commercially important penaeid species is starting to show results. It is not unreasonable to expect that most of the major species will be farm-raised by the end of the century.

There are some negatives, however. Shrimp farming uses a number of new technologies, which may not stand up to all the varied conditions that farmers meet over time. It is also concentrated in a number of poorer, mainly tropical countries where economic and political developments are always risky. Forecasts of ever-increasing production from these countries could easily be wrong due to political factors or simply to the shortage of expertise, which is a universal problem for this fast-growing industry. Diseases can and do strike shrimp farms just as they do any other farms. And diseases, especially viral ones, can destroy not just a few farms but an entire region's industry in a very short time, leaving water in farming areas which retains the infection and perhaps cannot be used again for shrimp culture for many years. Similar disasters have struck oyster farmers through the ages and their techniques are much less intensive than shrimp farming.

For the best information on a continuing basis about shrimp farming developments, subscribe to *Aquaculture Digest*. The address is 9434 Kearney Mesa Road, San Diego, CA 92126, telephone 619/271-0133.

SIERRA: See Kingfish

SILVERBRIGHT: A quality grade of chum salmon. See Salmon.

SIXTY-FORTY: Fancy Alaskan king and snow crab meat is specified as 60 percent body meat and 40 percent leg meat. This is often described as a 60/40 pack. Canadian and Japanese crabmeat is usually 70/30, giving only 30 percent of the more desirable legmeat. See Crabs.

SKATE *Scientific name: Raja spp.:* Also called rays, although rays are different fish. There are a number of species in both Atlantic and Pacific oceans. The edible part is the "wing" on each side, which may be packed as whole wings, as skinless wings or as fillets removed from the top and bottom of the wings. The top fillet has brown skin and is much thicker than the underside fillet which has white skin. The skin should be removed before cooking the fish. Whole wings may have the knuckle joint, which attaches the wing to the body of the fish, either attached or removed. Like sharks, skates do not have a urinary tract and build up a strong ammonia taint if not handled quickly and iced well.

There is no market in the U.S.A. for skate. A few upmarket restaurants may offer the fish, but this is highly specialized. In Europe, skate is popular and widely eaten. Export packed frozen product is available in 10kg or 28lb boxes. Wings or fillets should be individually wrapped and size graded. Small wings are between one-half and two pounds. Large wings may be 4lbs and up.

There is a widely held consumer belief that skate wings can be cut up and sold as scallops. This is nonsense, but it is a myth with staying power. If people believe that skate is good enough to pass for scallops, then they should be very willing to sample it for itself: it must be (and it is) a very good fish to eat.

SKIPJACK: See Tuna. The name is also used regionally for small bluefish. Headless, dressed ladyfish are sometimes called skipjacks.

SLIPPER LOBSTER: See Lobsters.

SMELTS: Also known as argentines, smelt herring and silversides. Small, silvery herring-like fishes. Different species come from the Atlantic, the Pacific and freshwater. Some are anadromous. All shoal in large numbers when spawning, making them easy and cheap to catch.

Canada is the largest supplier of smelts, from the Atlantic and from the freshwater lakes. There is a great variety of packs. Smelts may be whole eviscerated or eviscerated and breaded. There are many retail and institutional packs. The standard grading is as follows:

Mediums	4 to 5½ inches	15 per lb.
Number 1 (#1)	5½ to 7 inches	12 per lb.
Extras or extra large	7 inches up	7-9 per lb.

Eviscerated (dressed) smelts are usually number 1. Note that this refers to size and not to quality.

Smelts deteriorate quickly as they have a high oil content. Lake smelts are the most important supply and are considered superior because they are less oily than most marine smelts. Lake smelts are seldom more than 5 inches long and are eaten with the bones, which soften when cooked.

There are similar inexpensive fish in many parts of the world. Chile has started exporting smelts to the U.S. and there are numerous other possible sources.

SMOKED FISH: There is continuing and increasing interest in smoked seafoods. Most smoked fish can be frozen if it is properly prepared and packaged. Although smoking was originally a technique for preserving food, today's tastes are for lightly smoked product which is smoke-flavored and not preserved. Therefore, freezing is an important part of distributing and marketing smoked seafood. It is also important to remember that smoked fish and shellfish have about the same keeping quality as fresh, cooked product. Most smoking processes alone do not add to the shelf life.

Smoked seafoods generally need less salting or brining if they are to be frozen than if they are to be sold fresh. They also need careful packaging to protect the product from dehydration and to prevent the smell of the smoked product contaminating other items in storage. It is advisable to use packages which allow oxygen to penetrate: smoked fish can provide a breeding ground for botulinus organisms. These microbes are anaerobic, so allowing oxygen into the package will generally deter their growth.

Salting or brining is a necessary first step in smoking. Flavors, preservatives and colors can be added at this stage. Cold smoked products are processed so that the temperature of the product remains below 85°F. Most of these need to be cooked. Hot smoked products are cooked in the smoke, usually by

293

increasing the temperature of the fish to between 140°F. and 150°F. after an initial period of cold smoking.

Product loses a lot of weight during smoking: loss of up to 30 percent is possible. There are smoke dips which are sometimes used as an alternative to smoking. The texture of the product is different but the flavor can be good. There is no weight loss with a dipped product.

Finnans: A real "finnan haddock" is a medium-sized haddock, split down the back with the backbone left on, then brined and cold smoked. The U.S. market now calls any smoked cod or haddock product a finnan. Most of the product sold is filleted, some of it is processed with smoke dips and not smoked at all.

Kippers: Like finnans, kippers used to be split fish. Now, they are mostly fillets. Kippers are brined, cold smoked herring. The fish must have an oil content of at least 10 percent or the kipper will be dry and hard.

Smoked salmon is the most important smoked product, fresh or frozen. Fillets are smoked, not whole fish. The original European technique, still used in large quantities in Europe and the U.S.A., is heavy brine or salt, then lengthy cold smoking. In the Pacific northwest, hot smoking produces a cooked, drier product that is quite different, though every bit as enjoyable. It is sometimes called kippered salmon. Western smokers also produce small quantities of salmon jerky, which is heavily salted and cold smoked for very long periods so that it is dry and hard and keeps without refrigeration. Lox was originally salted salmon. The name now refers to lightly smoked salmon.

Smoking requires fat salmon. Atlantic, king, sockeye and coho are most favored. Chums are less desirable and pinks are seldom smoked. The best fish is ocean caught on hooks or farmed, so that bruising and other damage is minimized.

Smoked salmon must be trimmed and sliced before serving. Trimming involves cutting away edges and napes as well as the hard surface pellicle, which forms when the fish hangs to dry after brining. The pinbones must be removed individually. If salmon sides are frozen, they can be sliced on a machine so removing the pinbones may not be necessary. Packs include sides, trimmed sides, boneless trimmed sides, sliced and sliced and interleaved, all in both retail and institutional sizes.

Other smoked products: Almost any fish or shellfish can be smoked. In general, oilier fish make better smoked products. Sablefish, eel, whitefish, chub, trout, mackerel, tuna, turbot, bluefish, oysters and mussels are among the many species offered regularly.

SMOLT: Atlantic salmon when it leaves its home river for the first time to enter the sea.

SNAILS: Land snails – escargots – are sold both frozen and canned, with and without shells. The cleaned meats come mainly from France, which provides the best quality and type of product. Other, cheaper product is imported from Taiwan. See also conch and periwinkle.

SNAPPERS: This section is mainly about red snapper and similar fish. Small bluefish are sometimes called snappers, as are a species of turtle and cod, haddock or similar fish under 1½lb landed weight. Many fish are called snapper because the name has great market appeal. "Snapper" is probably misused almost as much as "scrod." Almost any fish with a reddish tinge to the skin is called snapper at some time or another, even a hybrid tilapia. The real thing is good eating, fairly scarce and invariably expensive. It is important to know what you are buying and eating.

Red snapper *Scientific name: Lutjanus campechanus:* Only this single Gulf species may be sold as red snapper in the U.S.A., although the F.D.A. has been giving consideration to calling *Lutjanus purpureus* "Caribbean red snapper." There are a number of other similar snappers fished in the same areas of the Gulf of Mexico and central Atlantic, most of which are good quality eating but have less attractive skin colors. There is no single identifying feature so that you can tell red snapper from other snappers. It is a red-colored fish growing as large as 35lbs, though most commercially available fish is under 10lbs. The premium size is between two and four pounds, which provide natural fillets of about 10 ounces. Red snapper has rose-red skin on top becoming lighter towards the underside. It has a longer pectoral fin than other snappers. However, distinguishing it from some of the other Gulf snappers requires a lot of experience.

Whole fish is usually graded in 2lb steps and packed in 25lb or 40lb boxes. Fillets are graded in 2oz steps and packed in 10lb or 25lb boxes. Most of this species is sold fresh and gutted. If it is filleted, natural fillets are the premium choice. Naturals are the whole fillets from one side of the fish. Larger fish produce bigger fillets that have to be cut. These are described as "cuts." Because they are thicker they are a little harder to cook and they look less attractive on the plate.

In 1980 the F.D.A. issued a "Compliance Policy Guide" 7108.04 to resolve concerns for selling Pacific coast rockfish (family Scorpaenidae) as red snappers. It stated:

BACKGROUND – The name "red snapper" has been preempted by many years of consistent consumer usage as meaning only fish *Lutjanus campechanus*. Because of the high esteem in which this fish is held by consumers, and the relatively limited catch, there have been numerous attempts to substitute other, less expensive fishes for this species. Substitutes of less desirable species have included members of the family Lutjanidae, groupers, a number of west coast rockfishes of the genus Sebastes, and other species. The west coast rockfishes have, until relatively recently, been distributed mostly locally, and thus have been beyond the reach of the Federal Food, Drug, and Cosmetic Act. Some of the states on the west coast have officially sanctioned "red snapper" as an alternative name for such members of the Sebastes genus, although these fishes are quite different in appearance, flavor, and texture, and are generally regarded by consumers familiar with *Lutjanus campechanus* as inferior.

POLICY – The labelling or sale of any fish other than *Lutjanus campechanus* as "red snapper" constitutes a misbranding in violation of the Federal Food, Drug, and Cosmetic Act.

Other snappers: The following table shows the species which may legally be called snapper.

Snappers: Market Names and Common Names

Market name	Common name	Scientific name	Location
Snapper, Caribbean red	Snapper, Caribbean red	*Lutjanus purpureus*	A
Snapper, Pacific	Snapper, Pacific	*Lutjanus peru*	P
Snapper, Pacific dog	Snapper, Pacific dog	*Lutjanus novemfasciatus*	P
Snapper, black	Snapper, black	*Apsilus dentatus*	A
Snapper, black and white	Snapper, black and white	*Macolor niger*	P
Snapper, blackfin	Snapper, blackfin	*Lutjanus buccanella*	A
Snapper, blacktail	Snapper, blacktail	*Lutjanus fulvus*	P
Snapper, blubberlip	Snapper, blubberlip	*Lutjanus rivulatus*	P
Snapper, bluestriped	Snapper, bluestriped	*Lutjanus kasmira*	P
Snapper, cardinal	Snapper, cardinal	*Pristipomoides macrophthalmus*	A
Snapper, colorado	Snapper, colorado	*Lutjanus colorado*	P
Snapper, crimson	Snapper, crimson	*Pristipomoides filamentosus*	P
Snapper, cubera	Snapper, cubera	*Lutjanus cyanopterus*	A
Snapper, dog	Snapper, dog	*Lutjanus jocu*	A
Snapper, emperor	Snapper, emperor	*Lutjanus sebae*	P
Snapper, golden	Snapper, golden	*Lutjanus inermis*	P
Snapper, gray	Snapper, gray	*Lutjanus griseus*	A-F
Snapper, humpback	Snapper, humpback	*Lutjanus gibbus*	P
Snapper, lane	Snapper, lane	*Lutjanus synagris*	A
Snapper, mahogony	Snapper, mahogany	*Lutjanus mahogoni*	A
Snapper, malabar	Malabar	*Lutjanus malabaricus*	P
Snapper, midnight	Snapper, midnight	*Macolor macularius*	P
Snapper, mullet	Snapper, mullet	*Lutjanus aratus*	P
Snapper, mutton	Snapper, mutton	*Lutjanus analis*	A
Snapper, onespot	Snapper, onespot	*Lutjanus monostigma*	P
Snapper, queen	Snapper, queen	*Etelis oculatus*	A
Snapper, red	Snapper, red	*Lutjanus campechanus*	A
Snapper, ruby	Snapper, ruby	*Etelis carbunculus*	P
Snapper, rufous	Snapper, rufous	*Lutjanus jordani*	P
Snapper, sailfin	Snapper, sailfin	*Symphorichthys spilurus*	P

Locations: A = Atlantic   P = Indo-Pacific   F = Freshwater
Source: F.D.A.

Market name	Common name	Scientific name	Location
Snapper, scarlet	Snapper, blood	*Lutjanus sanguineus*	P
Snapper, silk	Snapper, silk	*Lutjanus vivanus*	A
Snapper, spotted rose	Snapper, spotted rose	*Lutjanus guttatus*	P
Snapper, twinspot	Snapper, twinspot	*Lutjanus bohar*	P
Snapper, vermilion	Snapper, vermilion	*Rhomboplites aurorubens*	A
Snapper, yellowstriped	Snapper, yellowstriped	*Etelis coruscans*	P
Snapper, yellowtail	Snapper, yellowtail	*Ocyurus chrysurus*	A

Locations: A = Atlantic   P = Indo-Pacific   F = Freshwater
Source: F.D.A.

For comments on the differences between the more common Atlantic snappers, see *Fresh Seafood, the Commercial Buyer's Guide* from Osprey Books.

Brazil snapper: Yellowtail, mangrove and several other species are imported from Brazil and cost a lot less than red snapper. The fish is not distinguished by species but is sold generically as Brazil snapper. It commands a substantial and steady market because it is packed in a consistent and reliable way and is always available. Compared with the Florida snapper, the skin of most Brazil snapper is browner and the flesh darker.

Small quantities of gutted head-on fish are sold individually polywrapped in 40lb cartons, graded in pounds 1/2lb, 2/3lb, 3/4lb and so on. Most Brazil snapper is sold filleted and is always graded exact weights in ounces 3, 4, 5, through 18 oz. The preferred sizes are 7oz through 12 oz. Brazil packers ship "natural" and "cut" fillets. Cuts are seldom smaller than 9oz, since only natural fillets larger than about 18oz are divided – below that size they can be sold as naturals.

The straight weight gradings should not be interpreted to mean that every fillet in a box is the exact weight on the label. Obviously this would be impossible with a natural product. The technique used to grade in this way is as follows: A 10lb box contains 160oz of product. If the fillets are, say, 8oz, this means 20 fillets per box, all of closely similar size. The fillets are graded by eye so that they look very much the same. In practice, the weight of the individual fillet is not the deciding factor.

This gives the user the advantage of product which looks the same on the plate when portions are served. It also permits tighter inventory control since the number of portions in a carton is known. There are a defined number of pieces for each size. Since lobster and snapper are graded the same way, see Lobster for a listing. A similar grading applies for Brazilian lobster tails.

This grading pattern has been a major reason for the success of Brazil snapper in the U.S. market. Also, the item is standardized and generally of good quality. Problems are rare. Packing is always 4/10lb boxes, with the fillets individually polywrapped.

Thailand snapper: *Scientific name: Etelis coruscans:* Importers used to claim this as the same species as genuine red snapper. The fish is related to the ruby snapper, which is found throughout the Indo-Pacific's warmer waters and is called onaga in Hawaii, where it is an important species. Thailand snapper is often repacked as red snapper.

Fillets are imported in 4lb, 2kg, 5lb and 10lb boxes. All are individually wrapped. Grading is sometimes exact weights like Brazil snapper and sometimes in 2oz steps from 4/6oz upwards.

Some packers mix cuts with naturals. Others utilize the large number of big fish by cutting the fillet into three or more pieces, making strips as well as cut fillets, or dividing the naturals into tail cuts and frontal cuts to retain better shapes. Larger Thai snapper tends to have darker skin and this may cause it to be rejected by users who are looking for a cheaper alternative or substitute for red snapper.

Taiwan snapper *Scientific name: Lutjanus malabaricus,* or Malabar snapper, is a rather tough fish with reddish skin. It is unlike genuine red snapper and sells at much lower prices.

Dressed head-on Taiwan snapper is individually wrapped and packed in 50lb cartons, graded in pounds 1/2lb, 2/4lb and 4/6lb.

Fillets are graded in ounces, 4/6 oz, 6/8oz, 8/10oz, 10/12oz and 12/14oz. Largest and smallest sizes are least marketable. Standard packaging is individually wrapped fillets in 10lb boxes, 5 per master carton. As with all Taiwan seafood, marked weights are nominal and the fillets are heavily glazed. Always check the drained weight and claim from your supplier before you use the product.

Fillets may be whole (natural); one-cut meaning a single fillet cut in half; or chunks, which are pieces of much larger fillets and are usually described as cuts. Taiwan packers may mix these types, or may simply misdescribe what is in the boxes. Naturals, if you can get them, are easier to use and are worth more. Because of the frequent confusion on this aspect, your supplier may not know for certain what type of fillet he is selling.
Pacific snapper is a red skin perch and is discussed in the item Rockfish.

SNOW CRAB: Tanner crab; queen crab. See Crabs.

SOCKEYE: Red salmon; blueback. A small Pacific salmon, reaching 5-8lbs at maturity. It has the reddest flesh of all salmon and is the premium species for canning. See Salmon.

SODIUM PHOSPHATES: Also sodium triphosphates and sodium tripolyphosphates: See Dips.

SOFT CURE: Salt cured fish with moisture content over 40 percent after curing. See Curing.

SOFT-SHELL CRAB: Blue crabs which have just moulted and are eaten with the newly formed and still soft shell. See Crabs.

SOLDIER PACKS: Same as finger packs. Shrimp or other small items laid in rows in a block and frozen. This looks attractive and sometimes sells for a small premium.

SOLE: See Flatfish.

SPANISH MACKEREL *Scientific name: Scomberomorus maculatus:* A delicate, well-flavored fish with white meat in the mackerel family. It is caught mainly off the Gulf coast of Florida, although the fish ranges as far north as Rhode Island in summer. Spanish mackerel are generally between two and three pounds. Smaller fish are treated as pan fish, larger fish are filleted. It is easily distinguished by the golden spots on the sides. It lacks the lateral stripes of most other mackerels.

King mackerel (*Scomberomorus cavalla*) is similar but larger, reaching 100lbs (20lbs is more common for commercial fish). This fish is sometimes called cavalla. It is fatter than Spanish mackerel and is best when broiled.

Cero, also called pintada (*Scomberomorus regalis*), averages between five and ten pounds. This is also very similar to Spanish mackerel.

Frozen skin-on fillets of these fish are often available. They are excellent eating and usually good value.

SPECKLED TROUT: See Sea trout.

SPENT FISH: Fish which has recently spawned. Because much of the fish's reserves are put into the production of roe, the flesh of spent fish is soft and poor until the fish has had time to eat and recover for a period. The oil content of fat fish is at its lowest after spawning, making herring, for example, unsuitable for many smoking and curing uses.

SPIDER CRAB: Crabs with long spider-like legs, such as king, snow and red crab. The description spider crab is never used commercially.

SPLIT LEGS: King crab legs cut lengthwise. Some snow crab may also be processed this way. See Crabs.

SPOT *Scientific name: Leiostomus xanthurus:* A small Atlantic relative of the croaker, usually under 20 ounces, caught from Cape Cod to Mexico with most landings coming from the southern Atlantic states. It is used as a panfish and is usually sold whole or dressed. It has a rather strong flavor, which is improved if the dark lateral line is removed. The resource is large and many of these fish are caught by anglers. Frozen product is unusual, but should be cheap if offered.

SPRAT *Scientific name: Sprattus sprattus:* A small herring used for canning. Sometimes frozen whole, like sardines.

SQUETEAGUE: See Sea trout.

SQUID: Also called calamare and calamari. Cephalopod mollusc with ten arms and a tubular shaped body narrowing to a point and two fleshy wings along the rear part of the body. There are many species in all seas, ranging in length from one inch to the Chilean giant squid of six feet and 100lbs. Even larger monsters are thought to live in very deep water. Squid is an important marine resource and one capable of being utilized on a much larger scale. The U.S. market has only marginal interest in squid, although domestic resources on both coasts are substantial. Squid is not a name which attracts the consumer. Calamari does much better and markets are increasing as more people sample and like this "exotic" but inexpensive and nutritious seafood.

The edible parts of the squid are the tentacles, the whole body or mantle and the wings. The body and wings are covered with a thin, soft skin which is usually removed before cooking. The skin contains glands which allow the animal to change color as a protective device. The colors also change after the squid is caught and do not indicate spoilage. To avoid problems and to improve appearance, many packers bleach squid by soaking it in iced water before freezing. This whitens the skin and reduces the color changes that can occur even after freezing.

The body contains the viscera and a plastic-like strip called the pen which is the animal's shell or bone structure. Squid is cleaned by cutting off the head and tentacles and removing the viscera and pen through the neck opening. The remaining piece is called a tube and may be skinned; wings may be attached or removed. Tentacles are sometimes discarded or sometimes packed with tubes. Squid ink is available frozen in 1lb packs.

Squid tubes may be processed further into rings, which are slices cut through the tube. Strips, which resemble clam strips, should be cheaper because it is easier to clean squid if the tube is cut open and flattened out for strips to be made. Breaded squid strips are a popular prepared food in Spain and other parts of Europe, but are hardly known in the U.S.A. Breaded strips have also failed to find a market, although they offer a fairly inexpensive alternative to clam strips if properly processed. Steaks, circular pieces cut from the mantles of large squid and usually tenderized with a needle machine, are also produced as a retail trade alternative to expensive abalone steaks.

A great deal of squid is frozen whole for bait, used by both sportfishermen and commercial line fishermen. Whole frozen squid is also exported to Asian countries where it is processed using cheap local labor, refrozen and sold back to the U.S.A. Properly handled squid can be thawed and refrozen a number of times without noticeably losing texture or flavor.

There are numerous squid species throughout the world's oceans. The following are the major types found on the U.S. market. Bear in mind that there are many other squids, any of which might be sold here. For example, huge quantities of squid are caught off the Falkland Islands in the south Atlantic and sold in Asia and Europe. This resource has been fished for only a few years.

California market squid *Scientific name: Loligo opalescens:* Also called Monterey squid and San Pedro squid. These are small squid, caught seasonally inshore off central and southern California. As the names imply, the largest catches are taken in San Pedro (in winter) and Monterey (spring and summer). Monterey squid is preferred because it is close to 7 inches long. The San Pedro squid is around 3 to 4 inches tube length. Catches are uniform in size so are not graded. The squid is bleached and packed whole in 1½lb, 3lb and 5lb boxes, sometimes with windows in the boxes for retail sale. This is a cheap, standard reliable item. The size of the fishery varies in cycles, as does demand for the fish from overseas.

North Atlantic loligo *Scientific name: Loligo pealeii:* Also called long-finned squid and winter squid. It is caught at the edge of the continental shelf from November to March and inshore, when it is spawning, from April to July. Loligo has light colored flesh and is tender unless overcooked. It is mainly packed whole for export, domestic availability being surplus export packs. The best packs are graded according to tube length and layer packed in 10kg or 20kg boxes. Length grades should be clearly specified: some packers try to use small, medium and large designations. Others use letter grades designed for the Spanish market, but there is no uniformity in these. Japanese buyers also have complicated letter-names for size grades. Some cleaned loligo is available at very high prices. This species sells fresh throughout the east when available. Prices are more dependent on export contracts than on domestic supply.

As the domestic squid market increase, some packers are cleaning and processing loligo for home consumption. A wide range of processed products is available.

Illex squid *Scientific name: Illex illecebrosus:* Also called northern short-finned squid, winter squid and bait squid. It is very important to distinguish between these two types of squid landed in the northeast, since the illex variety sells for about one-fifth of the price of loligo. It is also available in much larger quantities. It is generally larger and darker than loligo and is much tougher. Packing is similar to that used for loligo when intended for export or human consumption. For the Japanese market, illex is size graded from 3S (under 50 grams) to 8L (over 700 grams). Large amounts are also packed in 50lb blocks for animal food or bait.

Canada catches and exports huge quantities of illex, both whole and cleaned. Some of this is exported to Taiwan and other Asian countries and reimported cleaned. This comes in two forms, either skinless cleaned tubes, or as skinless cleaned tubes with tentacles. If packed with tentacles, these are placed at one end of the block and constitute about 30 percent of the block weight. There is no regular price differential between the two packs.

In both packs, grading is dependent on tube length and is normally 3/5 inches, 5/8 inches and 8/12 inches. The two smaller sizes are usually packed 10/2/2½lb blocks – that is the 5lb inner carton is divided into two polywrapped blocks of 2½lb each – and the 8/12 inch size is normally packed 10/5lb. Price increases with size. Although squid is one of the more reliable products from Taiwan, you should expect that sizes and weights will be questionable.

Taiwan cleaned squid is used for retail as well as institutional sale. The wraps around the 2½lb inner blocks are usually color printed to facilitate retail use.

Other squid: New Zealand has large resources of arrow squid (*Nototodarus sloanii*) which is exported to many countries including the U.S.A. in a variety of prepared forms including steaks, rings and tubes. New Zealand also has broad squid (*Sepioteuthis bilineata*) which is a smaller resource. Argentina exports loligo species from Patagonia. Falklands loligo species are caught by vessels of many nations including Poland, Taiwan, Japan, Russia and Germany. Mexico giant squid is sold in California as steaks and strips. Thailand, Philippines and Indonesia all offer acceptable squid species. In fact, there are large quantities of squid available for exploitation throughout the world. This product is limited by its market, not by supply considerations.

STEAKS: Slices of fish with two parallel surfaces, subdivided as necessary. U.S. Grade Standards require halibut steaks to be at least two ounces and salmon steaks at least 2½ ounces, but commercially these would be too small. Steaks under six ounces for either are difficult to sell. Steaks are usually packed 10/5lb or 6/5lb boxes and should be in layers separated by paper or polyethylene film. Because of the large surface area exposed to dehydration, many users prefer to cut their own steaks from dressed fish.

STEELHEAD: Also called steelie, steelhead trout and steelhead salmon. An anadromous rainbow trout from the Pacific northwest. It is very similar in appearance and taste to Atlantic salmon. See Salmon.

STICKS: U.S. Grade Standards require fish sticks to be rectangular pieces of fish (not ground fish) weighing up to 1½oz including not more than 28 percent breading or batter. See Portions.

STOCKFISH: Hard dried unsalted fish, usually cod or similar species. It does not need refrigeration and is widely used in tropical countries. See Curing.

STORAGE TEMPERATURES: The maintenance of correct and stable temperatures for frozen product is vital to quality as well as to storage life. If the ideal level of $-20°F.$ is maintained, the product will keep at its best for the longest period. Fluctuations between say $-20°F.$ and $0°F.$, although not detectable since the product remains hard frozen, will shorten its life because of flexing of the cell walls. This affects the quality by destroying the texture, which becomes mushy and by squeezing oil and moisture to the surface of the product, leading to rancidity and drying.

Changes often occur during transportation. Product can deteriorate markedly while on a truck, especially if the refrigeration plant is not properly used, or the truck is making stops for deliveries, with doors opening and closing at each call. Refrigerated trucks carry an external thermometer showing the inside temperature and receiving staff should always record this on the bill. There are also recording devices (thermographs) which record fluctuations in temperature and fairly new technology that employs pigmented spots on a package. The spots change color at certain temperatures, showing whether the product has warmed beyond a certain point at any time.

Even in a modern warehouse, a location near a door, or even near product brought into the freezer at too high a temperature can affect storage life. The increased use of thermographs and of labels that change color if temperatures increase will help to reduce losses from these causes.

The worst part of the distribution chain for temperature maintenance is the retail outlet, where mishandling by both store personnel and customers can cause grave deterioration of product. Use of color-change labels is particularly valuable to monitor this stage.

Signs of defrost include frost and ice crystals inside a pack, distorted shape, clumping of I.Q.F. items and discoloration. Such signs show warming up to high levels – they do not reveal the insidious damage done by sub-zero fluctuations. These can only be controlled if product owners are willing to monitor temperatures and insist that warehouses, transporters and retailers keep product in the best possible condition at all times.

ST. PETER'S FISH: The French name for John Dory (*Zeus faber* and related species). See Dories. Its use for tilapia is not approved.

STRIPED BASS *Scientific name: Morone saxatilis:* Also called striper and rockfish. A game fish sometimes exceeding 50lbs originating on the Atlantic coast and now transplanted and living on both coasts. Atlantic striped bass is now protected in most of its range. The resource was first reserved for sport fishermen, then restricted further. Some states refuse to allow the sale of the fish even if it was caught legally on the west coast.

Striped bass has soft flesh with a large flake. It is oily and spoils quickly. Nevertheless, it is highly regarded as a food fish by many. To meet market demand, a farmed hybrid of striped and white bass has been developed. These fish look remarkably like striped bass. Laws preventing or permitting the sale of this hybrid vary in different eastern states and are changing. Check carefully before you use this fish.

STURGEON *Scientific name: Acipenser spp.:* A number of different species are found in the rivers, lakes and seawater of North America. The most commonly used commercially is the anadromous white sturgeon (*Acipenser transmontanus*) from the Columbia and other west coast rivers from Baja California to Cook Inlet. The largest fish recorded, from British Columbia, was 1800lbs. Fish over six feet long are now protected to conserve the breeding population, so this record will not be broken. White sturgeon are now being farmed with the long-term objective of growing them large enough to produce eggs for caviar.

Green sturgeon (*Acipenser medirostris*) is also a western species, caught mainly in the sea. Its flesh is dark red and strong tasting. It is barely edible unless smoked.

Sturgeon is mainly sold fresh. Headless, dressed fish with the spiny buttons removed from the sides are shipped. Sturgeon have cartilage, not bones. See also Caviar.

SUBJECT PASSAGE: All imported foodstuffs have to be cleared by the Food and Drug Administration before sale in the U.S.A. Product offered prior to F.D.A. examination is usually offered subject to approval, or "Subject Passage F.D.A." Product may be passed after inspection and approval, or passed without inspection on a green ticket. On this basis, the sale can only be completed if the product is passed.

This system can be abused by importers who may try to avoid commitments by claiming product was rejected. If this seems possible, ask for a copy of the rejection notice and check the date of import and the lot numbers from which samples were drawn. See also Rejection and Green ticket.

SUBSTITUTIONS: In this book, substitutions are defined as the dishonest use of a product purporting to be something of greater value. This must be carefully distinguished from an alternative product, which is one used with a correct description to cut costs or for some other legitimate reason. The key difference is in the use of correct descriptions.

Items which might be victims of substitution are mentioned throughout this book, but all are subject to price relationships. Cheaper product is sold as more expensive product, or the exercise has no point. As price relationships change, so do the common substitutions, therefore buyers must stay alert. See Economic fraud in the seafood business.

SUCKERS: Freshwater fish resembling catfish. In Canada they are sometimes marketed as mullet, which they do not resemble in the least.

SUJIKO: See Salmon eggs under Salmon entry.

SULFITES: Sulfites are used on many foods, not just seafoods. They are used to delay melanosis (blackening) on raw shrimp and are the most effective chemicals for achieving this. A number of common sulfiting agents, including sulfur dioxide, are on the G.R.A.S. list (Generally Recognized as Safe). However, because a small percentage of the population is allergic to sulfites and may suffer severe seizures from the substances, the F.D.A. carefully controls the residual amounts that may be present. The F.D.A. considers residues of more than 100 parts per million on the edible portion of shrimp to be evidence of abusive use. Note that the controversy over sulfites is in its early stages and the rules could change at any time.

SURIMI: Originally a Japanese product made from minced fish flesh. Used on an enormous scale in Japan, it is now the basis for an important seafood industry in the U.S.A. as well. Most surimi is made from Pacific pollock, but many other fish can be used, including cod, hake, whiting, croaker, barracuda, striped mullet and even cuttlefish.

Surimi is a raw material used for the manufacture of a wide range of food items. Imitation crabmeat, scallops, shrimp and even lobster tails are widely marketed. Salads, pasta products and other prepared foods are also made. The bulk of the market is imitation crab products, which include salad style meat, imitation leg meat and flake meats. The crab-style products may or may not include crabmeat in the ingredients.

Imported surimi is necessarily frozen and the products tend to contain large amounts of sugar, salt and preservatives to help stabilize and preserve the material. Domestic product may be shipped unfrozen, when fewer of these additional substances are needed. Frozen surimi tends to drip quite heavily when thawed, which looks unattractive and can be a problem in use.

There are a number of problems with surimi, only one of them major. Nutritionists note that surimi does not match the nutrition of the products it emulates. However, Americans are in no way undernourished, so this is not a problem for U.S. consumers. Additives can be quite heavy, although this is a problem shared with many highly processed foods. It is important, though, that the additives are listed accurately on the label.

Also essential for the label is the list of seafood ingredients. Some consumers are allergic to fish, others to shellfish. It is very important that people know what they are getting. If you serve someone who is allergic to fish a surimi product he thinks is crab, you may incur considerable liability.

The one major problem is the misrepresentation of surimi as the real seafood product it imitates. This hurts the industry in the long run by making consumers suspicious of what they are being sold, turning them away from seafoods altogether.

- Kamaboko is the food made from surimi and cooked by steam.
- Chikuwa are products of surimi that have been broiled.
- Satsuma-age are fried surimi products.

Most of the products sold in the U.S.A. are kamaboko, which has become the generic term for all surimi foods.

SUSHI: Raw fish and shellfish, thinly sliced and eaten. This is a Japanese word for a Japanese food ritual which has become enormously popular in the U.S.A. and has spread far beyond the specialized restaurants with trained sushi chefs. Sushi includes some raw fish and a number of smoked and cooked products. Tuna and clams are normally served raw. Octopus is cooked. Other seafoods are marinated. Although sushi is thought of as raw fish, many of the dishes in fact are not raw.

The fish and shellfish used must be top quality and extremely fresh. Nevertheless, eating fish raw involves the risk of consuming parasites such as tapeworm and roundworm. Most, if not all, of these parasites can be destroyed if the fish is frozen and stored for several days before being used. Use of top quality frozen fish is the best way to ensure that customers do not get parasites from your sushi.

SWORDFISH *Scientific name: Xiphias gladius:* A large fish, up to 1100lbs, with a distinctive sword on its head, found in all warm and temperate seas. Commercially, fish are usually caught between 50lbs and 400lbs. Most domestically caught fish is sold fresh, but as the season is mainly the warmer months, frozen swordfish can be sold readily in the winter and spring and is imported from many parts of the world.

Mako shark is sometimes used instead of swordfish. This has a slightly less solid texture and a rough skin, like sandpaper. Swordfish has a smooth feel to the skin. Because a number of shark species are substituted for swordfish, the appearance of the "grain" of the meat is not a reliable guide to which fish you have. However, all sharks have rough skin. This feature is distinctive.

A small amount of swordfish is harpooned, but most of it is caught on longlines. Harpooned fish is preferred by some buyers because the fish can be bled, giving whiter meat and better shelf life. However, the handling and processing of the fish is the most important factor in quality. This varies greatly among different origins and different packers.

Jelly sword is an occasional problem: the flesh is soft and jelly-like and the meat unusable. It appears to be caused by a micro-organism in the fish. Suppliers should not, of course, ship such product.

Swordfish is always used in the form of steaks, which are cut from the sides or slabs. Since larger fish can be cut more readily into similarly sized steaks and also give a higher yield of steaks, they are preferred to smaller fish. However, fish over approximately 200lbs are difficult to handle and some buyers dislike them. Frozen swordfish of this size is extremely difficult to manipulate on to a bandsaw for cutting. Very large frozen fish should be avoided.

Since swordfish retain mercury from their diet and larger fish have proportionately more in the flesh than smaller fish, importers of frozen swordfish prefer to buy fish under 100lbs as these are virtually certain to pass mercury inspection by the F.D.A. The current mercury limit is 1.0 part per million. See also Seafood safety.

Frozen swordfish is sold headless and dressed, as slabs or sides (which are fillets with the belly bone intact), as wheels (which are slices through the whole fish vertically across the backbone) or as steaks.

Headless dressed fish must be frozen carefully if it is to be good quality. The thickness of the fish makes freezing difficult, and either brine freezing or good quality blast freezing is required. Fish should be wrapped in polyethylene and cloth and each should be labelled with its true net weight. Small fish, pups between 20lb and 40lb, may be boxed. Transportation of headless swordfish is expensive because, without boxes, the fish is difficult to load and secure. Some packers will cut the fish into several chunks so that these can be boxed. Since the yield is better from the center cuts, make sure that you get a fair proportion of these. Boxing chunks helps to protect them and also makes handling easier.

Large slabs may be similarly wrapped and shipped loose, but these are more commonly chunked and boxed. The same consideration applies for getting a fair proportion of center cuts.

Wheels are less desirable because they expose considerable cut surface to the air and because they are harder to cut efficiently into steaks, as each wheel has a piece of the backbone.

Slices and steaks may be packed in almost any way. The important specification is the thickness of the slice, which should be 7/8 inch with a permitted variation of 1/8 inch either way. Steaks for retail or institutional use are best packed 6/5lb or 10/5lb boxes in the same way as salmon or halibut steaks.

The color of swordfish flesh varies from off-white through pink to brown. The color is determined by the fish's diet and is not an indication of quality. There are regional preferences and prejudices about swordfish color, which have to be taken into account although it all looks the same when cooked. In New England, pink flesh is generally liked and known as salmon sword while in parts of the west the pink fleshed fish is not accepted.

Swordfish sometimes have parasitic worms in the flesh which grow to substantial size. These are harmless, but sections of parasites found in steaks are aesthetically unpleasant and should be removed before the fish is cooked. Some buyers will reject fish with noticeable parasites.

When buying swordfish, look for parasites, for signs of dehydration and for any sign that it was frozen too slowly. This will be apparent near to the center of the fish, which may be soft or even decomposing. This problem is largely restricted to headless dressed fish. Slabs and slices do not suffer from slow freezing.

TAIL AND CLAW MEAT: Also expressed as "T and C." The top grade of Canadian lobster meat.

TAIL, CLAW AND KNUCKLE MEAT: Also expressed as "T.C.K." The second best grade of Canadian lobster meat.

TAIL-ON SHRIMP: Shrimp that is peeled except for the last (tail) segment. If not deveined, it is tail-on round. If deveined it is called butterfly. For further definitions, see Shrimp.

TARAKIHI *Scientific name: Nemadactylus macropterus:* A morwong found in the southern oceans from New Zealand to southern South America. It is called a jackass fish in Australia. It reaches about 2lbs. The flesh is off-white and reasonably firm. Frozen fillets are generally available.

TAUTOG *Scientific name: Tautoga onitis:* A wrasse from the east coast, caught by lobstermen in traps – the fish like to feed on the lobsters. It is known locally as blackfish. The flesh is excellent. The limited supplies are sold fresh.

TEMPURA: A light Japanese style batter becoming increasingly popular.

TERRAPIN: A type of turtle.

THAWING: See Defrosting methods and Economic fraud in the seafood business.

THERMOGRAPH: Recording thermometer. Sealed units continuously monitor the temperature and record the date on a paper strip, which can be used as evidence of proper or improper temperature maintenance inside trucks, containers or warehouses.

Since stable and correct temperatures are vital to the quality and storage life of frozen foods, it is surprising that these instruments are not used more often, especially on trucks. See also Storage temperatures.

THREAD HERRING *Scientific name: Opisthonema oglinum:* An Atlantic herring, usually low in oil so used mainly for fish meal or canning. There is a closely related Pacific coast species. The very similar *Opistonema libertate* from the Pacific coast of South America is a large resource used for canned products as well as fishmeal.

TILAPIA *Scientific name: Tilapia spp.:* A tropical freshwater fish introduced into the U.S.A. and now flourishing. The genus includes over 100 species. Hybrid tilapia is being touted as a major aquaculture resource for the future. The fish is extremely hardy, easy to grow and when added to fish ponds will survive without additional feed, serving also to clean up algae from the water. The fish is banned in many states because it displaces more desirable species in fresh water environments.

Tilapia sometimes sells under the illegal name of St. Peter's fish. Red-skinned tilapias have been offered as cherry snapper. The reason for marketing the fish under misleading names is that the meat is poor. It tends to have a muddy flavor and a rather unpleasant texture. Proponents claim that carefully farmed fish have better flavor but make absurd claims for it. Small fresh and frozen fillets are readily available and dressed fish up to about 2lb, usable as pan fish, can be bought. Supply is not a problem. The fish is easy to grow and farmers seem to have plenty of it. Marketing tilapia is so far much less successful.

TILEFISH *Scientific name: Lopholatilus chamaeleonticeps:* Also called ocean whitefish and golden tilefish. A deepwater fish growing to 35lbs which is popular fresh in the New York area. It is normally caught and marketed at between 6 and 8 pounds. It has firm flesh with a bland flavor and colorful skin distinguished by yellow spots. Tilefish are found along the entire east coast of the U.S.A. and as far south as Venezuela. There are several related species and similar species are found off Argentina. Tilefish are caught in exceptionally deep water and the resource fluctuates wildly.

Domestic tilefish is not normally frozen but some headless dressed frozen tilefish from South America reaches the market occasionally. Frozen pinbone-in fillets, both skin-on and skinless, as well as steaks, are available from Argentina and Mexico.

TOMALLEY: The lobster's fat, in effect its liver. It is a greenish mass found in the head part of the lobster. It is tasty and nutritious, but usually discarded by consumers who are unaware of its value.

TOMCOD *Scientific names: Microgadus tomcod* (Atlantic) and *Microgadus proximus* (Pacific): Small codlike fishes plentiful along the Pacific coast, but not much fished commercially because of their small size, which seldom exceeds 12 inches. A similar fish is caught along the New England and Canadian Atlantic coasts. If sold frozen tomcod is often mixed with other cod. Its appearance and taste are almost indistinguishable from the other cods.

TOPNECK: See Clams.

TRANSFER: An instruction to a public warehouse to give ownership of a particular product to a named party. The goods remain in storage with the seller paying storage charges until the next date when additional storage charges are due. See Delivery terms.

TRIGGERFISH: Highly colored reef fish, also called leatherjacket because of its tough skin, which must be removed before the fish can be filleted. Triggerfish is available from Florida, the Caribbean and the Gulf of Mexico. The meat is very good, similar to genuine turbot. Because it is difficult to process, it is not commonly available.

TRIPLOIDY: A technique for genetically altering animals so that they have two sets of female genetic material instead of the normal single set. Applied to oysters, the technique has given increased growth rates. It also results in sterile oysters. This means that the oysters can be harvested and sold year-round, including the months when they would normally be spawning (ripe oysters are considered less palatable). Triploid trout have also been developed and reportedly grow faster than fertile trout.

TRIPOLYPHOSPHATE: See Dips.

TROLL: A fishing technique; towing baited or lured hooks on lines behind the boat. Salmon caught this way is regarded as premium quality, partly because it is unbruised as it is handled individually by the fisherman, but also because troll-caught fish are gutted on the fishing boat which improves the quality of the meat by reducing spoilage.

TROUT: For striped, speckled, spotted, Mexican and other sea-trout, see Sea trout.

Rainbow, brook, cutthroat and brown trout are all different fish. Only rainbow trout is commercially available in frozen form in quantity. This section concentrates on rainbows. The less common "golden" trout is a rainbow variation that is colored by breeding and feed. It has yet to become popular and should not be confused with the rare fish of the same name found in northern California.

Anadromous trout are covered in Salmon.

Rainbow trout *Scientific name: Salmo gairdneri:* Rainbow trout is farmed on a large scale and can be bought fresh or frozen year round. Ninety-five percent of U.S. production is farm-raised and ninety percent of that comes from Idaho. Frozen rainbows are imported from Japan and Denmark, but are not always available because of disease problems and consequent import bans.

Frozen trout is always drawn and may be boneless, meaning that the ribs and backbone are removed through the belly cavity. Heads are invariably left on. Grading may be in 2oz steps or straight weights in ounces. Preferred sizes range between 5oz and 10oz. For institutional use, individually bagged trout packed 10/5lb cartons are usual. For retail use, there is a range of packs containing one or two trout, or up to three pounds, all in printed cartons. Fish with red or pink flesh sell at a slightly higher price.

Farmed trout is frequently sold ready stuffed or breaded. Smoked trout is a great delicacy and is becoming more widely known. Trout is a standard, branded product line with few problems.

TRUCKING CLAIMS: Reduce claims by purchasing product on a delivered basis and by selling ex-warehouse. Never sign for a shipment until you are convinced that you have the right amount of the correct product. Too bad if the driver is in a hurry – your money goes with your signature.

If you have a claim for lost or damaged goods; file promptly, keep copies of everything, write reminders every month, always use letters, not telephones and be patient, it will take many months to achieve a resolution. Buy a supply of Standard Forms for Presentation of Loss and Damage Claims (TOPS 3208) from your stationer. Follow the instructions on the form so the trucker has all the information he needs to resolve your claim quickly.

Never exaggerate prices in claims: truckers are often better informed than you are of market trends. Padding claims is fraud.

Truckers only compensate a nominal amount per pound of product, unless you have declared an additional value and paid an additional charge. Make sure you have insurance.

TULLIBEE: See Cisco.

TULLIES: Pale king salmon. The name applies to salmon very close to spawning. The flesh is very pale pink to grey and the skin is heavily watermarked. See Salmon.

TUNA: Tuna is a major seafood commodity. Although most of it is sold canned, fresh and frozen tuna is increasingly important. Giant bluefin is exported to Japan. Yellowfin and even albacore are regularly available in fish markets and restaurants in many parts of the country.

Albacore is canned as white meat tuna; yellowfin, bigeye and skipjack as light meat tuna. Bonito and frigate mackerel are not allowed to be called tuna. Almost all tuna species are found in all oceans. This is an oceanic fish unlike most of the fish that are hunted for food.

Fresh and frozen tuna are generally shipped as sides or loins. The fish is better if it is bled. Handling and packing is similar to swordfish or any other large, solid fish.

Burnt tuna syndrome (BTS) is a deterioration of the flesh in the central part of the body. The affected meat is pale and watery and has a sour or bitter taste and a chewy texture. It is caused by slow cooling and poor handling after the fish is caught. It is more common in large fish and much more likely in fish that are caught by sport fishermen. Commercial fishermen are aware of the importance of treating the fish properly. BTS can be detected only by cutting the fish in quarters. Some Japanese buyers take core samples of the flesh to avoid quartering the fish, but this method apparently only works when the fish is cooled to near-freezing temperatures. BTS is not a major or common problem.

Albacore *Scientific name: Thunnus alalunga:* This is the only species used for white meat tuna. It is found worldwide in warmer waters. Thanks to intensive marketing efforts in California, it is now accepted as a fresh or frozen fish as well as a canned staple.

Bigeye *Scientific name: Thunnus obesus:* This species grows to several hundred pounds and is used almost entirely for canning as lightmeat tuna. The meat is lighter than skipjack but darker than albacore.

Blackfin *Scientific name: Thunnus atlanticus:* Unlike most tunas, this species is found only in the Atlantic. It is a small fish, around ten pounds, frequently caught off Florida. The meat is dark, firm and well flavored. Fresh and frozen headless and dressed fish are available.

Bluefin *Scientific name: Thunnus thynnus:* Reaches 1500lbs as it swims north along the Atlantic coast in summertime. It is used fresh in New York and in sushi restaurants throughout the country. A substantial business has developed flying carefully handled fresh giant bluefin to Japan, under stringently controlled conditions. This is a highly specialized business and requires specific expertise.

Some bluefin is now being frozen very quickly to ultra-low temperatures. This appears to be an acceptable substitute for the fresh fish in the Japanese market where it is eaten raw. Freezing tuna destroys any parasites and is recommended, but it must be done properly. The huge fish take too long to freeze using normal equipment.

Bluefin meat is dark, almost red. There is a very dark and oily strip along the lateral line. Some of the smallest bluefin (the term is deceiving – this is a very large fish so even small bluefin are in the 100lb range) used to be canned as part of the lightmeat pack, but the fish is now too valuable for canning. The smaller fish are used domestically fresh and frozen. Giant bluefin are sold to Japan for sashimi. Sashimi grade bluefin is the fattest and freshest fish. If you do not need it for serving raw, lower grade fish is cheaper as well as milder when cooked.

Little tuna *Scientific name: Euthynnus alletteratus:* Also called tunny and little tunny, this is an Atlantic species growing to around 15 pounds. The flesh is dark and the flavor strong. In many Mediterranean recipes for tunny, the meat is brined before cooking to lighten the flavor. Tunny meat also smokes very well.

Skipjack tuna *Scientific name: Euthynnus pelamis:* Do not confuse the name skipjack with small bluefish, which are also called skipjacks. There is an older scientific name, *Katsuwonus pelamis*, which is still sometimes used when referring to this fish.

Skipjack is a small tuna, around seven to 12 pounds, found worldwide. It is a major part of the light meat tuna canned pack and is now well accepted by fresh and frozen markets. The meat is quite dark and can be used to replace bonito, horse mackerel and similar fish in recipes.

Yellowfin *Scientific name: Thunnus albacares:* Note the potential confusion of the scientific name, which does not refer to albacore. This species reaches 250 pounds, though most of the commercial catch is under 120 pounds. Found worldwide, it is an important California fishery which recently started selling to the fresh and frozen market instead of canneries. The meat is lighter than skipjack and darker than albacore. Restaurant and retail demand for yellowfin is strong.

TUNNY: This is little tuna (*Euthynnus alletteratus*). See Tuna.

TURBOT *Scientific name: Psetta maxima:* The same species is also classified as *Scophthalmus maximus*. A large flatfish from the North Sea and eastern Atlantic with fine quality, firm flesh. It is one of the most expensive of all fish, often selling for a higher price than salmon, halibut and other premium species. It is always the most expensive flatfish. Generally it is imported headless and dressed, graded in 1lb steps. Sizes under 3lb are not readily marketable. Fish between six and nine pounds are preferred. The market is small and specialized. Turbot is now being farmed successfully in Europe so may eventually become more plentiful.

It is most important to distinguish between real turbot and the Greenland turbot described in the next item.

TURBOT, GREENLAND *Scientific name: Reinhardtius hippoglossoides:* This is officially called Greenland turbot. It is also known, by the American Fisheries Society, as Greenland halibut. Other names include Japanese turbot, mock halibut, black halibut, blue turbot, Newfoundland turbot and Canadian turbot. Customers asking for turbot usually mean this, which has a large market throughout the U.S.A. It is a fairly large flatfish coming from the North Atlantic and the North Pacific. It seldom if ever comes from Greenland and is not a turbot. Neither is it a halibut.

Most supplies come from Japan and Korea. Substantial quantities are sold from eastern Canada. A few customers insist on turbot from Greenland and there are suppliers willing to create this for them by relabelling boxes. Canadian turbot is considered to be marginally better quality than Japanese origin fish, though the reasons for this distinction are unclear.

Greenland turbot is universally imported as skinless and boneless fillets. Normal size grading is 2/4oz, 4/8oz, 8/16oz and 16/32oz. Most Japanese product is individually wrapped and packed in 25lb boxes I.Q.F. Some Canadian fillets are packed similarly, in 10lb or 25lb boxes. Most Canadian turbot is layer packed in 10lb or 15lb units, four or five per master. Both Japan and Canada produce cello turbot.

Western Canada produces some turbot, but this is arrowtooth flounder, a very soft fish inferior to Greenland turbot. The naming is legal in Canada, but is most confusing for the U.S. market. This fish is best avoided.

Turbot is widely used instead of flounder and sole. It has a mild flavor and white meat and can best be described as bland and inoffensive. It is frequently repacked as sole when the price differential justifies such activity. Arrowtooth may be substituted for turbot or mixed with it. It is hard to distinguish the two fillets when they are frozen, though since arrowtooth falls apart when cooked it is obvious enough then. It is always worth checking turbot to make sure that this switch was not made.

Turbot fillets are often sold traypacked for retail use and the larger sizes enjoy a high and consistent volume of institutional sales. Turbot is a major seafood commodity, and it is important to know what it looks like and how it can be used.

TURTLES: Until the late 1970s there was a substantial market for frozen turtle meat. Since that time, most species of turtle have been placed on the endangered list under the Convention on International Trade in Endangered Species of Wild Flora and Fauna. The market for turtle meat and products has largely disappeared, although some domestic freshwater turtles may still be used.

If you insist on handling turtle product, ask the Fish and Wildlife Service of the Department of the Interior, Washington, D.C. and your State Fish and Game Department which species are legally usable, if any.

TUSK: European name for cusk.

UNIFORMITY RATIOS: See Shrimp.

U.S. GRADE STANDARDS: The U.S. Grade system for meat is well known to the consumer, if not always well understood; a similar program is available through the National Marine Fisheries Service for a small selection of fishery products. The system is voluntary and supported entirely by income from the fees it charges. The service covers a substantial part of the total output of seafood, but is concentrated heavily on mass-feeding and branded products such as breaded and battered portions. Mandatory inspection for all seafoods has been a political issue for many years. See Inspection.

Under the present system, inspection and quality grading of product is available for a fee, which means that if you have a quality dispute with a supplier or customer you can ask N.M.F.S. for an independent evaluation of the quality.

While useful, this is a marginal activity. The point of the inspection and grading system is to provide recognizable and widely used quality definitions, to increase consumer confidence in the value of seafood.

The standards formulated under Title 50 are reasonable and not onerous. These, and new standards that are being formulated for other products, are devised with the cooperation and participation of the industry. Seafood users should encourage wider use of the system, which would reduce greatly the number of quality disputes.

According to N.M.F.S.'s Food Fish Facts No. 51:

> **Grade A** means top or best quality. Grade A products are uniform in size, practically free of blemishes and defects, in excellent condition and possess good flavor for the species.
>
> **Grade B** means good quality. Grade B products may not be as uniform in size or as free from blemishes or defects as Grade A products. Grade B may be termed a general commercial grade, quite suitable for most purposes.
>
> **Grade C** means fairly good quality. Grade C products are just as wholesome and are generally as nutritious as higher grades. Grade C products have a definite value as a thrifty buy for use where appearance is not an important factor.

For retail use, only Grade A shields are normally displayed. Grade B and C products are more often sold without a grade designation printed on the pack.

VEIN: Also called the sandvein. This is the intestine of a shrimp or lobster. It runs the length of the tail. Its prominence varies according to the particular species and the food the individual has been eating. It is normal to remove the vein before eating shrimp or lobster, except in the case of very small shrimp where it is virtually undetectable. Freshwater crayfish are often purged of food before shipping to make the vein unnoticeable.

All crustacea have similar veins. They are not harmful to eat, but tend to look less than appetizing.

VISCERA: Guts, intestines.

VIVIPAROUS: A type of animal that bears its young alive. Most fish are oviparous, which means egg-laying.

VIVIPAROUS BLENNY: See Ocean pout.

WAHOO *Scientific name: Acanthocybium solanderi:* Called ono in Hawaii. A large tropical game fish in the mackerel family, related to tuna, reaching over 100lbs but normally sold at around 30lbs. It is found in all tropical seas. In the U.S.A. it is available off southern Florida, but is not abundant. It is a good food fish with the limited supplies selling fresh. Frozen wahoo is sometimes imported from India and other parts of Asia in steaks or fillets, but there is no regular market in the U.S.A.

WALLEYE: See Pike. For walleye pollock see Pollock.

WAREHOU *Scientific name: Seriolella spp.:* Southern species from New Zealand, Australia and South America. Fillets are available from New Zealand packers. Blue warehou is a large (about 8lbs) fairly soft fish colored like Atlantic pollock, which whitens when cooked. Silver and white warehou are both smaller (about 5lbs) with firmer texture and creamier meat.

WATERMARK: The changing skin colors of salmon as they swim upstream to spawn. The original silver color starts to fade. Reddish, grey and black patches and streaks appear. Some salmon may complete their journey with almost black skin, others with red skin.

Watermarking begins to appear along the back of the fish and spreads down towards the belly. An experienced salmon handler can estimate the flesh quality fairly accurately from the appearance of the skin, since the color of the skin and the texture and flavor of the meat deteriorate together.

WEAKFISH: See Sea trout.

WHELK: Seasnail. See Conch.

WHIPTAIL: See Hoki.

WHITEBAIT: Young or very small herrings, sardines and similar fish. Whitebait are eaten fried whole in Europe, but are little used in the U.S.A. Whitebait smelt is caught along the Pacific northwest coast and is used mainly for bait.

WHITEFISH *Scientific name: Coregonus clupeaformis:* Usually called lake whitefish; sometimes called humpback whitefish. Whitefish are found in lakes and rivers in the northern U.S.A. and throughout Canada. Most of the commercially available fish is two to three pounds and comes from Canada. It is shipped in a variety of packs including whole, dressed and pan-ready. It is also available as skin-on fillets and minced blocks. Whitefish is often smoked and is probably best known as a smoked product, sold from deli counters throughout the country.

Whitefish meat is white, sweet and delicate. Whitefish eggs are used as a caviar substitute.

For ocean whitefish, see Tilefish.

Whitefish is also a general term to indicate white-fleshed fish, in comparison to oily-fleshed fish such as herrings, or salmonids such as salmon or trout. Cod, flounder and all similar fishes are white fish. As the term is imprecise, it should be avoided.

WHITE KINGS: A race of king salmon from the Pacific northwest, with white instead of red flesh. It is well regarded for eating in areas where it is caught and almost impossible to sell in places unfamiliar with it, since consumers expect salmon to be red or pink.

WHITING: Whiting and hake are effectively the same fish in the U.S. market. The differences between them have to be related to commercial acceptance and usage rather than biological distinctions. Whiting is a preferred market name. In general, whiting looks like a small cod, to which it is related, and has soft, white flesh which has a large flake. Huge amounts are sold in the U.S.A. and a large proportion of supplies are imported.

Whiting is packed headless and dressed I.Q.F and in 5lb and 3lb blocks in boxes. Fillets may be skin-on or skinless, pinbone in or boneless. Many whiting fillets are deepskinned, since some species have a layer of subcutaneous fatty tissue which is better removed. Whiting blocks made from fillets and from minced fish are an important international commodity. Whiting is a huge volume commodity seafood and comes in almost every pack and form imaginable. Substantial amounts of whiting fillets made from dressed fish frozen at sea are produced in Asian countries. Such product is unlikely to be top quality.

The main commercial species are described in the following paragraphs:

Atlantic whiting *Scientific name: Merluccius bilinearis:* This species is also called silver hake. It is produced domestically in the northeast on a seasonal and erratic basis. From time to time very large quantities are landed. Other seasons produce very little fish. The fish average under a pound, giving dressed fish of about 8 ounces and fillets of under 3 ounces. Most of the catch is headed, dressed and packed into 5lb boxes, usually color printed for retail sale, 10 per master carton. Some packers use three pound boxes in dozens, but the industry standard is 10/5lb. There is also some I.Q.F. headless dressed whiting in bulk packs for traypacking and institutional use. Some domestic whiting is filleted, usually for cellos. Some whiting is landed in Canada, and treated similarly.

White hake *Scientific name: Urophycis tenuis:* This is the largest domestic hake or whiting. Most of the catch is about 2lbs, but the fish grow to as much as 25lbs. It is used for salting and for steaking in New England.

Red hake *Scientific name: Urophycis chuss:* Also called squirrel hake. This is another abundant northeast species, but is not much fished. The spawning fish which can be caught heavily in early summer has particularly soft flesh. It needs careful handling at all times.

Pacific whiting *Scientific name: Merluccius productus:* Also called North Pacific whiting. This fish was called hake until 1979, when the F.D.A. permitted the name change. It is a fairly large whiting, with soft flesh. It is found in the ocean, where the fish reach 19 to 26 inches. It is also found in Puget Sound where it is smaller, at 14 to 18 inches. The ocean fish are too large to fit into standard 5lb boxes, which is a problem. Most of the production is therefore I.Q.F. The fish needs to be deep-skinned if it is filleted.

Although the resource is large and many efforts have been made to exploit it, Pacific whiting is not fished very much because it is infested with a parasite which degrades the flesh very quickly once the fish dies. The effect is that the infested fish falls apart when cooked or smoked. The Puget Sound fish is not so badly affected, but the prospects for the resource are blighted unless the parasite problem can be solved.

Peru whiting *Scientific name: Merluccius gayi:* This is also called Chilean hake and Chilean whiting. It is the cheapest whiting. This fish is small, about 6oz headless dressed, and customarily packed in 10/5lb printed boxes. Peruvian and Chilean whiting has become a staple product for the retail trade. Layer pack and I.Q.F. fillets, skin-on and skinless, with and without pinbones are also produced by both Chile and Peru. Chile has a larger species, *Merluccius polyepsis*. Peru whiting is a very soft fish and is not usable for smoking, a problem since smoking is a major market for headless dressed whiting in the U.S.A.

Antarctic whiting *Scientific name: Merluccius australis:* This is sometimes called New Zealand whiting. It is also called Antarctic queen, by recent permission from the F.D.A. It is a larger whiting with firmer flesh than most. The flesh is white. Chile exports fresh and frozen fish and taps a premium price market for the species.

Argentine whiting *Scientific name: Merluccius hubbsi:* Argentina and Uruguay are major suppliers of this whiting. The fish is the same, but Uruguay packers tend to be a little less sloppy than their Argentine counterparts. Both countries supply large quantities of whiting blocks as well as defatted blocks. Headless and dressed whiting is usable for smoking, which is the main market for fish from these origins. Argentina and Uruguay do not pack in 5lb boxes, but prefer large blocks of various sizes, or I.Q.F. Smokers can use fish packed either way. Whiting fillets are shipped in both layer packs and I.Q.F., with or without skin and pinbones. Because the pinbones are small and soft, there is little point in buying boneless whiting. Grading from both Uruguay and Argentina tends to be uncertain and layer packs are seldom sufficiently separated with polywrap. From time to time, packs of unusual size are offered, usually the result of freezing at sea on non-standard equipment. These are fine if you can use them, but can be an inventory control problem.

South African whiting *Scientific name: Merluccius capensis:* This is probably the best of the whiting species after the European original. Fish of South African origin is not allowed into the U.S.A. at present, but factory trawlers from many other countries exploit the stock. The fish is quite large, white fleshed and has a large flake. It is sold in the U.S. at prices significantly higher than whiting from other origins and European buyers now take most of the catch.

Whiting *Scientific name: Merlangus merlangus:* This is the European whiting. It is not used in the U.S.A. It has soft, very white flesh with a delicate flavor and is caught throughout the eastern Atlantic as well as the Mediterranean.

Blue whiting is a different fish. See separate entry on it.

WING: Edible portion of a skate. See Skate.

WOLF FISH: Ocean catfish. See Catfish.

WORMS: See Parasites.

WRASSE: See Tautog.

WRECKFISH: Stone bass or grouper.

YELLOWFIN: See Tuna.

YELLOW PERCH: See Lake perch.

YELLOWTAIL *Scientific name: Seriola lalandei:* A large jack similar to amberjack caught off California and Baja California. A record fish weighed 80 pounds, but they are usually less than 30 pounds. The fish is taken mainly by sport fishermen and is sometimes available commercially as frozen fillets.

The Japanese yellowtail, *Seriola quinqueradiata*, is a very important farmed species, used for sashimi. It is an oily, delicate fish which fetches a high price. Small quantities are airfreighted fresh to California for high-ticket sushi shops.

For yellowtail snapper, see Snapper. For yellowtail flounder, see Flatfish.

YIELDS: A whole fish has head, tail, fins, viscera, skin and bones, all of which must be removed to yield the edible flesh. Yield is the percentage that is edible or saleable (not the same thing). Understanding yield is crucial to the sensible buying and using of seafood.

Yields from fresh cod are indicative of those from a wide selection of fish. Most cod is landed gutted with head on and the component parts weigh out as follows, for an average codfish of 6 to 7lbs:

head	25 percent
backbone	16 percent
fins and napes	12 percent
skin	4 percent
fillet	43 percent

These are rough and arguable averages that vary with the size of the fish, the season (yields are lower when a fish is full of roe, for example) and the skill of the individual processor. What it means is that if a fish is landed gutted head-on costing $1.00 per lb with a yield of edible fillet of 43 percent, then the raw material cost of that fillet, without accounting for the cost of labor or other processing, is $1.00 divided by 43 percent which is $2.33 per lb. If the fish is landed whole (since the guts are about 15 percent of the live weight, the yields in the table above will all be reduced by 15 percent. In this case the skinless fillet yield will be only 36½ percent. If this whole fish with guts sold dockside at $1.00 per lb, the raw material cost of the fillet from it would be $2.74 per lb.

To arrive at a reasonable fillet price, the costs of handling, filleting, packing and freezing must be taken into account. Distribution costs are additional. Yield varies substantially between different species, for example:

Cod, haddock, pollock etc, skinless fillets	40 percent
Ocean perch, skin on fillets	30 percent
Bluefish, skin on fillets	43 percent
Flounder and sole, skinless fillets	35 percent

King crab yields vary between 17 percent and 22 percent for meat from the live crab. If the dockside processor pays $4.00

per lb for the crab and the meat yield is 17 percent, the raw material cost of the king crab meat is $23.53 without processing or freight costs. At 22 percent yield the cost is $18.18 per lb, a very substantial difference.

Shrimp yields are less important to the user. Most shrimp intended for the shell-on market is landed domestically in shell-on tail form and is graded and packed for freezing. Peeled and deveined, this shrimp loses about 15 percent of its weight, but the markets for shell-on and peeled and deveined shrimp are often independent since users do not readily switch between them.

ZOOS AND AQUARIA: Some of these institutions, especially those with porpoises, polar bears, walruses or other large animals, use a great deal of fish. Most of what they buy is small whole fish such as herring, mackerel, blue runner, croaker or smelts. Sometimes they will buy head-on shrimp, which contain useful vitamins, or clams as a treat for a walrus, or other less usual items.

Remember that although zoos buy inexpensive fish, quality is of exceptional importance. Generally, fish should be at least good enough for human consumption and often should be of premium quality. A fully trained porpoise represents an investment of approximately one million dollars and will be pampered.

REFERENCES

BOOKS

1969. *Codex Alimentarius Commission: Recommended International Code of Practice - General Principles of Food Hygiene*, CAC/RCP 1-1969, Secretariat of the Joint FAO/WHO Food Standards Programme.

1970. *Codex Alimentarius Commission: Recommended International Code of Practice for Canned Shrimp or Prawns*, CAC/RCP 37-1970, Secretariat of the Joint FAO/WHO Food Standards Programme.

1976. *Codex Alimentarius Commission: Recommended International Code of Practice for Canned Fish*, CAC/RCP 10-1976, Secretariat of the Joint FAO/WHO Food Standards Programme.

1976. *Codex Alimentarius Commission: Recommended International Code of Practice for Fresh Fish*, CAC/RCP 9-1976, Secretariat of the Joint FAO/WHO Food Standards Programme.

1976. *Codex Alimentarius Commission: Recommended International Code of Practice for Quick Frozen Shrimps or Prawns*, CAC/RCP 92-1976, Secretariat of the Joint FAO/WHO Food Standards Programme.

1976, 1984. *Freshwater Fish Pond Culture and Management*, Superintendent of Documents, Government Printing Office.

1978. *Codex Alimentarius Commission: Recommended International Code of Practice for Frozen Fish*, CAC/RCP 16-1978, Secretariat of the Joint FAO/WHO Food Standards Programme.

1978. *Multilingual Dictionary of Fish and Fish Products*, Fishing News Books Ltd.

1981. *Code of Recommended Practices for the Handling and Merchandising of Frozen Foods*, Frozen Food Roundtable.

1981. *European Trade Fairs: A Guide for Exporters*, Superintendent of Documents, Government Printing Office.

1981. *Guide Book to New Zealand Commercial Fish Species*, New Zealand Fishing Industry Board.

1982. *Fishery Products from the Eastern United States Available for Export*, NMFS.

1983. *Federal Fisheries Management: A Guidebook to the Fishery Conservation and Management Act*, Ocean and Coastal Law Center, University of Oregon Law School.

1983. *NMFS Approved Quality Assurance Systems*, Fishery Products Inspection Manual, Pt. I, Chapt. 9, Sect. 01., U.S. Dep. of Commer., NOAA, NMFS.

1983. *Seafood Sense, Consumer Attitudes to Fish*, New Zealand Fishing Industry Board and Fishing Industry Training Council.

1984. *Fishes of the North-Eastern Atlantic and the Mediterranean (FNAM) Vol. I*, UNESCO Press.

1984. *Penaeid Shrimps — their Biology and Management*, Fishing News Books.

1985. *An Evaluation of the Role of Microbiological Criteria for Foods and Food Ingredients*, National Academy Press.

1985. *Common Carp 1. Mass Production of Eggs and Early Fry*, FAO.

1985. *Common Carp 2. Mass Production of Advanced Fry and Fingerlings in Ponds*, FAO.

1985. *Guide to the Preparation of Offers for Selling to the Mili-*

tary, Superintendent of Documents, Government Printing Office.

1985. *Seafood Exporting Opportunities for New York and New Jersey in the United Kingdom, Spain and Japan*, Bi-State Seafood Development Conference.

1985. *Seafood Marketing Guide*, Journal Publications, Seafood Business Report.

1986. *Code of Federal Regulations 50: Wildlife and Fisheries*, Part 200 to end. U.S. Government Printing Office, Office of Federal Register National Archives and Records Administration.

1986. *Fresh Ways With Fish and Shellfish*, Time-Life Books Inc.

1986. *Importing into the United States*, Superintendent of Documents, Government Printing Office.

1986. *National Shellfish Sanitation Programs Manual of Operations Part 1. Sanitation of Shellfish Growing Areas*, Interstate Shellfish Sanitation Conference.

1986. *Norwegian Salmon International Chefs' Recipes*, Gyldendal Norsk Forlag A/S.

1986. *Quality Handling of Hook-Caught Rockfish*, Marine Advisory Bulletin 20, Alaska Sea Grant College Program, University of Alaska.

1986. *Radiation, Doses, Effects, Risks*, UNIPUB.

1986. *Report on the Safety and Wholesomeness of Irradiated Food*, FAO/IAEA/WHO Expert Committee and the National Radiological Protection Board, HMSO Books and UNIPUB.

1986. *Seafood Marketing*, GAO/RCED-87-11BR. United States General Accounting Office.

1986. *Seafood Shipper's Guide*, Rhode Island Seafood Council.

1986. *U.S. Department of Commerce, A Basic Guide to Exporting*, U.S. Dept. of Commer.; Internat. Trade Admin.; U.S. and Foreign Commercial Service; U.S. Government Printing Office.

1987. *Code of Federal Regulations 21: Food and Drugs*, Parts 1 to 99. U.S. Government Printing Office, Office of Federal Register National Archives and Records Administration.

1987. *Code of Federal Regulations 21: Food and Drugs*, Parts 100 to 169. U.S. Government Printing Office, Office of Federal Register National Archives and Records Administration.

1987. *Code of Federal Regulations 21: Food and Drugs*, Parts 170 to 199. U.S. Government Printing Office, Office of Federal Register National Archives and Records Administration.

1987. *Codex Alimentarius Commission: Procedural Manual*, Secretariat of the Joint FAO/WHO Food Standards Programme.

1987. *Fishes of the North-Eastern Atlantic and the Mediterranean (FNAM) Vol. II*, UNESCO Press.

1987. *Fishes of the North-Eastern Atlantic and the Mediterranean (FNAM) Vol. III*, UNESCO Press.

1987. *International Trade 1985-86*, UNIPUB.

1987. *Pesticide Residues in Food —1985, Evaluations 1985, Part II — Toxicology*, UNIPUB.

1987. *Pesticide Residues in Food — 1986, Evaluation 1986, Part 1 — Residues*, UNIPUB.

1987. *The Seafood Handbook Series*, Journal Publications, Seafood Business.

1988. *Alaska Department of Fish and Game Observer Manual for Alaskan Crab Processors*, Alaska Department of Fish and Game.

1988. *Common and Scientific Names of Aquatic Invertebrates from the United States and Canada: Mollusks*, American Fisheries Soceity.

1988. *Recommended Marketing Names for Fish, A Practical Guide for Fish Marketing*, Australian Government Publishing Service.

1988. *USDC Approved List of Fish Establishments and Products* Vol 3., No. 1., U.S. Dept. of Commer.; NOAA; NMFS.

1989. *Approved Market Names for Fish*, FDA/USDC.

Allen, P.G., Bostsford, L.W., Schuur, A.M. and Johnston, W.E. 1984, 1988. *Bioeconomics of Aquaculture*, Elsevier Science Publishing Co, Inc.

Allsopp, W.H.L. 1985. *Fishery Development Experiences*, Fishing News Books Ltd.

Anderson, Robert. 1982. *Florida Saltwater Fish and Fishing, Sharks Included*, National Wildlife Publishing Inc.

Angell, C.L. 1986. *The Biology and Culture of Tropical Oysters*, The International Center for Living Aquatic Resources Management.

Annual. *Fisheries of the United States*, The National Marine Fisheries Service.

The Audubon Society Field Guide to North American Fishes, Whales and Dolphins, Alfred A. Knopf, Inc.

Ayling, Tony and Cox, Geoffrey J. 1982. *Collins Guide to the Sea Fishes of New Zealand*, William Collins Publishers Ltd.

Bayer, Robert and Juanita. 1987. *Lobsters Inside-Out. A Guide to the Maine Lobster*, Maine/New Hampshire Sea Grant College Program.

Beveridge, Malcolm C.M. 1987. *Cage Aquaculture*, Fishing News Books Ltd.

Bigelow, Henry B. and Schroeder, William C. 1953. *Fishes of the Gulf of Maine*, Museum of Comparative Zoology, Cambridge, MA.

Billington, G.C. 1983. *Fish for Food*, New Zealand Fishing Industry Board and the Fishing Industry Training Council.

Bird, K.T. and Benson, P.H., Editors. 1987. *Seaweed Cultivation for Renewable Resources*, Elsevier Science Publishing Co., Inc.

Boehmer, Raquel. 1982. *A Foraging Vacation. Edibles from Maine's Sea and Shore*, Down East Books.

Boyd, C.E. 1982, 1988. *Water Quality Management for Pond Fish Culture*, Elsevier Science Publishing Co., Inc.

Branyon, Max. 1987. *Florida Freshwater Fishing Guide*, Sentinel Communications Company.

Breder Jr., Charles M. 1929, 1948. *Marine Fishes of the Atlantic Coast*, G.P. Putnam's Sons.

Brown, E. Evan, Ph.D. and Gratzek, D.V.M., Ph.D. 1980. *Fish Farming Handbook*, AVI Publishing Company, Inc.

Bundy, Mark M. and Williams, John B. 1978. *Maryland's Chesapeake Bay Commercial Fisheries*, Maryland Department of Natural Resources, Tidewater Administration.

Bykov, V.P. 1983. *Marine Fishes Chemical Composition and Processing Properties*, NMFS, NOAA and National Science Foundation.

Castro, José I. 1983. *The Sharks of North American Waters*, Texas A & M University Press.

Chaston, Ian. 1984. *Business Management in Fisheries and Aquaculture*, Fishing News Books Ltd.

Chaston, Ian. 1988. *Managerial Effectiveness in Fisheries and Aquaculture*, Fishing News Books Ltd.

Chaston, Ian. 1983. *Marketing in Fisheries and Aquaculture*, Fishing News Books Ltd.

Chen, T.P. 1976. *Aquaculture Practices in Taiwan*, Fishing News Books Ltd.

Connell, J.J. *Advances in Fish Science and Technology*, Fishing News Books Ltd.

Connell, J.J. 1975. *Control of Fish Quality, 2nd Ed.*, Fishing News Books Ltd.

Costakes, James; Connors, Eugene; and Paquette, Gerald. *Quality at Sea, On Board Handling Procedures for Quality Developed Through the New Bedford Quality Project*, New Bedford Seafood Producers Association. New England Fisheries Development Foundation, Inc.

Davidson, Alan. 1972, 1981. *Mediterranean Seafood, 2nd Edition*, University of Louisiana.

Davidson, Alan. 1980, 1988. *North Atlantic Seafoods*, Harper and Row.

Davidson, Alan. 1976. *Seafood of South-East Asia*, Federal Publications.

Dore, Ian. 1984. *Fresh Seafood: The Commercial Buyer's Guide*, Osprey Books Ltd.

Dore, Ian. 1982. *Frozen Seafood: The Buyer's Handbook*, Osprey Books Ltd.

Dore, Ian and Frimodt, Claus. 1987. *An Illustrated Guide to Shrimp of the World*, Osprey Books Ltd. and Scandinavian Fishing Year Book.

Dore, Jennifer; Editor. 1988. *Seafood Quiz*, Osprey Books Ltd.

Doulman, David J. 1987. *The Development of the Tuna Industry in the Pacific Islands Region: An Analysis of Options*, East-West Center.

Dunfield, R.W. 1986. *The Atlantic Salmon in the History of North America*, UNIPUB.

Dupree, Harry K., and Huner, Jay V. 1984. *Third Report to the Fish Farmers*, U.S. Fish and Wildlife Service.

Ellis, Anthony E. 1985. *Fish and Shellfish Pathology*, Academic Press.

F.A.O. 1987. *Production of Fish Meal and Oil*, UNIPUB.

F.A.O. 1985. *Specifications for Identity and Purity of Certain Food Additives, Enzyme Preparations and Immobilizing Agents, Flavouring Agents, Flouring Agents, Flour Treatments Agents, Food Acids and Salts, Food Colours, Sweeteners, Thickeners and Miscellaneous Food Additives*, 29th Session of the Joint FAO/WHO Expert Committee on Food Additives, Geneva, 3-12 June 1985.

F.A.O. 1987. *World Agricultural Statistics 1986 — F.A.O. Statistical Pocketbook*, UNIPUB.

F.D.A. *The Food Defect Action Levels, Current Levels for Natural or Unavoidable Defects in Food for Human Use That Present No Health Hazard*, FDA 85-2199.

Fish Processing: Quality in the Plant. A Manual for In-Plant Quality Procedures, New England Fisheries Development Foundation, Inc.

Frimodt, Claus. 1988. *The European Fishing Handbook — Directory of the European Fish Trade*, Scandinavian Fishing Year Book.

Gall, Ken. *Handling Your Catch. A Guide for Saltwater Anglers*, A Cornell Cooperative Extension Publication Information Bulletin 203.

Gates, J.M., Matthiessen, G.C., and Griscom, C.A. 1974. *Aquaculture in New England*, Rhode Island Sea Grant.

Grey, D.L.; Dall, W.; and Baker, A. 1983. *A Guide to the Australian Penaeid Prawns*, Dept. of Primary Production of the Northern Territory.

Groves, Roy E. 1985. *The Crayfish, its Nature and Nurture*, Fishing News Books.

Hahn, Kirk O., Ph.D. 1988. *CRC Handbook of Culture of Abalone and other Marine Gastropods*, CRC Press, Inc.

Hallowell, E.R. 1980. *Cold and Freezer Storage Manual*, Avi Publishing Company, Inc.

Hara, T.J. 1982. *Chemorecption in Fishes*, Elsevier Science Publishing Co., Inc.

Hart, J.L. *Pacific Fishes of Canada*, Canadian Government Publishing Center.

Hibler, Jane Franke. 1984. *Easy and Elegant Seafood, An Everyday Guide to Buying and Cooking Seafood and Fish*, Frank Amato Publications.

Hoar, W.S. and Randall, D.J. 1983. *Fish Physiology, Vol. 9A*, Academic Press.

Hoar, W.S. and Randall, D.J. 1983. *Fish Physiology, Vol 9B*, Academic Press.

Hoar, W.S. and Randall, D.J. 1984. *Fish Physiology, Vol. 10A,* Academic Press.

Hoar, W.S. and Randall, D.J. 1984. *Fish Physiology, Vol. 10B,* Academic Press.

Horwitz, William. 1980 (13th edition). *Official Methods of Analysis of the Association of Official Analytical Chemists,* Association of Official Analytical Chemists.

Huet, Marcel. 1972, 1986. *Textbook of Fish Culture; Breeding and Cultivation of Fish,* Fishing News Books Ltd.

Huner, Jay V., Ph.D. and Brown, E. Evan, Ph.D. 1985. *Crustacean and Mollusk Aquaculture in the United States,* Avi Publishing Company,, Inc.

Hurlburt, Sarah. 1977. *The Mussel Cookbook,* Harvard University Press.

IAEA. 1985. *Food Irradiation Processing. Proceedings of an International Symposium on Food Irradiation Processing, Washington, D.C. March 4-8, 1985,* UNIPUB.

Iredale, David G. and York, Roberta K. 1983. *A Guide to Handling and Preparing Freshwater Fish,* Department of Fisheries and Oceans, Canada.

Jackson, Roy I. and Royce, Dr. William. 1986. *Ocean Forum, an Interpretative History of the International North Pacific Fisheries Commission,* Fishing News Books Ltd.

Jarvis, Norman R. 1987. *Curing of Fishery Products,* Teaparty Books.

Joseph, James, Klawe, Witold, and Murphy, Pat. 1988. *Tuna and Billfish, Fish Without a Country,* Inter-American Tropical Tuna Commission.

Jumonville, Bunny and Mounger, Joy. 1984. *The Louisiana Craw-fish Cookbook*, The Louisiana Crawfish Cookbook Inc.

Kinsella, John E. 1987. *Seafoods and Fish Oils in Human Health and Disease*, Marcel Dekker, Inc.

Korringa, P. 1976. *Farming Marine Orrganisms Low in the Food Chain*, Elsevier Science Publishers Co., Inc.

Korringa, P. 1976. *Farming the Cupped Oysters of the Genus Crassostrea*, Elsevier Science Publishing Co., Inc.

Korringa, P. 1976. *Farming the Flat Oysters of the Genus Ostrea*, Elsevier Science Publishing Co., Inc.

Kramer, Donald E. and O'Connell, Victoria M. 1988. *Guide to Northeast Pacific Rockfishes, Genera Sebastes and Sebastolobus*, Marine Advisory Bulletin #25, University of Alaska.

Kreuzer, Rudolf. 1974. *Fishery Products*, Fishing News Books, Ltd.

Laevastu, Taivo and Favorite, Felix. 1988. *Fishing and Stock Fluctuations*, Fishing News Books Ltd.

Lamb, Andy and Edgell, Phil. 1986. *Coastal Fishes of the Pacific Northwest*, Harbour Publishing Co.

Lands, William E. M. 1986. *Fish and Human Health*, Academic Press Inc.

Lannan, E., Smitherman, R.O., and Tchobanoglous, G. 1986. *Principles and Practices of Pond Aquaculture*, American Fisheries Society.

Lappin, Peter J. 1986. *Live Holding Systems*, Sea Plantations, Inc.

Lentz, Ginny. 1983. *Catch of the Day — Southern Seafood Secrets*, Lentz Enterprises.

Lockwood, Stephen J. 1988. *The Mackerel, its biology, assessment and management of a fishery*, Fishing News Books Ltd.

Love, R. Malcolm. 1988. *The Food Fishes, their intrinsic variation and practical implications*, Van Nostrand Reinhold Company.

Lutz, R.A.; Editor. 1980. *Mussel Culture and Harvest: A North American Perspective*, Elsevier Science Publishing Co., Inc.

Manchester, Alden. 1987. *Developing an Integrated Information System for the Food Sector*, Agric. Economic Report No. 575, U.S. Government Printing Office.

Manooch, Charles S. 1984. *Fishes of the Southeastern United States*, North Carolina State Museum of Natural History.

Marriott, Norman G. Ph.D. 1985. *Principles of Food Sanitation*, Avi Publishing Company,, Inc.

Martin, P.G., and Weatherwax, J. 1987. *Manuals of Food Quality Control 1. The Food Control Laboratory*, UNIPUB.

Martin, P.G., and Weatherwax, J. *Manuals of Food Quality Control 2. Additives, Contaminants, Techniques*, UNIPUB.

Martin, P.G., and Weatherwax, J. *Manuals of Food Quality Control 3. Commodities*, UNIPUB.

Martin, P.G., and Weatherwax, J. *Manuals of Food Quality Control 4. Microbiological analysis*, UNIPUB.

Martin, P.G., and Weatherwax, J. *Manuals of Food Quality Control 5. Food Inspection*, UNIPUB.

Martin, R.E., Flick, G.J., Hebard, C.E., and Ward, D.R. 1982. *Chemistry and Biochemistry of Marine Food Products*, AVI Publishing Company, Inc.

Martinson, Linda. 1986. *Simply Salmon: Fresh, Frozen & Canned*, Lance Publications.

Martinson, Linda. 1986. *Simply Shrimp: Fresh, Frozen & Canned*, Lance Publications.

McClane, A. J. 1977. *Encyclopedia of Fish Cookery*, Holt, Rinehart and Winston.

McClane, A.J. 1974. *McClane's Field Guide to Freshwater Fishes of North America*, Henry Holt and Company.

McClane, A.J. 1978. *McClane's Field Guide to Saltwater Fishes of North America*, Henry Holt and Company.

McClane, A.J. 1974, 1984. *McClane's New Standard Fishing Encyclopedia*, Henry Holt and Company.

McClane, A. J. 1981. *North American Fish Cookery*, Holt, Rinehart and Winston.

McDaniel, D. 1986. *Procedures for the Detection and Identification of Certain Fish Pathogens*, American Fisheries Society.

McVey, James P., PhD. 1983. *CRC Handbook of Mariculture Volume I: Crustacean Aquaculture*, CRC Press, Inc.

Migdalski, Edward C. and Fichter, George S. 1976, 1983. *The Fresh and Salt Water Fishes of the World*, Greenwich House.

Nelson, Joseph S. 1984. *Fishes of the World, 2nd edition*, John Wiley & Sons.

Nettleton, Joyce A. 1987. *Seafood and Health*, Osprey Books Ltd.

Nettleton, Joyce A. 1985. *Seafood Nutrition*, Osprey Books Ltd.

Niazi, Ph.D, S.K. 1987. *The Omega Connection*, Esquire Books, Inc.

Paquette, Gerald N. 1983. *Fish Quality Improvement — A Manual for Plant Operators*, Osprey Books Ltd.

Pillay, T.V.R. *Planning of Aquaculture Development, an introductory guide*, Fishing News Books.

Pullin, R.S.V. and Lowe-McConnell, R.H. 1982. *The Biology and Culture of Tilapias*, American Fisheries Society.

Rechcigl Jr., Miloslav. 1982. *CRC Handbook of Nutritive Value of Processed Food*, CRC Press, Inc.

Regenstein, Joe and Carrie. *Old Laws in a New Market, The Kosher Dietary Laws for Seafood Processors*, New York Sea Grant Institute.

Robinson, Robert H. 1983. *The Essential Book of Shellfish, How to Prepare, Dismantle and Enjoy Crabs, Lobster, Clams and Other Shellfish*, Liberty Publishing Company Inc.

Sacharow, M.A., S. 1979. *Packaging Regulations*, AVI Publishing Company, Inc.

Sacharow, M.A., S. and Griffin, M.S., R.C. 1980. *Principles of Food Packaging, 2nd Ed.*, Avi Publishing Company, Inc.

Sainsbury, John C. 1971, 1986. *Commercial Fishing Methods*, Fishing News Books Ltd.

Sainsbury, Keith J, Kailola, Patricia J., and Leyland, Guy G. 1984. *Continental Shelf Fishes of Northern and North-Western Australia, an Illustrated Guide*, Clouston & Hall and Peter Pownwall Fisheries Information Service.

Sanger, Claude. 1986. *Ordering the Oceans*, Zed Books Ltd.

Schmidt, R. Marilyn. 1982, 1986. *Seafood Secrets: A Nutritional Guide to Seafood*, Barnegat Light Press.

Schultz, H.W., Ph.D. 1981. *Food Law Handbook*, A.F.S. and Avi Publishing Company, Inc.

Seafood Products Resource Guide, Foundation Services.

Sedgwick, S. Drummond. 1988. *The Salmon Farming Handbook*, Fishing News Books Ltd.

Sindermann, C.J. and Lightner, D.V.; Editors. 1988. *Disease Diagnosis and Control in North-American Marine Aquaculture, 2nd Edition*, Elsevier Science Publishing Co., Inc.

Smith, Margaret M. and Heemstra, Phillip C. 1986. *Smiths' Sea Fishes*, Springer-Verlag.

Stevenson, John P. 1987. *Trout Farming Manual, 2nd. Edition*, Fishing News Books Ltd.

Stickney, Robert R. 1986. *Culture of Nonsalmonid Freshwater Fishes*, CRC Press, Inc.

Swift, Donald R. 1985. *Aquaculture Training Manual*, Fishing News Books Ltd.

Thorpe, J. 1980. *Salmon Ranching*, American Fisheries Society.

Tucker, C.S. 1985. *Channel Catfish Culture*, American Fisheries Society.

Veasy, E. Brian and Wallace, James L. 1986. *Export Packing: A Manual for Eight Northeast Seafood Species*, New England Fisheries Development Foundation.

von Brandt, Andres. 1984. *Fish Catching Methods of the World*, Fishing News Books Ltd.

Wagenvoord, James and Harris, Woodman. 1983. *The Complete Seafood Book, An Insider's Guide to Shopping, Preparing, and Enjoying the Harvest of the Sea*, Macmillan Publishing Co.

Walford, Lionel A. 1937, 1965. *Marine Game Fishes of the Pacific Coast from Alaska to the Equator*, Smithsonian Institution Press.

Walker, Charlotte. 1984. *Fish and Shellfish*, HP Books.

Webb, Tony, Lang, Tim and Tucker, Kathleen. 1987. *Food Irradiation. Who wants it?*, Thorsons Publishers, Inc.

Went, A.E.J. *Atlantic Salmon: its Future*, Fishing News Books Ltd.

Williams, Austin B. *Shrimps, Lobsters and Crabs of the Atlantic Coast of the United States, Maine to Northern Florida*, the Smithsonian Institution Press.

Williams, A.B. and Dore, Ian. 1988. *Lobsters of the World: An Illustrated Guide*, Osprey Books Ltd.

Yoshino, Masuo. 1986. *Sushi*, Gakken Co. Ltd.

Yuska, Joe and Ridlington, Sandy. 1985. *Underutilized Species and Seafood By-Products*, 5/22/85 workshop, Oregon Sea Grant.

Zinn, Donald J. 1975. *The Handbook for Beach Strollers from Maine to Cape Hatteras*, The Pequot Press.

PERIODICALS

Aquaculture Magazine. P.O. Box 2329, Asheville, NC 28802.

Austasia Aquaculture. P.O. Box 1275, East Victoria, W. Australia.

Australian Fisheries. Department of Primary Industry, Canberra, ACT 2600

Canadian Hotel and Restaurant. Maclean Hunter Business Publishing Company, 777 Bay Street, Toronto, Canada M5W 1A7.

Catering Today. P.O. Box 222, Santa Claus, IN 47579.

Catfish News. Aquacom, Inc. P.O. Box 4566, Jackson, MS 39296.

Chile Pesquero. Providencia 2286-A, Casilla 2508, Santiago de Chile.

Commercial Fisheries News. Fisheries Communications Inc., P.O. Box 37, Main Street, Stonington, ME 04681.

The Cook's Magazine. Pennington Publishing, 1698 Post Road East, Westport, CT 06880.

FAO Infofish Marketing Digest. INFOFISH. P.O. Box 10899, Kuala Lumpur 01-02, Malaysia.

FDA Consumer. Department of Health & Human Services, Public Health Service, Food and Drug Administration, Rockville, MD 20857.

Field & Stream. 1515 Broadway, New York, NY 10036.

Fisheries, A Bulletin of the American Fisheries Society. 5410 Grosvenor Lane, Bethesda, MD 20814.

Fisheries Product News. Fisheries Communications Inc., P.O. Box 37, Main Street, Stonington, ME 04681.

Fish Farming International. AGB Farringdon Lane, London, England EC1R 3AU.

Fishing News International. AGB Farringdon Lane, London, England EC1R 3AU.

Food Distributors Magazine (FDM). FDM, c/o Gro Com Group, P.O. Box 10378, Clearwater, FL 33517-8378.

Food Management. Harcourt Brace Jovanovich Publications, 7500 Old Oak Boulevard, Cleveland, OH 44130.

Foodservice Distributor, 1100 Superior Avenue, Cleveland, OH 44114.

Foodservice Product News. Young/Conway Publications Inc., 104 Fifth Avenue, New York, NY 10011.

Food Technology. Institute of Food Technologists, 221 N. LaSalle Street, Suite 2120, Chicago, IL 60601.

Frozen Food Digest: The Informative Magazine of the Frozen Food Industry. 261 Madison Ave, New York, NY 10016.

In-Fisherman, The. P.O. Box 999, 651 Edgewood Dr., Hwy. 371 No., Brainerd, MN 56401-1099.

Institutional Distribution. 633 Third Ave, New York, NY 10017.

Marine Fisheries Review. Scientific Publications Office, National Marine Fisheries Service, NOAA, 7600 Sand Point Way N.E., Bin C15700, Seattle, WA 98115.

Metro Foodservice. Metropolitan Restaurant News Inc., 104 Fifth Ave, New York, NY 10011.

National Fisherman. Journal Publications, 21 Elm St., Camden, ME 04843-0639.

Nations Restaurant News. Lebhar-Friedman Inc., 425 Park Ave., New York, NY 10022.

New Zealand Fishing Industry Board (FIB) Bulletin. Private Bag, Manners Street PO, Wellington, New Zealand.

Pacific Fishing. Salmon Bay Communications, 1515 N.W. 51st St, Seattle, WA 98107.

Prepared Foods. Gorman Publishing Company, 8750 West Bryn Mawr Ave., Chicago, IL 60631.

Progressive Grocer, The Magazine of Supermarketing. 1351 Washington Blvd., Stamford, CT 06902.

Quick Frozen Foods. 7500 Old Oak Boulevard, Cleveland, OH 44130.

Quick Frozen Foods International. E.W. Williams Publications Co., Division of Pioneer Assoc., Inc., 80 Eighth Avenue, New York, NY 10011.

Restaurant Business Magazine. 633 Third Ave., New York, NY 10017.

Restaurant Exchange News. P.O. Box 473, New City, NY 10956.

Restaurants & Institutions. Cahners Plaza, 1350 E. Touhy Ave., P.O. Box 5080, Des Plaines, IL 60017-5080.

Revista de Circulación Mundial PESCA. PESCA, Publicaciones S.A., P.O. Box 877, Lima 1, Avida José Pardo No. 138, Of. 301, Miraflores, Lima.

Salmonid. 515 Rock St., Little Rock, AR 72202.

Seafood Business. 120 Tillson Ave., P.O. Box 908, Rockland, ME 04841.

Seafood International. AGB Heighway Ltd., Cloister Court, 22-26 Farringdon Lane, London, England EC1R 3AU.

Seafood Leader. Waterfront Press Co., 1115 N.W. 46th St., Seattle, WA 98107.

Seafood Magazine. Borghouts Publishers, Postbox 84055, 2508 AB, The Hague, Netherlands.

Seafood Supplier. Seafood Business, Journal Publications, 120 Tillson Ave., P.O. Box 908, Rockland, ME 04841.

Shoreline: Rhode Island Fishermen's News. 11 School Street, Wakefield, RI 02879.

Southeastern Seafood Magazine. 312 East Georgia St., Tallahassee, FL 32301.

Supermarket Business Magazine. Sosland Publishing Co., 25 West 43rd Street, New York, NY 10036.

Supermarket News. Capital Cities Media Inc., 7 E. 12th Street, New York, NY 10003.

Water Farming Journal. CT&A, Inc., 3400 Neyrey Dr., Metairie, LA 70002.

World Fishing, IPC Industrial Press Ltd., Quadrant, Sutton, Surrey SM2 5AS.

NEWSLETTERS

Aquafarm Letter. 3400 Neyrey Drive, Metairie, LA 70002.

At Sea. University of Delaware Graduate College of Marine Studies, Newark, Delaware 19716.

Australian Fishing Industry Directory. The Australian Fisheries Service, Department of Primary Industry, Edmund Barton Building, Barton ACT 2600.

Cameron's Foodservice Promotions Reporter. P.O. Box 1160, Williamsville, NY 14221.

Commercial Fishing Newsletter. Sea Grant Communications, Virginia Institute of Marine Science, Gloucester Point, VA 23062.

Environmental Nutrition. P.O. Box 3000, Dept. BBB, Denville, NJ 07834.

Erkins Seafood Letter, The. P.O. Box 108. Bliss, ID 83314.

Florida Aquaculture Association, P.O. Box 3989, Tallahassee, FL 32315-3989.

The International Institute of Fisheries Economics and Trade. Office of International Research and Development, Oregon State University, Corvallis, OR 97331.

LMR Shrimp Market Report. LMR Fisheries Research Inc., 11855 Sorrento Valley Rd., Suite A, San Diego, CA 92121.

Marine Resource Bulletin. Marine Advisory Services, Virginia Institute of Marine Science, Gloucester Point, VA 23062.

Market News Reports: New York Report: U.S. Department of Commerce — NOAA National Marine Fisheries Service, Utilization & Development Branch, 201 Varick Street, Room 1145, New York, NY 10014-4897.

Boston Report: U.S. Department of Commerce — NOAA National Marine Fisheries Service, Utilization & Development Branch, 408 Atlantic Ave., Room 141, Boston, MA 02210-2203.

New Orleans Report: U.S. Department of Commerce — NOAA National Marine Fisheries Service Fisheries Development, Analysis Branch, World Trade Center, 2 Canal Street, Suite 400-H, New Orleans, LA 70130-1206.

Terminal Island Report: U.S. Department of Commerce — NOAA National Marine Fisheries Service Industry, Analysis & Information Section, 300 South Ferry Street, Box 3266, Room 2016, Customs House, Terminal Island, CA 90731.

Seattle Report: U.S. Department of Commerce — NOAA National Marine Fisheries Service, F-NWR-23 Statistics & Market News Office, 7600 Sand Point Way, N.E., Bin C15700, Seattle, WA 98115-0070.

MAS Note. University of Delaware Sea Grant Marine Advisory Service, College of Marine Studies, University of Delaware, 700 Pilottown Road, Lewes, DE 19958.

Osprey's Seafood Newsletter. 6 West 18th Street, Huntington Station, NY 11746.

Pacific Seafood Chronicle, The. West Coast Fisheries Development Foundation, 812 S.W. Washington, Suite 900, Portland, OR 97205.

Practical Aquaculture and Lake Management. AAS, Dept. N., Rt. 3, Box 299-B, Raleigh, NC 27603.

Seafood Price-Current. Urner Barry Publications Inc., P.O. Box 389, Toms River, NJ 08753.

Seafood Trend. Seafood Trend Associates, 8227 Ashworth Avenue North, Seattle, WA 98103.

Sea Grant Abstracts. P.O. Box 125, Woods Hole, MA 02543.

Shrimp Notes: A Market News Analysis. Shrimp Notes Incorporated, 417 Eliza Street, New Orleans, LA 70114.

Washington Sea Grant Newsletter. Marine Advisory Services, 3716 Brooklyn Ave, N.E., Seattle, WA 98105.

INDEX

Abalone 12, 17
Acanthocybium solanderi 322
Acipenser spp. 307
additives 13
Aden tails 14, 156
ahi 14
Alaska plaice 100
albacore 316
Albula vupes 25
alewife 14
alligators 14
Allocyttus spp. 79
Alosa pseuoharengus 14
Alosa spp. 263
Alpodinotus grunniens 80
amarelo 67
amberjack 15, 134
American Shrimp Canners Association 84
ammonia 292
ammonia in shark meat 264
anadramous 14
anadromous fish 15
anaerobic bacteria 15
Anarhichas denticulatus 34
anchovy 16
anglerfish 16, 164
Anguilla spp. 87
Anoplopoma fimbriia 237
antibiotics 16
anti-oxidants 13
A.O.A.C. 17
aquaculture 17
Archosargus probatocephalus 268
Arctica islandica 40
Arctic char 18
Arctic surfclam 41
argentine 292
Argopecten circularis 252
Argopecten gibbus 251
Argopecten irradians 250
Aristaeomorpha foliacea 284
Aristeus antennatus 285
Arius felis 34
arrowtooth flounder 100
arrowtooth sole 100
Astacus astacus 64
Atheresthes stomias 100
atka mackerel 19
aureomycin 16
Auxis thazard 26, 100

Baby lobster 156
bacalao 48, 68
backfin 53
bacteria 19
Bahama conch 50
bairdii 20, 61
barracuda 20, 37
barramundi 21, 31
bass 21
bass, channel 227
bass, red 227
bass, striped 230
batter 22

battered 22
bay scallops 22
bellyburn 22
bellyclams 38
bellyfish 164
bellyflaps 78
belon 22, 205
bigeye 316
billfish 22
biological filters 76
bird-eye 61
bisque 22, 50
bivalve 164
blackback 101
blackback flounder 101
blackcod 237
black drum 80
blackmouth 240
black oreo dory 79
black sea bass 21
black spot 161
blanks 23, 209
blast freezing 107
blind robins 23
bloaters 23
block frozen 209
blocklisting 23
blowfish 224
blown 206
blueback 240, 242
blue crabs 53
blue fin 70, 317
bluefish 24, 25
blue runner 134
bone 25
bonefish 25
boneless fillets 25
bonito 26, 109, 316
borax 26
Boston bluefish 25, 218
botulinus 15
botulism 16, 261
Brachyplatysoma vaillanti 31
Brama spp. 219
branco 67
breaded shrimp 27
breading 27
bream 27
Brevoortia tyrannus 162
brill 27
brine 108
brining, salting and 248
broken shrimp 272
brokers 27
bronze bream 28
Brosme brosme 68
buckling 28
buffalo 28
bugs 258
bulldozer lobster 156
bumber 134
Busycon carica 51
Busycotypus canaliculatus 51
butterfish 28, 237

butterfly fillets 29, 90
butterfly shrimp 30

C & F 74
calamare 30, 302
calamari 30
calico scallop 30, 71
Callinectes sapidus 53
Cancer spp. 61
Cancer magister 54
canned salmon 71
capelin 30
Caranx hippos 66
Caribbean conch 50
carp 16, 30
catadromous 21, 87
catadromous fish 31
catfish 16, 31
catfish, spoonbill 213
Catostomus commersoni 166
cavalla 66, 137
caviar 35
cello 23, 47
cellophane 209
cello wraps 209
Centropristis striata 21
cephalapod 35, 164
cero 35, 137, 301
Cervimunida johni 143
cestodes 214
channel bass 227
Chanos chanos 164
cherrystone 39
chikuwa 309
chinook 240
Chionecetes spp. 20, 61
Chlamys delicatula 253
Chlamys islandica 251
Chlamys opercularis 251
Chlamys purpuratus 252
chlorination 76
cholesterol 123
chopped clams 41
chowders 36, 50
chub 35, 70
chums 243
chum, dark 69
C.I.F. 74
C.I.F.R. 74
ciguatera 15, 21, 36, 261
ciguatoxin 261
cisco 36, 37, 70
clam 18, 22, 37, 36, 74
clam cakes 44
clam juice 43
clam strips 43
class A shrimp 273
cleaned shrimp 272
clean tail 44
clumping 45
Clupea harengus 123
clusters 45, 62
coalfish 218
cobbler 219
cobia 45, 145
cockle 45

cocktail claws 53
cod 17, 45
cod cheeks 49
Code of Federal Regulations 71, 85, 96
Codex Alimentarius 50, 272
coho 50, 242
coley 50, 218
colors and types of shrimps 277
contaminants 259
cooked and peeled shrimp 273
coonstripe 52
concentrates 50
conch 50
conger eel 52
Conger oceanicus 52
consignment 74
Coregonus clupeaformis 323
Coregonus spp. 36, 37
corvina 21, 52, 80
Coryphaena hippurus 160
Coryphaenoides acrolepsis 116
crabs 52
crabs, stone 63
crabs, others 63
Crangon crangon 223
Crangon franciscorum 278
Crassostrea gigas 205
crayfish and crawfish 17, 63
credit and credit control 65
crevalle jack 66, 134
croaker 67, 80
crustacea 67
cryogenic freezing 108
Ctenopharyngodon idella 31
curing 67
cusk 68
cusk-eel 138
cutlassfishes 13, 35, 69
Cyclopterus lumpus 158
Cynoscion spp. 263
Cynoscion nebulosus 262
Cynoscion nobilis 21
Cyprinus carpio 30
cysts 70

Dab 100, 101, 218
dainty lobster 156
dark chum 69
decomposition 70, 130
deep sea tails 14
defatted 32, 69
defect action level 70
defrosting methods 71
dehydration 105, 112
Delaney clause 73
delivery terms 73
depuration 74
devein 77
Diagramma pictum 213
Dicentrachus labrax 21
dips 77
dogfish 78, 257, 264
dog shark 78
dollar fish 28
Dolly Varden 79
dolphin 79

dolphin fish 79, 160
dorado 160
doré 216
dories 79
Dover sole 102
Dover sole, genuine 80
Dover sole, Pacific 80
drum 21, 137, 80
drum, red 227
dry salting 67
Dublin Bay prawn 156
dungeness crab 54

Eastern oysters, size definitions 205
E. coli 19
economic fraud in the seafood business 81
eel 31, 87
eelpout 203
eel, slime 119
Elops saurus 143
elver 88
English sole 88, 102
Engraulis spp. 16
Eopsetta jordani 103
Epinephelus itajara 116
Eptatretus stouti 119
Erimacrus eisenbecki 63
Escherichia coli 19
Esox spp. 217
Etelis Coruscans 299
Euphausia superba 141
Euthynnus spp. 318

Fair packaging act 141
fall 67
fantail 30
F.A.O. 50
F.A.S. 73
fat fish 88
F.D.A. 22, 23, 17, 19
F.D.A. action levels for poisonous or deleterious substances in
    seafood 260
Federal grade standards 25
Federal inspection 88
feeder claw 56
fillets 89
fillets, married
filter feeders 75, 90
finger packs 90
finished counts 90
finnans 90, 294
fish blocks 90
fish block/ grade A blocks 47
fisheries management 91
fish farming 17
Fishlist, the: approved market names for fish 168, 170
fish meal and fish by-products 93
fish oil
fish protein concentrate 93
fish sticks 94, 305
flake 78, 94
flake meat 53
flatfish 94
flatfish: market names and common names 97

flat lobster 156
fletch 89, 104, 121
flounder 94
flounder, arrowtooth 100
flounder, blackback 101
flounder or sole? 96
fluke 94, 102,
F.O.B. 73, 74
Food, drug and cosmetic act 71
formed fillets 105
F.P.C. 93
freeze-drying 105
freezer-burn 105
freezing at sea 105
freezing processes 106
fresh water herring 70
fried clams 43
frigate mackerel 26, 109, 316
frill 94
frogfish 164
frog legs 109
frozen hardshell clam products 41
fryers 38
fugu 224

Gadus spp. 45
gag 116
gaping 110
gaspareau 14
gaspe 67
gefilte 112
gemfish 112
Genypterus spp. 138
geoduck 37, 41
giant sea bass 21
gibbed 112
glass eels 87
glaze 105, 112, 200
glazed seafoods 71
glazing 154
globefish 224
Glyptocephalus cynoglossus 103
Glyptocephalus zachirus 103
goatfish 113
gonads 113
good manufacturing practice 113
goosefish 16, 164
grade A 25, 321
G.R.A.S. 113, 308
gravadlax 114
gravlax 114
gray sole 103
green headless 114
green headless shrimp 269
Greenland halibut 319
Greenland turbot 100, 114, 319
greenling 19, 146
green-lipped mussel 167
green runner 134
green sheet 114
green ticket 115
grenadier 115
grouper 22, 116
gurry 118

Haddock 118
hagfish 119
hake 23, 119, 323
halibut 94, 119
Haliotis spp. 12
H and G 121
hard cured 121
hardhead 34, 67
hard smoked 121
harvestfish 28
hatchery salmon 121
Hazard Analysis of Critical Control Points
    (H.A.C.C.P.) 89, 127
head meat 121
health 122
herring 23, 28, 123
herring, fresh water 70
hind 116
Hippoglossoides platessoides 101
Hippoglossus spp. 120
histamines 125
hoki 25, 116, 125
Homarus americanus 146
Homarus gammarus 147
Hoplostethus atlanticus 204
horse crevally 66
horse mackerel 126, 160
humpback salmon 126
huss 78, 126
hydrolized fish proteins 93

Ictalurus spp. 31
Ictiobus spp. 28
Illex illecebrosus 304
inconnu 70, 126
Individually Quick Frozen (I.Q.F.) 107, 131, 211
ink 126
inkfish 69, 126
inspection 126
interleaved 131, 212
ipswich clams 38
I.P.W. 131
irradiate 110
irradiation 131
iso-electric focussing 81, 133

Jack 15, 134, 160
jack crevalle 66
jack mackerel 126,160
jacks: market names and common names 135
j-cut 89
jelly 102
jewfish 116
John Dory 79, 306
jonah crab 61
jumbo cod 136
jumbo lump 53
jumbo shrimp 137

Kamaboko 309
Kathetostoma giganteum 165
kegani crabmeat 63
kench 67, 68
kg 137
killer claw 56, 57
kilogram 137

king crab 55
kingfish 137
kingfish, southern 137
kingklip 138, 145
king mackerel 35, 137, 301
king salmon 138
king whiting 137, 138
kipper 138, 294
kippered fish 139
klipfish 68
Korean hair crab 63
kosher 139
krill 140

Labelling 141
labelling, nutrition
labrador (cure) 68
lacey act 142
ladyfish 143
lake herring 36, 37
lake perch 143
langostinos 143
langoustines 144, 156
largemouth bass 21
Lates calcarifer 21
Lates niloticus 200
layerpacks 47, 212
lean fish 144
leatherjacket 314
left-eyed fish 94
legs and claws 56
Leiostomus xanthurus 123, 301
lemon sole 101, 145
Lepidopsetta bilineata 103
letter of credit 145
Limanda spp. 104
ling 145
lingcod 19, 146
Linuparus trigonus 227
Lisa 165
listeria 146
Listeria monocytogenes 146
Lithodes antarctica 55
littlenecks 39
Littorina littorea 216
liver 314
lobster 18. 22. 146
lobsterette 14, 156
lobster, red rock 227
locos 12
locust lobster 156
Loligo spp. 303
Lophius spp. 16, 164
Lopholatilus chamaeleonticeps 313
lotte 157, 164
lox 157
lump 53
lumpfish 35, 158
lump meat 158
Lutjanus spp. 295

Mackerel 26, 158
mackerel, horse 126
mackerel: market and common names 159
Macrobrachium rosenbergii 285
Macrozoarces americanus 203

Macruronus novaezelandiae 125
Mactromeris polynyma 41
mahi-mahi 15, 79, 160, 125
mako 264, 310
Mallotus villosus 30
manila clam 40
marine toxins 261
marlin 22
married fillets 161
masu 161
may proceed 115
melanin 161
Melanogrammus aeglefinus 118
melanosis 64, 77, 161
menhaden 162
Menticirrhus spp. 137
Mercenaria mercenaria 39
mercury 162
Merlangus merlangus 326
Merluccius spp. 119, 324
merus 59, 162
Metanephrops spp. 156
Metapenaeus spp. 281
metric weights and measures 162
Microgadus spp. 314
Micromesistius spp. 25
Micropogonias undulatus 67
Microstomus pacificus 80, 102
milkfish 17, 164
milt 113, 164
minced clams 41
molluscs 35, 164
molluscs, bi-valve 37
Molva molva 145
monkfish 16, 164
monoclonal antibodies 82
Morone saxatilis 22, 306
mother-in-law fish 214
Mugil cephalus 165
mullet 165
muskellunge 217
mussels 18, 74, 164
Mustelus canis 78
muttonfish 203
Mya arenaria 38
Mytilus edulis 166

N-3 122, 167
names 167
National Fisheries Institute, the 200
Nemadactylus macropterus 312
nematodes 71, 214
Nephrops spp. 144, 156
Nephrops norvegicus 223
net salmon 200
net weights 200
net weight of frozen seafoods 71
New England conch 51
New Zealand whiting 125
N.F.I. 200
Nile perch 200
nobbing 200
non-kosher fishes 139
Norway lobster 156
Nototodarus sloanii 304
Nova salmon 200

nuggets 34
nutrition 122, 201
nutrition labelling 201

Ocean blowfish 164
ocean catfish 34
ocean perch 27, 70, 227, 230
ocean pout 203
ocean quahog 40
ocean run 57, 203
ocean whitefish 313
octopus 35, 203
oily fish 88
omega-3 fatty acids 122
O. mykiss 239
Oncorhynchus masou 161
Oncorhynchus mykiss 239
ono 322
Ophiodon elongatus 146
opilio 61
Opisthonema oglinum 125, 313
orange roughy 138, 204
Ostrea edulis 22
Ostreola spp. 205
oxidation 225
oysters 17, 18, 22, 74, 205, 314
ozone 76

P.C.B. 25, 88
P.P.M. 223
P.S.P. 227, 261
Pacifastacus lenivesculus 63
Pacific oysters: meat counts 205
Pacific littlenecks 40
Pacific pompanpo 29
Pacific snapper 230
packing 208
packing styles 209
paddlefish 213
Pagrus pagrus 221
painted sweetlips 213
Palaemon serratus 223
pale kings 214
palometa 29, 220
pan-ready 214
Pandulus spp. 278
Pandulus borealis 223
Panopea abrupta 41
Paralichthys albigutta 104
Paralichthys californicus 120
Paralichthys dentatus 102
Paralichthys lethostigma 103
Paralithodes spp. 55
Paralytic shellfish poisoning 227
Parapenaeus longinostris 283
parasites 29, 214, 259, 310
Parophrys vetulus 88, 102
pasteurizing 216
Patinopecten caurinus 251
Patinopecten yessoensis 252
Pecten maximus 250
Pecten novaezealandiae 253
peeled and deveined shrimp 271
peeled, deveined and split 272
peeled from counts 216
peeled shrimp 271

peeled, tail-on 272
Penaeus spp. 279
Peprilus spp. 28, 29
Perca flavescens 143
perch 230
perch, lake 143
perch, Nile 200
perch, ocean 27,70, 227, 230
periwinkle 216
permit 220
Perna canaliculis 167
petrale sole 27, 103
phosphates 13, 77, 83
pickle cure 68
picowaving 131
pieces 272
pike and pickerel 216
pike-perch 216
pilchard 217
pillow pack 217
pinbones 25, 34, 217
pintada 301
Placopecten magellanicus 249
plaice 101, 218
plaice, Alaska 100
plankton 140
plate freezing 107
Platichthys stellatus 104
Pleoticus spp. 284
Plesionika edwardsii 283
Pleurogrammus spp. 19
Pleuroncodes spp. 143
Pleuronectes quadrituberculatus 100
Pogonias cromis 80
pogy 162, 218
Pollachius virens 218
pollack 23, 24, 26, 218
polyethylene 209
Polyodon spathula 213
Pomatomus saltatrix 24
pomfret 219
pompano 134, 219
porgy 27, 221
porpoise 79
portions 221
portion pack 222
potassium pyrophosphate 77
prawn 223
prawn balls 273
prawn, ridgeback 235
pre-cooked 224
preservatives 13
Procambarus spp. 63
product forms of frozen shrimp 270
products of Atlantic cod 47
products of king crab 56
products of Pacific cod 49
Prototheca staminea 40
Psetta maxima 318
Psettichthys melanostictus 103
Pseudocyttus maculatus 79
Pseudopleuronectes americanus 101
puffer 224
pulpo 203
pumpkins 39

Quahogs 36, 39
queen crab 61
quinnat 225
quinnault 240

Rachycentron canadum 45
raddapertization 132
radicidation 132
radurization 132
Raja spp. 292
rancidity 225
random pack 226
Ranidae 109
rat-packing 86, 226
rattail 115
rays 292
recall 226
red bass 227
red crab 60
red drum 227
redfish 27, 227, 230
red rock lobster 227
red snapper 295
red tide 12 261, 227
Reinhardtius hippoglossoides 114, 120, 319
rejection and rejection insurance 228
release 230
retail fillet packs 230
rex sole 103
Rexea solandri 112
Rhombus laevis 27
rice meat 59
ridgeback prawn 235
right-eyed fish 94
rigor mortis 111, 230
ripe fish 230
river herring 14
rock cod 230
rock crab 61
rock lobster 150
rock salmon 78
rock shrimp 234
rock sole 103
rockfish 230, 306
roe 30, 113, 235
roundworms 214

Sablefish 29, 237
sailfish 22
saithe 218
Salmo spp. 239
Salmo gairdneri 315
salmon 17, 18, 22, 238
salmon, canned 71
salmon, king 138
salmon, rock 78
salmonella 110, 133, 247
saltfish 68
salting and brining 248
Saltonstall-Kennedy 248
Salvelinus alpinus 18
Salvelinus malma 79
sand pike 217
sand sole 103
sandvein 321

sarda spp. 26
sardine 123, 248
Sardinella spp. 249
Sardinops sagax 248
satsuma age 309
sauger 217
scad 126
scallops 17, 249
scallops, calico 30, 71
scamp 116
scampi 156
schillerlocken 78, 257
schrod 27, 257
Sciaenops ocellatus 227
scientific names 256
Scomber spp. 158
Scomberomorus spp. 300
Scomberomorus cavalla 137
Scomberomorus regalis 35
scombroid poisoning 125, 261
Scophthalmus maximus 318
scrod 27, 46, 257
scungili 51
scup 27, 221
sea bass 116, 262
sea bream 219, 221
sea catfish 34
sea devil 164
sea egg 263
sea perch 116
sea pout 203
sea run 262
sea squab 224
sea trout 80, 262
sea urchin 263
seabob 286
seafood safety 258
Sebastes spp. 231
semibright 243
sepia 69
Sepioteuthis bilmeata 304
Seriola dumerili 15
Seriola spp. 326
Seriolella spp. 322
seviche 263
shad 263
shark 264
sharks: market names and common names 265
shatterpack 213
sheepshead 268
Shellfish Sanitation Program 37, 166, 228, 268
shigella 20
shore (cure) 68
short weight or short shipment 82
shovel-nosed lobster 156
shrimp 17, 18, 22, 70, 223, 269
shrimp aquaculture 290
shrimp, rock 234
shrimp counts 287
shrimp quality 275
Sicyonia brevirostris 234
sierra 137
silver 242
silver dollar 28
silverbright 243
silverbrite 243

silversides 292
skate 292
skipjacks 143, 316
slime eels 119
slimehead 204
slipper lobsters 156
smallmouth bass 21
smelts 292
smelt herring 292
smoked fish 293
smoked salmon 294
smolt 295
smooth oreo dory 79
snails 295
snappers 24, 295
snappers: market names and common names 297
snow crab 61
sockeye 240
sodium pyrophosphate 77
sodium tripolyphosphate 77
soft (cure) 68
softshell clams 38
softshell crabs 53
soldier packs 300
sole 94
sole, arrowtooth 100
sole, lemon 101
Solea vulgaris 80
somali tails 156
southern flounder 103
Spanish lobster 156
Spanish mackerel 300
spearfish 22
spent fish 301
spent salmon 121
Sphoeroides spp. 224
Sphyraena spp. 20, 21
spider crab 301
spiny lobster 150
Spisula solidissima 40
split legs 58
split tails 271
spoonbill catfish 213
spot 123, 301
sprat 301
Sprattus sprattus 301
spring 240
Squalus acanthias 78
squeteague 263
squid 13, 30, 35, 302
St. Pierre 79
St. Peter 79
St. Peter's fish 306, 313
Staphylococcus aureus 20
starry flounder 104
steaks 305
steamers 38
steelhead 239
Stenodus leucichthys 126
Stenotomus chrysops 221
Stereolepis gigas 21
sticks 305
Stizostedion canadense 217
Stizostedion vitreum 216
stockfish 48, 68, 305

stone crabs 63
stones 64
storage temperatures 305
striped bass 22, 230, 306
striper 306
Strombus gigas 50
stuffed clams 44
sturgeons 35, 307
subject passage 307
substitutions 95, 307
suckers 308
sujiko 236
sulfites 77, 308
surf clam 40
surimi 67, 162, 219, 308
sushi 309
swordfish 22, 310

T & C 149
T.C.K. 149
T.D. 286
tail, claw and knuckle meat 312
tail and claw meat 312
tail meat 60
tanner 61
tapeworms 214
tarakihi 312
tarpon 143
tautog 312
Tautoga onitis 312
tele 286
tempura 312
ten-pounder 143
terramycin 16
terrapin 312
tetracycline 16
thawing methods 84
Thenus orientalis 156
Theragra chalcogramma 219
thermographs 306, 312
thread herring 125, 313
Thunnus spp. 317
tide runner 263
tilapia 306, 313
Tilapia spp. 313
tilefish 313
tomalley 314
tomcod 314
topnecks 39
toro 66
toxins 36
Trachinotus spp. 219, 220
Trachurus symmetricus 160
transfer 314
trash fish 19, 29
trematodes 214
trevally 134
triggerfish 314
triploidy 314
troll 245, 315
trout 17, 18, 315
trucking claims 316
true bass 21
tullibees 37, 70
tullies 214, 316
tuna 14, 26, 316

tunny 318
turbot 17, 27, 94, 318
turbot, Greenland 100
turtles 320
tusk 68, 320
tyee 240

Ultra-violet 76
uniformity ratios 288
univalves 164
Urophycis spp. 119, 324
U.S. Grade Standards 320
V-cut 89, 218
vein 321
Venerupis japonica 40
Vibrio spp. 20
viscera 322
viviparous 322
viviparous blenny 203

Wahoo 322
walleye 218
warehou 322
warsaw 116
watermark 322
weakfish 262, 263
western style 272
W.H.O. 50
whelk 322
whiptail 125
white amur 31
white kings 323
white seabass 21
white sucker 166
whitebait 16, 323
whitefish 35, 323
whitefish, freshwater 70
whitings 69, 323
whiting, king 137, 138
whiting, New Zealand 125
whole cooked shrimp 273
wing 292
witch 103
wolffish 34

Xiphias gladius 310
Xiphopenaeus kroyeri 286

Yellow pickerel 216
yellow walleye 217
yellowfin 14, 316
yellowfin sole 104
yellowpout 203
yellowtail 15, 326
yellowtail flounder 104
yields 327

Zenopsis ocellata 79
Zeus faber 79, 306
Zoarces vivparus 203
zoos and aquaria 328